F. A. Davis's
Practice Guide for the
RADIOGRAPHY
EXAMINATION

F. A. Davis's
Practice Guide for the
RADIOGRAPHY
EXAMINATION

Jennifer Thomas, MS, RT(R)(MR)

Program Coordinator
School of Radiologic Technology
Jefferson Regional Medical Center
Pine Bluff, Arkansas

CONTRIBUTOR
Joseph R. Bittengle, MEd, RT(R)(ARRT)
Chair and Assistant Professor
Department of Radiologic Technology
University of Arkansas for Medical Sciences
Little Rock, Arkansas

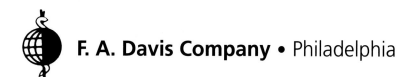

F. A. Davis Company • Philadelphia

F. A. Davis Company
1915 Arch Street
Philadelphia, PA 19103

Printed in the United States of America

Last digit indicates print number: 10 9 8 7 6 5

Publisher, Health Professions: Jean-François Vilain
Senior Editor: Lynn Borders Caldwell
Developmental Editors: Sharon Lee, Crystal Spraggins
Production Editor: Stephen D. Johnson
Cover Designer: Louis J. Forgione

As new scientific information becomes available through basic and clinical re-search, recommended treatments and drug therapies undergo changes. The au-thor and publisher have done everything possible to make this book accurate, up to date, and in accord with accepted standards at the time of publication. The au-thor, editors, and publisher are not responsible for errors or omissions or for con-sequences from application of the book, and make no warranty, expressed or im-plied, in regard to the contents of the book. Any practice described in this book should be applied by the reader in accordance with professional standards of care used in regard to the unique circumstances that may apply in each situation. The reader is advised always to check product information (package inserts) for changes and new information regarding dose and contraindications before ad-ministering any drug. Caution is especially urged when using new or infrequently ordered drugs.

Library of Congress Cataloging-in-Publication Data

Thomas, Jennifer, 1963–
    F. A. Davis's practice guide for the radiography examination / Jennifer Thomas.
        p.   cm.
    Includes bibliographical references (p.).
    ISBN 10: 0-8036-0460-2 (alk. paper) ISBN 13: 978-0-8036-0460-5
    1. Radiography, Medical—Examinations, questions, etc.
    2. Radiologic technologists—Examinations, questions, etc.   I. Title: Davis's practice guide for the radiography examination.   II. Title: Practice guide for the radiography examination.   III. F.A. Davis Company.   IV. Title.
    RC78.15.T48 1999
    616.07′572′076—dc21   99-043605
                                                           CIP

This book is dedicated to my loving husband, Mike, and our children, Jessica and Jacob.

PREFACE

To the Student:

F. A. Davis's Practice Guide for the Radiography Examination is intended to measure your comprehension of practical radiological skills. Although a brief review will not dramatically change the abilities you have gained from past formal education, use of this book may help you to evaluate strengths and weaknesses and to identify areas for further study before taking a certification or licensure examination.

This review book contains five practice tests and a CD-ROM that includes multiple reviews of the questions from the book as well as a totally new 220-question test modeled on the American Registry of Radiologic Technologists' recently instituted computerized exams. Both the questions in the book and the questions on the CD-ROM simulate typical certification and licensure examinations and were designed to follow the latest format recommendations.

Also included in this book is a review section describing ways to prepare for an examination, as well as sample questions of the most commonly used formulas seen on radiography examinations.

In writing questions, a conscious effort was made to use references that are familiar to most radiographers. As needed, multiple sources for each question were also used to come as close as possible to simulating material that may be on an actual examination. Having a variety of references should enable the reader to see a concept from a different perspective.

This review book is not intended to:
- Be a guide to the practice of radiologic technology, or to take the place of formal education,
- Replicate a particular examination or any of the questions on an examination, or
- Guarantee that a student will pass the examination.

This review book is intended for:
- Advanced-level radiography students or graduates of accredited programs preparing to take a certification or licensure examination.
- Identifying strengths and weaknesses in the knowledge of radiologic science.
- Introducing the student to the format of questions used on certification and licensure examinations.
- Helping students organize and set priorities for study time.

To the Instructor:

Although this book may be purchased by an individual desiring to study on his or her own, it is also an invaluable tool in the assessment of a student's knowledge during a radiography examination preparatory course.

Each test is intended to simulate the actual radiography certification and licensure examinations and follows the format recommendations. As an instructor of this course, you may choose to review some of the physics exposure and protection formulas listed in the review chapter as a lecture guide. There are also tips in the first chapter on how to review for a certification or licensure examination and more importantly *what* to review.

Each instructor may have his or her own method of teaching a comprehensive course such as this. My suggestion would be to give the students the first simulated examination at the beginning of the course to identify any major areas of concern for each student, as well as any general weaknesses that the entire class may have.

This early assessment will give you an idea of which subjects most need review. After several review lectures, you may then choose to give each additional examination approximately 2 weeks apart, allowing students ample time to review their weak points. The instructor may also choose to go through the entire test question by question to demonstrate to the students why errors were made. Make sure that references are available as you review the test to reinforce a particularly difficult concept.

To make scoring easier for the instructors, each examination has been separated into five separate sections. Students should be given a breakdown of *their* individual scores. Likewise, class averages in each section can also demonstrate program strengths and weaknesses.

Located after each simulation examination in this book are score sheets, which may be used by the instructor; these include class average score, content average score for each student, and scaled score.

If you have adopted this textbook for your students, you should also receive an Instructor's Guide on CD-ROM. The Instructor's Guide is meant to help direct the instructor through a registry review course. It includes a course outline, a syllabus, and lesson plans. It also contains samples of overheads for use during lectures for review of positioning and related anatomy, radiation protection, equipment operation and maintenance, and image production and evaluation.

The Instructor's Guide also has score sheets that your program may use to evaluate student performance in each section. Finally, the IG contains its own original simulated examination to be given to the students at the end of the course. This should give your program a good estimate of how students may perform on the actual credentialing examination.

ACKNOWLEDGMENTS

Although my name is listed as the author of this textbook, it would not have been possible without the assistance, support, and professional expertise of many individuals. My gratitude and sincere appreciation go to the students, faculty, and radiographers of the Jefferson Regional Medical Center School of Radiologic Technology. I would especially like to thank the graduates from the classes of 1996, 1997, 1998, and 1999 for their support and input for this project, and also to members of the class of 2000 who are continuing to encourage me. My thanks and great admiration to all of the faculty and clinical educators involved with the JRMC Radiologic Technology program.

I also owe much to the institutions that contributed illustrations, radiographs, charts, and photographs. I wish to thank the University of Arkansas Medical Center in Little Rock, Arkansas, as well as the Jefferson Regional Medical Center in Pine Bluff, Arkansas.

Special thanks go to those who helped review questions and material throughout this project for their comments and suggestions. Among those deserving special acknowledgment are Joseph Bittengle, my contributor, from the University of Arkansas for Medical Sciences Radiologic Technology program, whose professional expertise and contributions were invaluable; reviewers Michael Fugate and Ronald Becker, whose honest input and professional knowledge have given this project credibility; Rick Carlton, for his suggestions on professional writing and publishing; Nadia Bugg and all the faculty of Midwestern State University, for helping me to develop writing skills and for their publishing expertise; and Sharon Lee, Crystal Spraggins, Stephen Johnson, and Lynn Borders Caldwell at F. A. Davis Company for all their input and knowledge.

I owe an additional debt of gratitude to Ronald Becker for offering to put together the Instructor's Guide that accompanies this text. It would not have been possible to complete it had it not been for his commitment.

Of course, many thanks go to my family, especially my husband for his encouragement and patience during the production of this book that took much quality time away from him and our children. I am very fortunate to be blessed with wonderful, supportive parents and an unselfish and giving husband. Without all of you, this project would not have been possible. Each of you has contributed in a special way to this book, and I will keep you all in my thoughts and prayers.

REVIEWERS

Many thanks to the following individuals for reviewing this textbook. If not for their valuable input and professional expertise, this textbook would not have been possible.

Ronald Becker, MS, RT(R)
Program Director
Shadyside Hospital
Pittsburgh, Pennsylvania

Paul Creech, RT(R), MPH
Program Director
Capital Community—Technical College
Hartford, Connecticut

Eugene D. Frank, MA, RT(R), FASRT
Assistant Professor
Radiography Program
Mayo Clinic Foundation
Rochester, Minnesota

Michael L. Fugate, MEd, RT(R)
Lead Didactic Faculty
Radiography Program
Santa Fe Community College
Gainesville, Florida

Sheryl D. Steeg-Murray, ARRT(R)
Instructor and Clinical Coordinator
John Peter Smith Hospital of Radiology
Ft. Worth, Texas

Wanda E. Wesolowski, RT, MEd
Professor and Chairperson
Department of Radiography
Community College of Philadelphia
Philadelphia, Pennsylvania

CONTENTS

PART 1

PREPARING FOR THE EXAMINATION

TEST-TAKING TIPS

On the following pages are suggestions for the use of this review book. To obtain the maximum benefit, try following these steps:

1. Take the first test; then using the sheets provided at the end of the text, score it. Be sure to obtain both a percentage score and a scaled score.
2. Read the review material on pages 9 to 15.
3. Work through the first test, question by question, with the explanations to determine why errors were made.
4. Take the second test, score it, and compare these scores with your scores on the first test, noting any persistent areas of weakness.
5. Again review the sample questions and explanations specifically related to the sections in which you have answered questions incorrectly. Be sure to take note of the references listed in the explanations to help guide your further study.
6. When you are ready, take the third test. The scores you earn on this attempt are good estimates of what your performance might be if you were to take a certification or licensure examination in the near future. For more practice, take the remaining examinations in the book and on the accompanying CD-ROM.

EXAMINATION STRATEGIES

Students' test-taking strategies may dramatically affect the score achieved on the certification or licensure examination. Some individuals who have equal knowledge or ability may have better grades because they have superior test-taking skills.

There are various strategies for mastering the different types of test formats. As you are probably aware, most certification and licensure examinations use the same format as other standardized tests. That format is the multiple-choice question.

Although this format may not be the best way to determine your level of knowledge, it is by far the easiest and most cost-efficient one to score. Because the exact format is known, it becomes easier to hone your test-taking skills for the multiple-choice examination.

As is true for every multiple-choice test, the answer to *every* question is printed right beneath the question. All you have to do is recognize it.

Recognizing the answer to a question is vastly simpler than trying to come up with the answer off the top of your head. Here are two types of physics questions that demonstrate what I mean. Try them both and see which one is easier to answer:

1. What is the System of International Units (SI) equivalent of 1 roentgen? _____

2. The SI equivalent of 1 roentgen is:
   A. 100 ergs/g
   B. 2.58×10^{-4} C/kg
   C. 2.09×10^9 electrostatic units (ESU)
   D. 1 J/kg

Even a physics expert may find that the second question is much easier than the first. The correct answer to both is 1 R = 2.58×10^{-4} C/kg. But to answer the first question correctly, you would have needed to memorize all of the *precise* numbers used in the SI unit that correspond to exactly 1 roentgen. In contrast, all you needed to know to answer the second question correctly was that the SI system uses the unit coulomb (C) per kilogram as its measure for exposure.

The key to unlocking the multiple-choice format is the process of elimination!

In approaching the second question above, you did not need to know the *exact* answer ahead of time to find it among the choices. Instead, it could be found by eliminating the three choices that are known to be incorrect. This is known as the process of elimination and is a very effective tool.

Looking for Wrong Answers

As all examination creators can tell you, multiple-choice questions are the most tedious to write because not only do the item writers have to come up with the question *and* the correct answer, they also have to make up pertinent but definitely *incorrect* answers. These incorrect answers are known as *distracters*.

In writing questions for a specific course, I have found that the best method for assessing a student's knowledge of a particular subject is to use a variety of questions for unit tests, such as fill-in-the-blank, essay, matching, and short answer. However, for all final examinations, I use multiple-choice questions and some of the students' incorrect answers from the unit tests as distracters. This format is not only easiest for me to grade, but it seems to be the most comprehensive.

The Importance of Distracters

A good distracter, or incorrect choice, will distract less knowledgeable students away from correct choices on questions they do not understand. By using the process of elimination to spot these distracters, you will be able to greatly improve your chances of passing a certification or licensure examination. On difficult questions, distracters or wrong answers are usually easier to spot. And once the wrong ones are found, the correct answer is usually obvious. Thus, learning to recognize wrong answers is a key to success in a multiple-choice format.

The good news is that most certification and licensure examination questions have only four possible choices: A, B, C, or D. If you can eliminate a single distracter, you now have increased the odds to one in three of finding the correct response. If two choices are eliminated, you have a 50 percent chance of selecting the correct answer.

Sometimes the distracters will be so obvious that they will literally seem to jump off the page. Many students have told me that they had mixed emotions after completing a certification or licensure examination. Some of the more "test-wise" students said it seemed easy because even if they were not sure of the answer, the other choices were so obviously incorrect that the process of elimination worked every time. Many students felt unsure of their performance because they felt that the test was not as difficult as they had anticipated, and they therefore assumed that there must have been many "trick" questions thrown in to confuse them.

Trick questions are simply not the case. If a question seems easy, it probably is because you are prepared and know the correct response instinctively. It is not the intention of the certification or licensure agency to purposely confuse a qualified technologist. It is the responsibility of the certification or licensure agency to find out who is and who is not qualified. Virtually every question has the same goal: *to accurately test the knowledge of the examinee.*

What You Will Not Find on Most Certification or Licensure Examinations

Because it is not the intention of the certification or licensure agency to confuse examinees, you will not find certain types of questions on the radiography examination. These types are:

1. **Negative questions:** For example:

    I. When a radiographer obtains an abdominal radiograph, which of the following will *not* have a detrimental effect on image quality?
       A. Poor patient-technologist communication
       B. Developer temperature of 38°C
       C. Use of rare earth screens
       D. A 3-second exposure time

    A question that is much more likely to be asked is:

    II. When a radiographer obtains an abdominal radiograph, which of the following will have a detrimental effect on image quality?
       A. Use of rare earth screens
       B. Developer temperature of 38°C
       C. An extremely short exposure time (<100 milliseconds)
       D. Use of a compression device

    The second question is a "positive" question and is much less confusing and more appropriate in testing the knowledge of an examinee. The answer to Question I is C, and the answer to Question II is B. Negative questions are more likely to confuse a knowledgeable student and, in fact, may give a "test-wise" student—but not necessarily a knowledgeable student—an unfair advantage.

2. **Overlapping ranges:** Any legitimate test maker will not put itself at risk by having questions with

more than one possible response. This situation could arise if the writer of a test item submits a question with all of the responses presented as a range of possibilities. These ranges *absolutely* must not overlap. Most certification or licensure agencies discourage these types of questions from their item writers. Here is an example:

   I. The normal range of diastolic blood pressure for an average adult should be between:
   A. 40–60 mm Hg
   B. 50–70 mm Hg
   C. 60–80 mm Hg
   D. 70–90 mm Hg

3. **All of the above questions:** Most certification and licensure examinations do not use this type of question because a very knowledgeable student may answer "A" because it is correct, without looking at the remaining options.

What You Will Find on Most Certification and Licensure Examinations

1. **Multiple-response format:** What you *will* find on the certification and licensure examination instead of the "all of the above" question is what is called the "multiple-response format." Actually these questions should be much easier to answer by using the process of elimination method.

   Unfortunately, these questions are often the pitfall of many examinees. When approaching these types of questions, it is best to simply treat them as "True" or "False." Here is an example:

1. Examples of somatic effects of radiation would include which of the following:

   I. An individual who had been radiated 20 years previously and gave birth to a baby with Down syndrome
   II. An individual who had been exposed to a high dose of fluoroscopic radiation and experienced skin erythema
   III. An individual who had been employed as a radiographer and through an accumulated dose experienced cataracts.

   A. I and II only
   B. I and III only
   C. II and III only
   D. I, II, and III

   *Even if you know nothing about "somatic" effects, an examinee could probably still eliminate number I because it is most definitely a "genetic" effect. By eliminating number I all possible responses (A, B, and D) except C, which is the

correct answer, are now eliminated. This is why most certification and licensure agencies frown upon this type of question, because a very "test-wise" student—but not necessarily knowledgeable student—could easily find the answer to this type of question. However, there still are quite a few of these questions that will show up on your examination, so it is a good idea to learn how to tackle them.

2. **Charts, diagrams, and illustrations:** Asking students questions that refer to a chart, diagram, or illustration is probably the *best* method of using the multiple-choice format. These types of questions are very fair, accurately test the knowledge of the examinee, and are easy to write. Expect to see many of these on the certification or licensure examination. Examples would include (1) identifying anatomy, artifacts, and various positions on a radiograph, (2) determining various types of quality control (QC) test tools used in radiography, (3) labeling parts of the x-ray tube, (4) tube rating charts, and (5) monitoring the processor (sensitometry), just to name a few.

CONTENT SPECIFICATIONS: YOUR STUDY GUIDE

The certification and licensure agencies do not keep secret what is going to be asked on their examinations. It is all spelled out very clearly in the content specifications located in the respective examination application handbook.

   For example, since 1995, the radiography examination has consisted of questions covering the following content areas:
   Radiation Biology and Protection
   Physics of Equipment Construction, Operation, and Maintenance
   Production and Evaluation of Radiographic Images
   Radiographic Procedures
   Radiographic Anatomy and Terminology
   Patient Care during Radiographic Procedures
Most certification and licensure agencies take a step further and identify what particular topics in each of the content areas may be asked on the examination. Use these content specifications as a study guide. If a particular area listed in the content specifications is troublesome to you, then study that subject using the available references.

The "Scaled" Score

The score that is received from the certification or licensure agency is usually based on a scaled score, not a raw percentage score. The reason is that some versions of the examination may be easier or more difficult than previous examinations. Therefore, each test is graded on a different scale.

In some instances, the scaled score may be adjusted as much as 8 percentage points. In other words, if the overall raw score were 70 percent, you would receive a "scaled" score of 78. Because a scaled score of only 75 is needed to pass the examination, the scaled score helps to elevate the percentage score for the more difficult examinations.

I have included in the back of this review book a graph for calculating the scaled score. To make it easier, all five simulated examinations in this book have been given the same scale. The column on the left in white indicates the number of questions that were answered correctly, and the column on the right in gray indicates the corresponding scaled score. Be sure to also calculate the raw percentage score.

THE DAY OF THE EXAMINATION

1. **Be prepared:** Make sure that you have familiarized yourself with the exact location as well as the best route to take to get there. You will need to arrive at least 30 minutes early to find parking and register.

   You may need to sign an entrance pass and staple a 2 × 2 inch passport-quality photograph to the front of it. You may also need an additional photo identification (ID) (driver's license, state ID card, etc.) to verify your identity. Examinees without these items may *not* be allowed into the test site. It is also a good idea to bring a pencil, a watch, and a nonprogrammable calculator (programmable calculators may be prohibited and may be confiscated before entry into the test site).

   Finally, you should dress in layers so that your clothing may be adjusted, as necessary, to the environment. A cold or warm room could prove to be a distraction while taking the examination. You do not need this added distraction. Anticipate both scenarios and wear layers.

2. **Prepare your body as well as your mind:** During the week of the examination, be sure to get plenty of rest, especially the night before. Last-minute "cramming" is usually not going to help at this point and may produce unnecessary stress. It is advisable to eat well the day of the examination, starting with a balanced breakfast and avoiding stimulants. Coffee or caffeinated sodas may make you feel energized for the moment, but the ultimate effect will be a sluggish performance when you least desire it.

   Odds are you will grow increasingly nervous as the examination date nears. This reaction is perfectly normal. Realizing that your preparation

to take the examination is adequate and reassuring yourself of this fact is a comfort. Many experts believe that a little anxiety may actually improve performance in some individuals. So think of this extra nervous energy as an ally and use it to your advantage. If at any time during the examination an overwhelmed feeling or loss of concentration occurs because of increased nervousness, try closing your eyes and taking some slow deep breaths. Too much stress can create a condition of anoxia in vital organs of the body. Breathing correctly will not only help you to relax, but it will also help deliver oxygen to the brain, where it is needed the most. Above all, be confident in your level of preparation to take this examination.

3. **Review the test packet prior to starting the examination:** The test center should supply every examinee with scratch paper for use with the computerized examination. Be sure to have your pen/pencil and a calculator handy.

4. **Pace yourself:** One of the main goals of this review book is to provide a means of practicing how to pace yourself for a "timed" examination. Each simulation should be completed within 3 hours. Within this time frame, 200 multiple-choice questions are to be answered. The goal should be to complete at least 67 questions per hour. By understanding the format of the test and budgeting your time, you can work more efficiently through the questions in the allotted time. If questions remain incomplete within the last 10 minutes of the examination, use discretion to select one letter and answer *all* of the remaining questions with that letter. (Remember, for most certification or licensure examinations, there is no penalty for guessing, only for leaving questions unanswered.) Avoid wasting time by looking frequently at the clock.

5. **Write notes as needed on the scratch paper provided to use the process of elimination in a computerized examination:** Feel free to jot down as many notes, symbols, or formulas as needed throughout the test. For uncertain answers, make an educated guess after eliminating one or two of the possible choices. Again, there is no penalty for guessing, only for leaving questions unanswered.

6. **When you use the same letter for more than three answers in a row, double check the questions to verify each answer.** Most multiple-choice examinations will usually break up strings of four or more of the same letter or answer. This format is usually set so that three of the same letters in a row are the maximum run of correct responses. If four or more of the same

letters in a row are marked, and if time allows, it may be beneficial to recheck your answers. Save this task for the very end of the examination. You will be allowed to go back and change answers on the computerized version of the examination.

7. **Use key techniques to help select the correct answer:**
   a. **Follow your instincts:** If you have properly prepared and studied for the examination, your brain will instinctively know the correct responses among the choices. Do not try to "second guess" yourself; simply learn to trust your instincts, because the majority of the time, they are correct. Never go back and change answers at the end of the examination unless you know for certain that they are absolutely incorrect.
   b. **Ask, "What is this question asking?"** If you are unsure of what a question is asking, look for key words, and try not to be distracted by peripheral information. By determining what the question is asking, you will be more likely to choose the correct response.
   c. **Anticipate the answer:** If distracters can easily sway you, try this technique: Cover the responses after reading through the question and determine the answer without looking at the responses. Once again, if this choice is among the responses, this is by far the best response. Do not be influenced by those tempting distracters.
   d. **Use the process of elimination:** Sometimes, you will find that the first answer that pops into your mind instinctively is not among the list of options. In this case, you should revert back to the process of elimination. For example, while taking an examination, you may know instinctively that the centering point for a lateral view of the sella turcica is $3/4$ inch anterior and $3/4$ inch superior to the external auditory meatus (EAM). Unfortunately, this response may not be among the list of choices. The only response that comes close is 1 inch anterior and 1 inch superior to the EAM. If the right answer cannot be found, finding the wrong ones may invariably bring you to the correct choice.

CONCLUSION

As you go through this review book, remember these tips on test-taking strategy and practice using them with difficult questions. The tips that have been provided here are not all-inclusive. You may have found your own techniques for taking examinations that have proved successful. You should select only the tips that you feel comfortable using and then practice using these techniques while working through the simulations.

REFERENCES

American Registry of Radiologic Technologists Examinee Handbook. ARRT, Mendota Heights, MN, 1995.

American Registry of Radiologic Technologists Item Writers Manual. ARRT, Mendota Heights, MN, 1990

Anderson, DN, et al: The Occupational Therapy Examination Review Guide. FA Davis, Philadelphia, 1996.

GRE: Practicing to Take the General Test. Warner Books, New York, 1994.

Princeton Review of the Graduate Record Examination. Random House, New York, 1994.

REVIEW OF RADIOGRAPHIC EQUATIONS AND APPLIED PRINCIPLES

This review is not meant to be an exhaustive list of every formula used in radiologic technology. I know that your time is limited, so I tried to zero in on those particular concepts that seem to give every radiography student difficulty on examinations.

From my experience in talking with various graduates who have recently completed a certification or licensure examination, the test seems to focus mainly on applied knowledge, that is, concepts used in daily practice. Common examples include performing film critique, adjusting exposure factors to obtain optimum results while reducing the exposure risk to the patient and radiographer, providing proper care for a patient while in the radiology department, differentiating between normal and abnormal vital signs, and properly disposing of contaminated linens. Because of the renewed importance of quality assurance, other questions focus on making sure that your equipment, especially your processor, is working properly.

Concepts that are good to know, but are outside of the scope of practice, are typically not asked on certification or licensure examinations. For example, knowing the exact percentage of iodine content in a particular contrast material or being able to recognize unusual pathology on an image receptor is not gener-ally within the scope of practice. Although such knowledge may make you a very valuable employee, you can expect that very few questions at this difficulty level will be encountered on the examination.

Many of my students said that they concentrated much of their study efforts on the mathematical principles. Be sure to note the percent weighting for each section. Realize that if your weak points are radiation protection and radiographic equipment, both of these sections together may only comprise 30 percent of the entire examination. Although it would be desirable to score well in all sections, scoring high in the radiographic procedures and patient care sections, which may account for 45 percent of the examination, will greatly improve your chances of passing.

THE TWO MOST COMMON RADIOGRAPHIC FORMULAS

There are two formulas that have consistently shown up on simulated examinations. It is important for you to have a thorough understanding of both and be able to differentiate between the two, because they are very similar.

Inverse-square Law

Realize that the inverse-square law is an equation used routinely as a part of the *Radiation Protection* section of the examination. It is a formula that deals with properly protecting the patient and the technologist from overexposure. Because the intensity of the x-ray beam decreases with the square of the distance, distancing yourself from the radiation source will greatly reduce your occupational dose. It is for this reason that *distance is the No. 1 protection for an occupational worker!* The formula is set up as follows:

$$\frac{I_1}{I_2} = \left(\frac{D_2}{D_1}\right)^2$$

> **EXAMPLE:** If an occupational worker stood at a distance of 300 cm from a source and received a dose of 100 mR, what would the intensity be at a distance of 900 cm from the source?

$$\frac{100}{x} = \frac{900^2}{300^2}; \frac{100}{x} = \frac{810,000}{90,000}; 9x = 100;$$

$$x = \frac{100}{9}; x = 11.11 \text{ mR}$$

Milliamperage-seconds (mAs)–Distance Formula

Many students get this formula and the inverse-square law confused. Remember that this formula would only be used in instances where you need to alter your technique. The inverse-square law is an equation used routinely in questions pertaining to radiation protection, not in determining your knowledge of varying technical factors, such as milliamperage-seconds. However, because the intensity decreases with the square of the distance, it stands to reason that you would need to adjust your technique whenever a change of source-image receptor-distance (SID) is necessitated for the same patient's body part. The formula is as follows:

$$\frac{mAs_1}{mAs_2} = \frac{D_1{}^2}{D_2{}^2}$$

> **EXAMPLE:** A technologist was called to the postoperative area to take a mobile chest radiograph on a critically ill patient in the recumbent position. The maximum distance achievable was 40 inches. The technologist set a technique of 70 kVp at 2.5 mAs. Later when the patient was sent to his or her room, another mobile chest radiograph was ordered. This time the patient was sitting up in bed. The technologist took the radiograph at a distance of 72 inches. What new technique was necessary?

First of all, you should reasonably assume that more mAs is needed at a greater distance. Before be-

ginning to calculate for a change in technical factors, take a quick look at the possible choices. Those choices that are less than or the same as the original milliamperage-seconds should immediately be eliminated. When it becomes necessary to alter the SID, milliamperage-seconds should be the *only* controlling factor, not kVp!

$$\frac{2.5 \text{ mAs}}{x} = \frac{40^2}{72^2}; \frac{2.5 \text{ mAs}}{x} = \frac{1600}{5184}$$

$$2.5 \text{ mAs} = 0.308x; x = \frac{2.5}{0.308}; x = 8.1 \text{ mAs}$$

Exercises

As you work through the following problems, determine what is being asked and which formula needs to be used. Look for key words and weed out peripheral information.

1. If a radiographer is being exposed to 250 mR/h at a distance of 3 m from a source during a fluoroscopic procedure and then moves to a distance of 1 m to better care for the patient, what is the radiographer's exposure now?_____

2. If an examination requires a technique of 70 kVp, 400 mA, and 0.1 second at a distance of 100 cm from the source, what new technical factors would be required if it became necessary to adjust the SID to 250 cm?_____

3. When using a technique of 80 kVp and 40 mAs, a patient's entrance skin exposure measured 150 mR at 40 inches SSD. Using the same technical factors, what would this patient's exposure be at a 30 inches SSD?_____

4. A chest radiograph was taken using 75 kVp and 5 mAs at 72 inches SID. What technique would be required if the radiograph were to be taken with the patient in the recumbent position at a 50 inches SID?_____

RADIOGRAPHIC QUALITY "CHECKLIST"-TYPE QUESTIONS

There will be many of these questions asked in the Image Production and Evaluation section and possibly in the Radiation Protection section. Because these can be very time-consuming, it is important to establish a strategy for tackling these types of questions.

Here is an example:

I. Which of the following sets of technical factors would provide the greatest radiographic density?

	mA	Time	kVp	Screen Speed	Grid Ratio
A.	400	200 ms	90	200	12:1
B.	300	500 ms	70	400	8:1
C.	800	100 ms	80	100	10:1
D.	600	300 ms	80	200	6:1

Questions like these are extremely challenging because they combine an abundance of information in a single question. Thus, they are an easy way for the certification or licensure agency to establish your overall knowledge of a particular aspect of radiographic quality and factors affecting it such as density, contrast, and image blur.

First ask, "What is this question asking?" Well, it is asking the result of a variety of technical factors and their influence on *radiographic density*. Radiographic density is affected by all of the factors listed in the previous question, requiring you to put your knowledge of all of these aspects together to solve the problem (knowledge of screens, grids, milliamperes, and kilovolt [peaks]).

NOTE: Sometimes, these questions *will* include factors that have no influence on the elements in question. For instance, a question dealing with the effect of geometric blur on an image may throw in the factors of milliampere and kilovolt (peak) along with the factors most affecting blur, which include SID, object-image receptor-distance (OID), and focal spot size. Be careful not to include the erroneous factors.

Assuming you already possess the knowledge to solve this problem, a fast and easy way to do this is as follows:

1. First solve for milliamperes (mA × time)
2. Next assign a number to each factor in the list according to its effect on density. For example, if there are four different milliampere settings for the four choices, assign a 1 to the milliampere-seconds that would create the least radiographic density and a 4 to the milliampere-seconds that would create the greatest radiographic density. Do this for each of the factors listed that affect radiographic density.
3. Finally, add up all of the numbers from each factor for each item across the row. The item with the highest sum will be the radiograph with the greatest density.

Here is an example using this question:

I. Which of the following sets of technical factors would provide the film with the greatest radiographic density?

	mA	Time	mAs	kVp	Screen Speed	Grid Ratio
A.	400	200 ms	80^1	90^3	200^2	$12{:}1^1$
B.	300	500 ms	150^2	70^1	400^3	$8{:}1^2$
C.	800	100 ms	80^1	80^2	100^1	$10{:}1^1$
D.	600	300 ms	180^3	80^2	200^2	$6{:}1^3$

The answer would be D using this method because it contains the highest sum from each of the contributing factors (A = 7, B = 8, C = 5, D = 10).

Bear in mind that this method has been found to be correct only 75 percent of the time. Therefore, you may have to find the answer the long way by using all of the radiographic quality rules that were learned (15 percent rule, new grid and old grid, old screen and new screen, etc.). You will feel much more relaxed knowing that you can spend very little time on each of these questions and still be confident choosing the correct answer.

If there is time at the end of the examination, it would not hurt to go back and recheck the answers to ensure that each has been calculated correctly. It is easy to get confused using the shortened method because you may have inadvertently assigned a "1" to one contributing factor and a "4" to another, both of which will have the greatest effect on density. Be careful not to do this. If this method does not work, stick to a method that does. Whatever method used, just remember to *practice and practice* solving these questions and they will become easier.

RADIOGRAPHIC FORMULAS AND CALCULATIONS WITH SAMPLE QUESTIONS

The following is a list of the most common prefixes and the most frequently used formulas in radiography. It is not important to be an expert in calculating all of these formulas to be successful on the examination. However, having the analytical ability to understand the application of these formulas will help you to understand some of the basic concepts of radiation protection, radiation physics, radiographic technique selection, and quality assurance.

1. Numerical Prefixes

Prefix	Scientific Notation	Corres. No.
mega (M)	10^6	1,000,000
kilo (k)	10^3	1,000
centi (c)	10^{-2}	1/100
milli (m)	10^{-3}	1/1000
micro (μ)	10^{-6}	1/1,000,000
nano (n)	10^{-9}	1/1,000,000,000
angstrom (Å)	10^{-10}	1/10,000,000,000
pico (p)	10^{-12}	1/1,000,000,000,000

EXAMPLE 1: 1 millirem (mrem) = 1/1000 of a rem

EXAMPLE 2: 1 megavolt (MV) = 1 million volts (V)

SAMPLES:

70,000 V = _____ kilovolts (kV)

511 kV = _____ MV

10^{-11} m = _____ nm = _____ Å

50 mSv (5000 mrem) = _____ rem

5000 mSv (mrem) = _____ mSv (mrem) = _____ Sv

For the following formulas, the subscript 1 stands for the original factor in the equation, and the subscript 2 is the change, or new technical factor:

2. Milliampere-second Conversions

$$\frac{mA_1}{mA_2} = \frac{Time_2}{Time_1} \qquad mA \times time = mAs$$

3. Milliampere-second–Distance Formula

$$\frac{mAs_1}{mAs_2} = \frac{D_1^2}{D_2^2}$$

a. Time-distance Formula

$$\frac{t_1}{t_2} = \frac{D_1^2}{D_2^2}$$

b. Milliampere-distance Formula

$$\frac{mA_1}{mA_2} = \frac{D_1^2}{D_2^2}$$

4. Inverse-square Law

$$\frac{I_1}{I_2} = \frac{D_2^2}{D_1^2}$$

5. Grid Conversion Factors (factors most accepted by certification or licensure examinations)

Grid Type	Factor
No grid	1
5:1	2
6:1	3
8:1	4
10:1 & 12:1	5
16:1	6

$$\left(\frac{\text{Grid Conversion Factor}_2}{\text{Grid Conversion Factor}_1}\right) \times mAs_1 = mAs_2$$

EXAMPLE: If a technologist used 80 kVp at 50 mAs using an 8:1 grid while performing a mobile examination, what new milliampere-seconds would be needed in a 12:1 Bucky grid?

$$\left(\frac{5}{4} = 1.25\right) \times 50 = 62.5 \text{ mAs}$$

6. Grid Ratio (R = h/d)

EXAMPLE: If the height of the lead strips is 2.5 mm, the thickness of the strips is 0.2 mm, and the distance between them is 0.25 mm, what is the grid ratio?

$$\frac{2.5}{0.25} = 10:1$$

SAMPLE: If the height of the lead strips is 3.6 mm, the thickness of the strips is 0.15 mm, and the distance between them is 0.3 mm, what is the grid ratio?_____

7. mR/mAs

EXAMPLE: Exposure equals 150 mR at 50 mAs.

$$\frac{150}{50} = 3 \text{ mR/mAs}$$

SAMPLE: If a radiographic x-ray tube is calibrated to have a dose of 5 mR/mAs, what would be the dose if a technique of 50 mAs were used?

_____

8. Entrance Skin Exposure (fluoroscopy)

At 2.1 rad/mA per minute at 80 kVp

EXAMPLE: What is the exposure at 2.5 mA, 80 kVp for 3 minutes?

$2 \times 2.5 \times 3 = @15$ rad skin dose

SAMPLE: What would be the approximate skin dose for a patient if the fluoroscopic unit were set at 3 mA, 80 kVp for 4 minutes?

_____

9. Fifteen Percent Kilovolts (peak) Rule

Increase kilovolts (peak) by 15 percent: must compensate with a 50% reduction of the mAs to maintain density.
Decrease kilovolts (peak) by 15 percent: must compensate by doubling the milliampere-seconds to maintain radiographic density.

EXAMPLE: If an original technique set at 70 kVp, 40 mAs demonstrated adequate radiographic density but a decrease in contrast was desired, what new technique would increase contrast while maintaining proper radiographic density?

$70 \times 0.15 = 10.5; 70 + 10.5 =$
81 kVp at ½ mAs, or 20 mAs

SAMPLE: If an original technique set at 80 kVp, 50 mAs demonstrated adequate radiographic density but poor contrast, what new technique would demonstrate higher contrast while maintaining proper radiographic density?

_____

10. Heat Units (HU)

kVp $\times$ mA $\times$ Time $\times$ 1 for single phase
kVp $\times$ mA $\times$ Time $\times$ 1.35 for 3-phase, 6-pulse
kVp $\times$ mA $\times$ Time $\times$ 1.41 for 3-phase, 12-pulse
kVp $\times$ mA $\times$ Time $\times$ 1.45 for high frequency

11. Screen Conversion

$$\frac{\text{Old screen (RS)} \times \text{Old mAs}}{\text{New screen (RS)}} = \text{New mAs}$$

or

$$\frac{\text{mAs}_1}{\text{mAs}_2} = \frac{\text{(RS) Screen speed}_2}{\text{(RS) Screen speed}_1}$$

12. Ohm's Law

$$V = IR$$

13. Calculation of Power

$$P = IV \ or \ P = I^2R$$

14. Maximum Number of Electrons in Shells of Atom ($2n^2$)

K $= 2$	2×1^2
L $= 8$	2×2^2
M $= 18$	2×3^2
N $= 32$	2×4^2
O $= 50$	2×5^2
P $= 72$	2×6^2

15. Magnification Factor (MF)

$$\frac{\text{SID}}{\text{SOD}} \ or \ \frac{\text{SID}}{\text{SID} - \text{OID}} \ or \ \frac{\text{Image size}}{\text{Object size}} = \text{MF}$$

16. Magnification (%)

$$\frac{\text{SID}}{\text{SOD}} - 1 \times 100$$

EXAMPLE:

$$\frac{40}{36} = 1.11 - 1 = 0.11 \times 100 = 11\%$$

17. Transformer Law

$$\frac{V_s}{V_p} = \frac{N_s}{N_p}$$

18. Voltage-Amperage Relationship

$$\frac{V_s}{V_p} = \frac{I_p}{I_s}$$

19. Dose-equivalent Limits (cumulative exposure)

1 rem $\times$ Age of worker

or

10 mSv $\times$ Age *or* 1 cSv $\times$ Age

EXAMPLE: A 50-year-old technologist working for 20 years should have a total cumulative lifetime limit of 50 rem, or 500 mSv.

20. Unit Conversions

a. Exposure: $1 R = 2.58 \times 10^{-4} C/ kg$ of air

PROBLEMS:

$$25 R = \text{_____} C/kg$$
$$440 mR = \text{_____} C/kg$$
$$1 C/kg = \text{_____} R$$

b. Absorbed dose: $1 rad = 10^{-2} Gy$

$$1 Gy = 100 rad$$

PROBLEMS:

$$85 rad = \text{_____} Gy$$
$$\text{_____} rad = 6.25 Gy$$
$$2400 rad = \text{_____} Gy$$

c. Dose equivalent: rad $\times$ quality factor (QF) = rem

$1 rem = 0.01 Sv$; $1 rem = 10 mSv$; $1 rem = 1 cSv$

$$1 Sv = 100 rem$$

PROBLEMS:

$$16 rem = \text{_____} Sv$$
$$\text{_____} rem = 0.60 Sv \text{ or } 60 cSv$$
$$512 rem = \text{_____} Sv$$

21. Brightness Gain (fluoroscopy)

$$\text{Minification gain} = \frac{\text{Input phosphor}^2}{\text{Output phosphor}^2}$$

$$\text{Brightness gain} = \text{Minification gain} \times \text{Flux gain}$$

EXAMPLE: What is the brightness gain for a 17-cm image-intensifier tube having a flux gain of 120 and an output phosphor of 2.5 cm?

$$\frac{17^2}{2.5^2} \times 120 = 46 \times 120 = 5548$$

22. Energy-wavelength Relationship

$$E = \frac{12.4}{\lambda} \qquad \lambda = \frac{12.4}{E}$$

As energy increases, wavelength decreases for all electromagnetic (EM) radiation. Because 12.4 is a constant (Planck's constant), the relationship is inversely proportional.

23. Wavelength-frequency Relationship

$c = \nu\lambda$; Speed of light in the SI system = Frequency $\times$ Wavelength
As frequency goes up, wavelength goes down for all EM energy, because the velocity is con stant.
(Inversely proportional!)

24. Speed of Light

$$\text{MKS system (SI)} = 3 \times 10^8 \text{ m/s}$$
$$\text{CGS system} = 3 \times 10^{10} \text{ cm/s}$$
$$\text{English system} = 186,400 \text{ miles/second}$$

25. Energy-frequency Relationship

$$E = h\nu$$

As energy of an EM photon increases, so does its frequency according to Planck's constant. (Directly proportional!)

26. Field-size Coverage

$$\frac{F_1}{F_2} = \frac{D_1}{D_2}$$

EXAMPLE: When radiographing an image at a distance of 40 in., the x-ray beam covers a field size of 10×12. What would the field size be at a 20-in. SID?

$$\frac{10 \times 12 \text{ in.}}{x} = \frac{40 \text{ in.}}{20 \text{ in.}} ; \frac{10 \times 12 \text{ in.}}{x} = 2;$$

$$\frac{10 \times 12 \text{ in.}}{2} = x$$

$$x = 5 \times 6 \text{ in.}$$

27. Spinning Top Test and Oscilloscope

a. $$\frac{\text{No. of dots}}{\text{No. of pulses}} = \text{time}$$

(Half-wave rectified = 60 pulses/s)

(Full-wave rectified = 120 pulses/s)

or

No. of pulses $\times$ time = No. of dots

EXAMPLE: When performing a spinning top test on a single-phase, half-wave rectified machine, how many dots would you expect to see for an exposure time of $\frac{1}{10}$ second?

60 × 1/10 = 6 dots

SAMPLE: What if the machine were a full-wave rectified unit?_____

b. For 3-phase equipment, no dots will appear on the radiograph because voltage never drops to zero. You will simply measure the arc angle made by the oscilloscope:

$$\frac{Arc\ (°)}{360°} = time$$

or

$$360° × time = Arc\ (°)$$

EXAMPLE: When performing a timer test on a 3-phase machine using an exposure time of ½₀ second, what would the resultant QC film look like?

$$360° × \tfrac{1}{20} = 18°\ arc$$

28. Geometric Blur

$$\frac{OID}{SOD} × FSS = blur$$

SID-OID

EXAMPLE: Which of the following sets of technical factors would provide the image with the least geometric blur (greatest unsharpness)?

mAs	kVp	SID	OID	FS
A. 50	75	100	20	1
B. 65	84	140	40	2
C. 75	65	180	30	2
D. 60	70	140	30	1

20/80 × 1 = 0.25 = least blur
40/100 × 2 = 0.8
30/150 × 2 = 0.4
30/110 × 1 = 0.27

REVIEW OF MATHEMATICS SKILLS

Now, try the following sample questions:

1. A technique of 85 kVp, 500 mA at 0.012 second would result in what milliampere-seconds setting? _____

2. The wavelength of an x-ray photon measures 0.5 A. What is its equivalent in meters? _____

3. A technique of 32 mAs at 60 kVp would be equivalent to 16 mAs at what kVp? _____

4. A radiograph of the knee is taken using 65 kVp, 8 mAs at tabletop with no grid. If the image needs to have better contrast and is placed in the Bucky tray with a 10:1 grid, what new mAs would be necessary to maintain density? _____

5. A patient's skin dose at a 60-cm SSD is approximately 156 mR. What would be the approximate skin dose if the SSD were changed to 120 cm? _____

6. A technique chart recommends using 15 mAs, 70 kVp at a 40-in. SID for a particular procedure. Because of patient limitations, only a 35-in. SID is possible. What new mAs should be used? _____

7. Using a 40-in. SID, an object is placed 4 in. from the image-receptor. What would be the magnification factor for this image?
_____

8. If the object in the previous question measured 5 cm, what would be the image size?
_____

9. Using this same magnification factor, what if the image size measured 9.435 cm. What would the size of the object?
_____

10. Calculate the heat units for a 3-phase, 12-pulse machine when five rapid exposures of 70 kVp, 1000 mA at 32 ms are taken?
_____

ANSWERS TO SAMPLE QUESTIONS

Milliampere-Seconds–Square Law versus Inverse-Square Law
1. 250 × 9 = 2250 mR; *inverse-square law*
2. 40 mAs × 6.25 = 250 mAs; *mAs-square law*
3. 16/9 × 150 mR = 266.66 mR; *inverse-square law*
4. 0.48 × 5 = 2.4 mAs; *mAs-square law*

Prefix Conversions
1. 70,000 V = 70 kV
2. 511 kV = 0.511 MeV
3. 10^{-11} m = 10^{-2} nm = 10^{-1} A
4. 5000 mrem = 5 rem
5. 5000 mSv = 5,000,000 μSv = 5 sV

Grid Ratio
1. 3.6 mm/0.3 mm = 12:1 grid ratio

mR/mAs Formula
1. 5 mR/mAs × 50 mAs = 250 mR total exposure

Entrance Skin Exposure
1. 2.1 R/3 mA/4 min = 2.1 × 3 × 4 = 24 rad

15 Percent Kilovolts (Peak) Rule
1. 80 kVp × 0.15 = 12; 80 − 12 = 68 kVp at mAs = 25 mAs
New technique: 68 kVp at 25 mAs to produce superior contrast

Dose Unit Conversions
1. 25 R = 25 × 2.58 × 10^{-4} C/kg = 64.5 × 10^{-4} *or* 6.45 × 10^{-3} C/Kg
2. 440 mR = 0.44 R = 0.44 × 2.58 × 10^{-4} C/kg = 1.132 × 10^{-4} C/kg
3. 1 C/kg = 1/2.58 × 10^{-4} R = 1/0.000258 R = 3876 R
4. 85 rad = 0.85 Gy
5. 6.25 Gy = 625 rad
6. 2400 rad = 24 Gy
7. 16 rem = 0.16 sievert
8. 60 rem = 0.60 Sv
9. 512 rem = 5.12 Sv

Spinning Top Test
1. 120 pulses for full-wave; 120 × 1/10 = 12 dots

ANSWERS TO REVIEW OF MATHEMATICS SKILLS

1. 6 mAs
2. 5 × 10^{-11} meters
3. 69 kVp
4. 8 × 5 = 40 mAs
5. 156/4 = 39 mR
6. 15 × $35^2/40^2$; $7^2/8^2$; 49/64 × 15 = 11.48 or 12 mAs
7. 40/36 = 1.11
8. 5× 1.11 = 5.55
9. 9.435/1.11 = 8.5 cm
10. 70 × 1000 × 0.032 × 1.41 × 5 = 15,792

PART 2

SIMULATION
EXAMINATIONS

SIMULATION EXAMINATION 1

QUESTIONS

Directions: (Questions 1 to 200) For each of the following items, select the best answer among the four possible choices (A, B, C, or D). For ease of scoring, it is suggested that you use the bubble sheet provided in the back of this examination. Make sure to answer all questions. You should allow yourself a maximum of 3 hours to take this examination.

Refer to the scale in the back of the book to determine a passing score in each section. It is not necessary that you pass each section, but you must receive a total "scaled" score of 75 to pass the examination.

SECTION I: RADIATION PROTECTION AND RADIOBIOLOGY

1. If a male patient were exposed to a dose of 0.3 Gy (30 rad) or more while undergoing a fluoroscopic procedure, what is the most likely *early* biologic response the patient may experience?
   A. Temporary sterility
   B. Cataractogenesis
   C. Decreased blood count
   D. Skin erythema

2. Which of the following statements would be *most* important for a pregnant radiographer?
   A. "Don't wear a lead apron to assure an accurate fetal dose."
   B. "Don't switch dosimeters between the collar and waist level."

C. "Make sure you are assigned to high-radiation areas only."
   D. "Find temporary alternative employment outside of radiology."

3. Which of the following would best demonstrate free air in the abdomen of a 3-year-old child with the least risk to the patient?
   A. Upright anteroposterior (AP) projection with a grid
   B. Decubitus projection without a grid
   C. Recumbent AP projection with a grid
   D. Recumbent AP projection without a grid

4. Which of the following are considered in the calculation of the monthly dosimetry reading?
   1. Natural background radiation
   2. Nuclear fallout
   3. Occupational dose

   A. 1 only
   B. 1 and 2 only
   C. 2 and 3 only
   D. 3 only

5. While radiographing the lumbar vertebrae of a geriatric patient, an optimal radiograph requires a technique of 70 kilovolts (peak) (kVp) and 40 mAs. What kind of changes could one make in technique while maintaining adequate radiographic density to reduce exposure to the patient?
   A. Increase kilovolts (peak) by 15 percent.
   B. Increase milliamperage-seconds by 30 percent.
   C. Increase kilovolts (peak) by 15 percent with a

50 percent decrease in milliamperage-seconds.

D. Increase milliamperage-seconds by 30 percent with a 15 percent decrease in kilovolts (peak).

6. When using the C-arm mobile unit, which of these choices will best reduce patient dose?
   A. Placing the x-ray tube as close as possible to the patient
   B. Placing the intensification tower as close as possible to the patient
   C. Properly placing the tower drape on the C-arm mobile unit
   D. Properly placing the shadow shield in the beam

7. In the third trimester, what is the recommended monthly dose-equivalent limit for the fetus?
   A. 0.5 mSv (0.05 rem)
   B. 5 mSv (0.5 rem)
   C. 50 mSv (5 rem)
   D. 0 mSv (0 rem)

8. Which of the following methods of detecting radiation is the most useful for measuring radiation exposure in air?
   A. Scintillation
   B. Ionization
   C. Biologic
   D. Chemical

9. What is the recommended minimum source-skin distance (SSD) on a mobile fluoroscopic unit?
   A. 30 cm (12 in.)
   B. 38 cm (15 in.)
   C. 45 cm (18 in.)
   D. 60 cm (24 in.)

10. Which of the following will be accomplished by the proper use of beam-limiting devices?
    1. Improved image quality
    2. Reduced patient dose
    3. Reduced scatter radiation production

    A. 1 only
    B. 1 and 3 only
    C. 2 and 3 only
    D. 1, 2, and 3

11. If a radiographer receives a dose of 68 mR/h while standing at a distance of 40 inches from the radiation source, what would the new exposure be if the radiographer moves to a distance of 60 inches from the radiation source?
    A. 30 mR/h
    B. 45 mR/h
    C. 90 mR/h
    D. 150 mR/h

12. Which type of personnel monitor measures radiation through a chemical change or reaction?
    A. Film badge
    B. Thermoluminescent dosimeter (TLD)
    C. Blood count
    D. Pocket dosimeter

13. To protect both the patient and the radiographer, at a distance of 1 m from the source, leakage radiation should not exceed:
    A. 10 mR/h
    B. 100 mR/h
    C. 10 mR/min
    D. 100 mR/min

14. If a patient were to undergo a fluoroscopic procedure for 5 minutes at 3 mA and 80 kVp, the maximum skin dose would be approximately:
    A. 15 cGy (15 rad)
    B. 30 cGy (30 rad)
    C. 45 cGy (45 rad)
    D. 60 cGy (60 rad)

    [handwritten: time x mAX 2.1
    5 x 3 x 2.1
    15
    2.1   31.5
    ——
    315 *]*

15. What is the acronym used in radiobiology for the genetic load on a population following gonadal exposure?
    A. ALARA
    B. GSD
    C. RBE
    D. LET

16. What is the most likely potential hazard involved in working in diagnostic radiology?
    A. Aplastic anemia
    B. Cataractogenesis
    C. Skin erythema
    D. Carcinogenesis

17. What is the recommended minimum amount of filtration in a fluoroscopic unit?
    A. 1.5 mm aluminum (Al) equivalent
    B. 2 mm Al equivalent
    C. 2.5 mm Al equivalent
    D. 3 mm Al equivalent

18. The main property of x-radiation that makes it potentially hazardous is its ability to:
    A. Travel at the speed of light
    B. Scatter
    C. Ionize
    D. Cause fluorescence

19. Which of the following sets of exposure factors would provide the least patient exposure?

mA	Time	kVp	Screen Speed	Grid
A. 200	0.4	70	100	12:1
B. 400	0.2	80	200	8:1
C. 800	0.1	90	400	6:1
D. 600	0.2	70	200	5:1

20. According to current standards, a radiation worker's cumulative dose-equivalent limit is determined by:
    A. (Age − 18) × 5 mSv (0.5 rem)
    B. (Age − 18) × 50 mSv (5 rem)
    C. Age × 100 mSv (10 rem)
    D. Age × 10 mSv (1 rem)

21. The x-ray interactions with matter that cause ionization of the irradiated material include:
    1. Photoelectric effect
    2. Compton scattering
    3. Pair production

    A. 1 and 2 only
    B. 2 and 3 only
    C. 1 and 3 only
    D. 1, 2, and 3

22. What is the active component of the TLD?
    A. Cesium iodide
    B. Zinc cadmium sulfide
    C. Lithium fluoride
    D. Sodium iodide

23. Which unit of measure would be most appropriate for stating the quantity of radiation exposure as measured by an ionization chamber?
    A. Coulomb (C) per kilogram (roentgen)
    B. Sievert (rad)
    C. Gray (rem)
    D. Curie (becquerel)

24. Which of the following types of human tissue cells is considered to be the most radioresistant?
    A. Neuroblast
    B. Erythrocyte
    C. Lymphocyte
    D. Spermatogonia

25. Which of the following types of radiation effects would be considered a deterministic effect?
    A. Genetic defects
    B. Cataractogenesis
    C. Leukemia
    D. Thyroid cancer

26. The occupational radiation dose-equivalent limit for stochastic effects of the whole body is now determined to be:
    A. 0.5 mSv (0.05 rem)
    B. 5 mSv (0.5 rem)
    C. 50 mSv (5 rem)
    D. 500 mSv (50 rem)

27. If a radiographer sets a technique of 75 kVp and 50 mAs for an AP projection of the abdomen but was asked to reduce the dose to the patient, the radiographer could:
    A. Use a detail speed screen with a comparable change in milliamperage-seconds

B. Use a decrease in kilovolts (peak) with a comparable change in milliamperage-seconds
C. Use a higher speed screen with a comparable change in milliamperage-seconds
D. Use an increase in milliamperage-seconds with a comparable change in kilovolts (peak)

28. Added filtration in a diagnostic x-ray machine is used for the main purpose of reducing radiation dose to the
    A. Radiographer/operator
    B. Patient's gonads
    C. Patient's skin
    D. Patient's bone marrow

29. Which type of personnel monitor may be worn for the longest period of time?
    A. TLD
    B. Pocket dosimeter
    C. Film badge
    D. Cutie pie

30. Which of the following groups benefit from the as low as reasonably achievable (ALARA) principle as set forth by the National Council on Radiation Protection and Measurement (NCRP)?
    1. General public
    2. Patient
    3. Radiographers/operators

    A. 2 only
    B. 3 only
    C. 2 and 3 only
    D. 1, 2, and 3

SECTION II: EQUIPMENT OPERATION AND MAINTENANCE

31. The reduction in resolution often seen with the use of higher tube currents in single-focus tubes is a phenomenon called:
    A. Off-focus radiation
    B. Blooming
    C. Line focus principle
    D. Characteristic radiation

32. In a modern image intensifier, what purpose does the photocathode serve?
    A. Converts exit radiation to light photons
    B. Converts light photons to electrons
    C. Converts electrons to light photons
    D. Converts electrons to x-radiation

Using the diagram in Figure 1–1, answer questions 33 and 34.

33. Identify the part of the x-ray tube labeled 5:
    A. Cathode
    B. Focusing cup

C. Rotor
D. Stator

34. Identify the part of the x-ray tube labeled 2:
    A. Filament
    B. Focusing cup
    C. Anode
    D. Stator

35. Which type of generator would incorporate a DC chopper in order to convert 60 Hz AC to pulsed DC?
    A. Full-wave rectified
    B. 3-phase, 12-pulse
    C. 3-phase, 6-pulse
    D. High-frequency

36. In a series circuit, the total resistance is calculated by the reciprocal of each of the individual resistors. The unit used to measure resistance is the
    A. Farad
    B. Ampere
    C. Ohm
    D. Watt

37. Where is the exposure timer located in a typical x-ray circuit?
    A. On the primary side of the step-up transformer
    B. Between the secondary side of the step-up transformer and the x-ray tube   meter
    C. On the primary side of the step-down transformer
    D. Between the secondary side of the step-down transformer and the x-ray tube

38. In an image intensifier, the squared ratio of the area of the input screen to the output screen is defined as:
    A. Brightness gain
    B. Minification gain
    C. Intensification factor
    D. Automatic brightness control

39. What is the typical frame size of most spot film (photospot) cameras used for diagnostic imaging?
    A. 16 to 35 mm
    B. 40 to 60 mm
    C. 70 to 105 mm
    D. 110 to 125 mm

40. Where should the ionization chamber be located if it is to be used as an efficient automatic exposure timer?
    A. On the primary side of the autotransformer
    B. Between the x-ray tube and the patient
    C. Between the patient and the image receptor
    D. Behind the image receptor

41. What must be done to x-ray film to make it compatible with a rare earth phosphor intensification screen?
    A. Use silver oxysulfide in place of silver halide in the film emulsion.
    B. Use a rare earth component in the x-ray film emulsion.
    C. Add a light-absorbing dye in the x-ray film emulsion.
    D. Use a rare earth component in the x-ray film base.

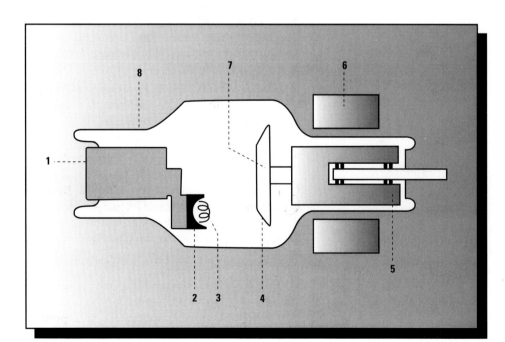

FIGURE 1–1. Diagram of x-ray tube.

42. To emit electrons from its surface, the x-ray tube filament must be heated sufficiently to cause:
    A. Phosphorescence
    B. Incandescence → *heating of filament*
    C. Luminescence
    D. Fluorescence

43. To ensure proper light field to radiation field alignment, the deflecting mirror must be situated at a _____ angle to the x-ray beam.
    A. 30°
    B. 45°
    C. 75°
    D. 90°

44. If you were using an automatic exposure control (AEC) device to make an exposure, which of these would be adjusted to ensure a proper optical density from patient to patient?

    1. Set time
    2. Set field detector
    3. Set density compensation

    A. 1 and 2 only
    B. 1 and 3 only
    C. 2 and 3 only
    D. 1, 2, and 3

45. Which device in the typical x-ray circuit is adjusted to select the kilovoltage?
    A. Autotransformer
    B. Step-up transformer
    C. Step-down transformer
    D. Rectification system

46. How many pulses per cycle are found in a single-phase, full-wave rectified x-ray machine?
    A. 1
    B. 2
    C. 4
    D. 6

47. What is the typical voltage ripple in a high-frequency generator?
    A. 100 percent
    B. 13.5 percent
    C. 4 to 5 percent
    D. <4 percent

48. What is the primary factor affecting the brightness of the fluoroscopic image?
    A. Field size
    B. Magnification factor
    C. Density of the anatomic part
    D. Source-image receptor-distance (SID)

49. What is the minimum suggested schedule for testing lead aprons and gloves for inadequate shielding?
    A. Weekly
    B. Monthly
    C. Semiannually
    D. Annually

For questions 50 and 51, refer to the graph in Figure 1–2:

50. What is the maximum exposure time that may be used with 90 kVp, 400 mA, and a small focal spot size (FSS)?
    A. 10 milliseconds
    B. 50 milliseconds
    C. 100 milliseconds
    D. 500 milliseconds

51. What is the maximum milliampere station that can be used for a 0.5-second (500-millisecond) exposure with 70 kVp and a large FSS?
    A. 200-mA station
    B. 300-mA station
    C. 400-mA station
    D. 500-mA station

52. Images are being produced with excessive blurring at the edges when certain cassettes are used. What quality control device should be used to evaluate this blur?
    A. Pinhole camera *focal spot*
    B. Wire-mesh → *film screen contact*
    C. Star test pattern *focal spot*
    D. Oscilloscope *timer of 3 phase*

53. What result is indicated by evaluating the radiograph in Figure 1–3?
    A. Inaccurate timer
    B. Faulty milliampere output
    C. Insufficient kilovolt (peak) output
    D. Incorrect light/x-ray field alignment

54. What component of the image intensifier accelerates electrons toward the output phosphor?
    A. Electrostatic lenses
    B. Focusing cup
    C. Electron gun
    D. Photocathode

55. What type of artifact will result on a radiograph from dirt or dust on an intensification screen?
    A. An area of increased film density
    B. An area of decreased film density
    C. An area of geometric unsharpness
    D. An area of decreased contrast

56. Underexposed radiographs produced while using an AEC device might result from:
    A. Using high-speed screens when the device has been calibrated for medium screens
    B. Having the Bucky chamber set while taking exposures in the chest unit
    C. Having an insufficient backup time set for a very large patient
    D. Having the density setting set at a positive level, instead of at zero or a normal level

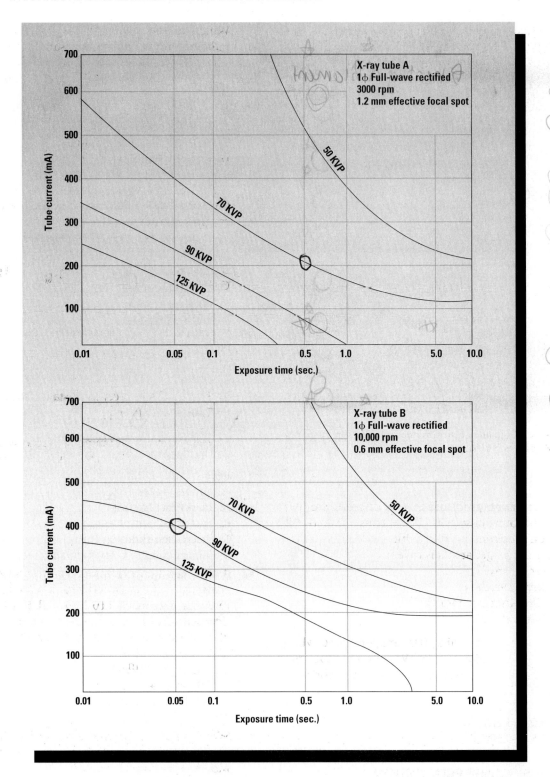

FIGURE 1–2. X-ray tube rating charts.

57. An older x-ray tube that has evaporated tungsten deposited on the tube window may cause one or more of the following problems:

1. Decreased tube output
2. Decreased half-value layer (HVL)
3. Arcing of the tube current

A. 1 and 2 only
B. 2 and 3 only
C. 1 and 3 only
D. 1, 2, and 3

58. What is the maximum number of electrons that may be found in the L shell of an atom?

A. 2
B. 4
C. 6
D. 8

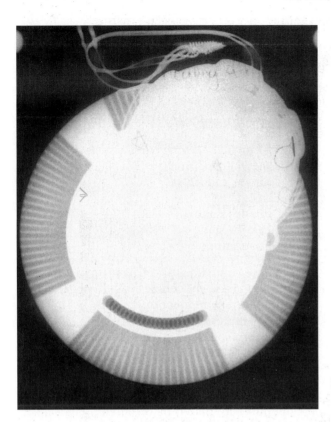

FIGURE 1–3. Radiograph of a synchronous spinning top. (Courtesy of JRMC Engineering Department.)

59. The radiation produced at very discrete energies of approximately 69 kiloelectron volts (keV) when electrons interact with the K shell of the tungsten target atoms is called:
    A. Grenz rays
    B. *Bremsstrahlung*
    C. Characteristic radiation
    D. Photoelectric

60. How many heat units (HU) are generated when setting a technique of 75 kVp, 400 mA, 250 milliseconds, on a 3-phase, 12-pulse generator?
    A. 7500 HU
    B. 10,125 HU
    C. 10,575 HU
    D. 75,000 HU

SECTION III: IMAGE PRODUCTION AND EVALUATION

61. Which one of the following sets of exposure factors would result in an image with the greatest optical density?

	mA	Time	kVp	Screen Speed	Grid Ratio	SID
A.	400	100 ms	70	200	12:1	100 cm
B.	200	400 ms	75	400	6:1	200 cm
C.	300	200 ms	80	800	8:1	100 cm
D.	800	100 ms	65	200	8:1	200 cm

62. Which of the following may be used by the radiographer to help compensate for the varying densities of anatomic structures on a routine posteroanterior (PA) projection of the chest?
    A. Rare earth intensifying screen
    B. Trough filter
    C. Line voltage compensator
    D. Compensating wedge filter

63. When performing magnification radiography, if the SID is 40 in. (100 cm) and the object-image receptor-distance (OID) is 6 in. (15 cm), how much would the object be magnified?
    A. ×0.85
    B. ×1.18
    C. ×1.35
    D. ×1.50

    $40/40-6 = 40/34 = 1.18$ $1.176\sim$

64. Which of the following would affect shape distortion?
    A. SID
    B. OID
    C. Source-object receptor-distance (SOD)
    D. Tube angulation

65. All other factors remaining the same, what effect does *excessive* filtration have on a radiographic image?
    A. Reduced contrast
    B. Increased density
    C. Increased contrast
    D. Decreased sharpness

66. A chest radiograph is taken with the patient erect against the chest Bucky with a 12:1 grid using technical factors of 110 kVp and 5 mAs. What new technical factors should be used on a dedicated chest unit that has an 8:1 grid?
    A. 110 kVp, 4 mAs
    B. 110 kVp, 6.25 mAs
    C. 100 kVp, 4 mAs
    D. 100 kVp, 6.25 mAs

    $8:1/12:1 = 4/5 \times 5 = 4$ mAs

67. Which of the following advanced pathological conditions would require an *increase* in the technical factors normally used?
    A. Osteomyelitis
    B. Pneumothorax
    C. Bowel obstruction
    D. Ascites

68. Using the line focus principle to gain sharper images will enhance a side effect known as:
    A. Parallax effect
    B. Anode heel effect
    C. Shape distortion
    D. Size distortion

69. Which of the following should be considerations when using an AEC device?
    1. Proper selection of time
    2. Proper selection of ionization chamber(s)
    3. Precise positioning over the desired chamber(s)
    A. 1 and 2 only
    B. 2 and 3 only
    C. 1 and 3 only
    D. 1, 2, and 3

70. At what minimum distance should the safelight be positioned above the processor shelf to avoid fogging the radiograph?
    A. 1 foot
    B. 2 feet
    C. 3 feet
    D. 5 feet

71. Which of the following sets of technical factors would result in an image with the greatest recorded detail?

mA	Time	kVp	SID	OID	FSS
A. 200	0.01 s	80	100 cm	20 cm	1 mm
B. 400	0.05 s	70	200 cm	60 cm	2 mm
C. 500	0.02 s	75	150 cm	25 cm	1 mm
D. 600	0.01 s	65	180 cm	30 cm	2 mm

72. What is the milliampere setting if the desired milliamperage-seconds are 40 and if the time setting is 50 milliseconds?
    A. 200 mA
    B. 400 mA
    C. 600 mA
    D. 800 mA

73. Contrast can be measured from a characteristic curve by finding the tangent of which of the following?
    A. Toe
    B. Shoulder
    C. D-max
    D. Straight-line portion

74. What new exposure factors should be used to create a longer scale of contrast without altering the radiographic density if the original radiograph is produced using exposure factors of 300 mA, 1/10 second, and 60 kVp?
    A. 300 mA, 1/20 second, and 70 kVp
    B. 400 mA, 1/10 second, and 66 kVp
    C. 600 mA, 1/20 second, and 70 kVp
    D. 100 mA, 1/10 second, and 66 kVp

75. Which of the following radiographic procedures typically requires an image demonstrating a long scale of contrast?
    A. Thoracic vertebrae
    B. Chest
    C. Myelography
    D. Barium enema (BE)

76. All other factors being equal, which of the following body types will produce the greatest subject contrast?
    A. Sthenic
    B. Asthenic
    C. Hyposthenic
    D. Hypersthenic

77. Which of the following types of static does pulling the sheet of film from the film bin or the film box too rapidly cause?
    A. Tree static
    B. Smudge static
    C. Ringlike static
    D. Photon static

78. The most numerous silver halide molecules that are found in the emulsion of modern radiographic film are those of:
    A. Silver bromide
    B. Silver iodide
    C. Calcium tungstate
    D. Gadolinium oxysulfide

79. About what percentage of radiographic density is due to light emitted by an intensifying screen's phosphors?
    A. 5 to 8 percent
    B. 10 to 15 percent
    C. 45 to 60 percent
    D. 95 to 98 percent

Refer to the characteristic curve diagrammed in Figure 1–4 to answer questions 80 and 81:

80. Which of the films will have the longest scale of contrast?
    A. Film A
    B. Film B
    C. Film C
    D. All are the same

81. Which of the films would result in the greatest density if identical technical factors were used?
    A. Film A
    B. Film B
    C. Film C
    D. All are the same

82. Which of the following sets of technical factors will result in the image with the shortest scale of contrast?

mAs	kVp	Screen Speed	Grid Ratio	SID	OID	FSS
A. 100	75	200	8:1	100 cm	25 cm	1 mm
B. 200	80	400	12:1	200 cm	40 cm	0.5 mm
C. 200	70	400	16:1	200 cm	20 cm	2 mm
D. 400	66	100	6:1	150 cm	15 cm	1 mm

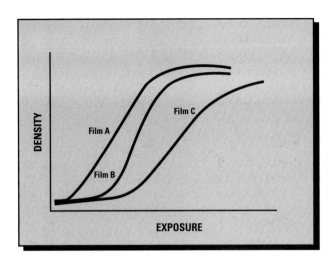

FIGURE 1–4. Characteristic curve.

83. The film processing system responsible for the greatest amount of artifacts is the:
    A. Replenisher system
    B. Dryer system
    C. Recirculation system
    D. Transport system

84. The shoulder portion of the characteristic curve is principally controlled by the automatic processor reducing agent termed:
    A. Hydroquinone
    B. Sodium thiosulfate
    C. Potassium bromide
    D. Glutaraldehyde

85. Developer temperature in an automatic processor should be measured by:
    A. Digital external indicators
    B. A dryer thermostat
    C. An immersed stem thermometer
    D. A glass-enclosed mercury thermometer

86. Which of the following sets of technical factors would result in the radiograph with the least density?

	mA	Time	kVp	*Screen* Speed	Grid	SID	OID	FSS
A.	200	0.05	70	200	8:1	200 cm	20 cm	1 mm
B.	100	0.02	80	400	5:1	100 cm	10 cm	2 mm
C.	400	0.50	90	200	16:1	200 cm	5 cm	0.5 mm
D.	800	0.001	80	100	12:1	150 cm	10 cm	2 mm

87. If a radiograph demonstrates excessive size distortion, which of the following corrections should be made before repeating the radiograph?
    A. Increase the OID.
    B. Decrease the SID.
    C. Decrease the tube angulation.
    D. Increase the SID.

88. If a radiographer failed to correctly mark a radiograph that subsequently resulted in a faulty diagnosis, he or she may be guilty of a tort under the doctrine *res ipsa loquitur,* which means:
    A. Let the master answer
    B. Captain of the ship
    C. The thing speaks for itself
    D. Assault and battery

89. What type of device would increase the diagnostic quality of a radiograph of the dorsoplantar projection of the foot?
    A. Trough filter
    B. Wedge filter
    C. Densitometer
    D. Sensitometer

90. Which of the following test tools would be used to measure FSS?
    A. Wire mesh
    B. Spinning top
    C. Wisconsin test cassette
    D. Star test pattern

91. Which of the following would demonstrate off-focus grid cutoff?
    A. Top of the film is underexposed.
    B. Both sides of the film are underexposed.
    C. One side of the film is underexposed.
    D. Bottom of the film is underexposed.

92. One of the first signs of chemical contamination or excessive oxidation of the developer is the reduction of the darker regions of film density. This is caused by a lack of:
    A. Sodium carbonate
    B. Potassium bromide
    C. Hydroquinone
    D. Glutaraldehyde

93. What is the ratio of a grid whose lead strips are 0.25 mm thick, 1.6 mm high, and are separated by 0.10-mm aluminum spacers?
    A. 6:1
    B. 8:1
    C. 12:1
    D. 16:1

94. Many transport problems or damp films exiting from the automatic processor are associated with exhausted
    A. Glutaraldehyde
    B. Water
    C. Sodium carbonate
    D. Sodium sulfite

95. Sensitometric measurements in a quality assurance program are:
    A. The results of monitoring replenishment rates
    B. A running total of chemical use in an automatic processor

C. The responses of film to exposure and processing

D. A weekly requirement

96. What effect does using a compression band have during the production of a radiograph?

1. Reduced scatter radiation
2. Reduced patient motion
3. Decreased radiographic contrast

   A. 1 and 2 only
   B. 1 and 3 only
   C. 2 and 3 only
   D. 1, 2, and 3

97. Ensuring that the radiographic film is sensitive to the color of light emitted by the intensifying screen phosphor is referred to as:
   A. Conversion efficiency
   B. Intensification factor
   C. Spectral matching
   D. Line focus principle

98. Which of the following x-ray interactions with matter is primarily responsible for radiographic contrast?
   A. *Bremsstrahlung* radiation
   B. Photoelectric effect
   C. Compton scatter
   D. Photodisintegration

99. Phosphorescence or afterglow is a property of intensifying screens that:
   A. Enhances resolution
   B. Reduces screen speed
   C. Tends to increase image blur
   D. Absorbs excess scatter radiation

100. As the field size is increased with all other factors remaining constant, the scale of radiographic contrast will:
   A. Be shortened
   B. Be lengthened
   C. Be unaffected
   D. Increase with high kilovolts (peak), but decrease with low kilovolts (peak)

101. With a table Bucky device, the appearance of grid lines on the radiograph could indicate that:
   A. The kilovolts (peak) are too low
   B. The milliamperage-seconds are too high
   C. The exposure time is too short
   D. The grid frequency is too low

102. Which of the following would decrease the production of scatter radiation?
   A. Use of a grid
   B. An increase in SID
   C. An increase in milliamperage-seconds
   D. A decrease in kilovolts (peak)

103. During latent image formation, the concentration of metallic silver in the exposed crystal occurs in the region of the sensitivity speck. This explanation of the formation of the image is referred to as:
   A. Einstein's theory of relativity
   B. Law of conservation of energy
   C. Gurney-Mott theory
   D. Faraday's law of induction

104. A densitometer film density measurement of 3 corresponds to approximately _____ of the light from a viewbox being transmitted through the film.
   A. 100 percent
   B. 10 percent
   C. 1 percent
   D. 0.1 percent

105. For all dedicated chest units whose tube potential routinely exceeds 90 kVp, the minimum recommended grid ratio is:
   A. 6:1
   B. 8:1
   C. 12:1
   D. 16:1

106. Which of the following radiographs would benefit most from the use of the anode heel effect?
   A. Dorsoplantar projection of the foot
   B. AP projection of the femur
   C. Lateral projection of the cervical spine
   D. Lateral projection of the hand

107. Which of the following chemicals prevents the developer from reducing unexposed silver bromide crystals in an automatic processor?
   A. Sodium sulfite
   B. Hydroquinone
   C. Potassium bromide
   D. Ammonium thiosulfate

108. What is the color of light emitted by lanthanum oxybromide rare earth intensifying screens?
   A. Amber
   B. Blue
   C. Green
   D. Yellow

109. The number of grid lines per inch or centimeter defines:
   A. Grid focusing distance
   B. Grid ratio
   C. Grid frequency
   D. Conversion efficiency

110. According to quality assurance programs, how often should the chemicals be changed in an automatic processor?

A. Once a day
B. Once a week
C. Once a month
D. Once a year

SECTION IV: RADIOGRAPHIC PROCEDURES AND RELATED ANATOMY

111. Which of the following radiographic methods are used to demonstrate the intercondylar fossa?

    1. Holmblad (PA axial)
    2. Danelius-Miller (axiolateral)
    3. Camp-Coventry (PA axial)

    A. 1 and 2 only
    B. 1 and 3 only
    C. 2 and 3 only
    D. 1, 2, and 3

112. If the patient places the back of the right hand against the right thigh, the humerus will be in:
    A. The oblique position
    B. External rotation
    C. Recumbent position
    D. The lateral position

113. To demonstrate the apophyseal joints of the lumbar vertebrae with an AP projection, the patient rotation is:
    A. 30°
    B. 45°
    C. 50°
    D. 55°

114. Which number in the radiograph in Figure 1–5 corresponds to the greater wing of the sphenoid bone?
    A. 1
    B. 2
    C. 3
    D. 4

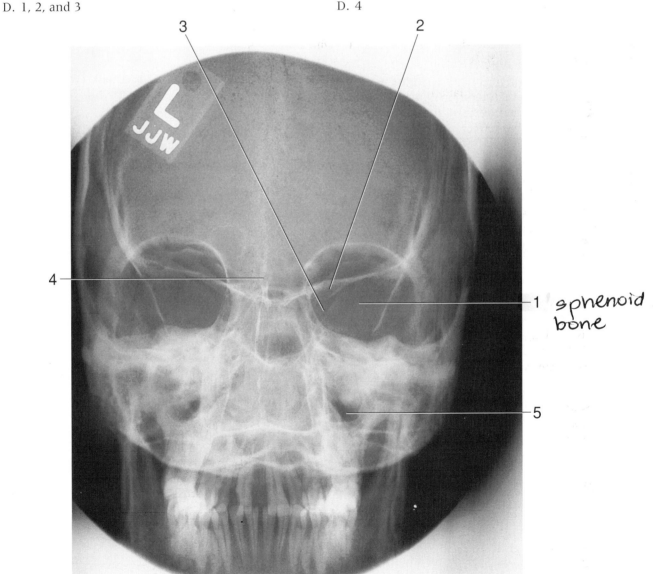

FIGURE 1–5. PA (Caldwell) projection skull radiograph. (Courtesy of JRMC Radiology Department.)

115. Which of the following radiographic positions will demonstrate the duodenal bulb and loop in profile during a gastrointestinal (GI) procedure?
    A. Prone position
    B. Right anterior oblique (RAO) position
    C. Left posterior oblique (LPO) position
    D. Right lateral position

116. What is the main reason for instructing a patient to swallow a thick barium contrast agent prior to obtaining a radiograph of several projections of the chest?
    A. To diagnose cardiac hypertrophy
    B. To demonstrate mediastinal shifts
    C. To rule out inguinal hernia
    D. To evaluate for mitral valve stenosis

117. For which type of body habitus will the diaphragm be at the highest position?
    A. Sthenic
    B. Asthenic
    C. Hyposthenic
    D. Hypersthenic

118. How should the patient's hands be positioned for an erect lateral projection of the sternum?
    A. Raised over the head
    B. Relaxed at the patient's side
    C. Clasped behind the patient's back
    D. Held at a 90° angle straight out in front of the patient

119. Which radiographic projection of the shoulder joint will demonstrate the glenoid cavity in profile?
    A. AP oblique (Grashey method)
    B. Transthoracic lateral (Lawrence method)
    C. Superoinferior projection (curved cassette)
    D. Inferosuperior projection (Clements modification)

120. Where should the contrast media be injected for a lumbar myelogram?
    A. Subdural space
    B. Epidural space
    C. Subarachnoid space
    D. Conus medullaris

121. Which of the following anatomic structures pumps oxygenated blood into the aorta?
    A. Right ventricle
    B. Left ventricle
    C. Inferior vena cava
    D. Superior vena cava

122. How many degrees is the patient's face rotated from the lateral position for the single-tube angulation axiolateral (Law) method of demonstrating the mastoid process?

    A. 10° to 12°
    B. 15°
    C. 35° to 40°
    D. 45°

123. How much will the kidneys move when changing the patient from the recumbent to the erect position?
    A. 1 inch
    B. 2 inches
    C. 3 inches
    D. 4 inches

124. The anatomic organ used for phonation is called the
    A. Uvula
    B. Epiglottis
    C. Pharynx
    D. Larynx

125. Which of the following methods for obtaining a radiograph of the hip should be performed when a fracture is suspected?
    A. Chassard-Lapine method
    B. Danelius-Miller method
    C. Lauenstein-Hickey method
    D. Cleaves method

126. What may be demonstrated on a tangential projection of the patella (Settegast method)?
    1. Transverse fractures of the patella
    2. Patellofemoral articulation
    3. Longitudinal fractures of the patella

    A. 1 and 2 only
    B. 1 and 3 only
    C. 2 and 3 only
    D. 1, 2, and 3

127. How many degrees and in which direction should the central ray be directed for an AP projection of the sacrum?
    A. 10° caudal
    B. 10° cephalad
    C. 15° caudal
    D. 15° cephalad

128. The bone identified in Figure 1–6 is the
    A. Tibia
    B. Talus
    C. Cuboid
    D. Navicular

129. Which of the following joints may be examined by arthrography?
    1. Wrist
    2. Temporomandibular joint (TMJ)
    3. Shoulder

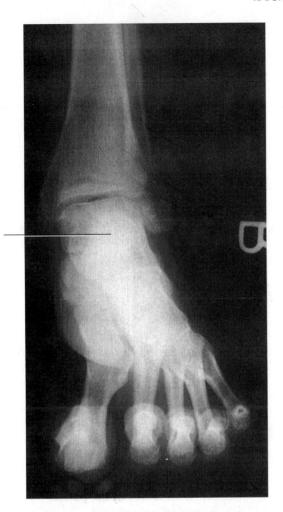

FIGURE 1–6. AP projection of the ankle. (From McKinnis, LN: Fundamentals of Orthopedic Radiology. FA Davis, Philadelphia, 1997, p 291, with permission.)

A. 1 and 2 only
B. 1 and 3 only
C. 2 and 3 only
D. 1, 2, and 3

130. Determination of radiological bone age is most frequently applied to the
   A. Spine
   B. Hand and wrist
   C. Lower limbs
   D. Femurs only

131. The plane of the body that divides the thorax into equal anterior and posterior parts is called the
   A. Transthoracic plane
   B. Midsagittal plane (MSP)
   C. Midtransverse plane
   D. Median coronal plane

132. The ampulla of Vater empties its contents into the duodenum through the structure called the
   A. Gallbladder
   B. Wharton's duct
   C. Sphincter of Oddi
   D. Duct of Wirsung

133. Which part of the rib articulates with the transverse process of the thoracic vertebrae?
   A. Shaft
   B. Head
   C. Tubercle
   D. Neck

134. When radiographing the multiple-trauma patient who is incapacitated, what rule of thumb should be observed to provide greatest diagnostic benefit for the patient?
   A. Remove all splints carefully and proceed quickly.
   B. Move the patient immediately to the x-ray table.
   C. Obtain two views, 90° apart, of all traumatized anatomy.
   D. Be sure to include an oblique view of the cervical spine to rule out fracture.

135. In the lateral position, how far posterior does the sacrum lie from the median coronal plane?
   A. 2 inches
   B. 3 inches
   C. 4 inches
   D. 5 inches

136. What is the name of the opening through which the spinal nerves pass after branching from the spinal cord?
   A. Vertebral foramen
   B. Intervertebral foramen
   C. Transverse foramen
   D. Obturator foramen

137. What radiographic baseline should be parallel to the image receptor for a submentovertical (SMV) projection of the paranasal sinuses?
   A. Orbitomeatal line
   B. Infraorbitomeatal line
   C. Acanthomeatal line
   D. Glabellomeatal line

138. Which imaging study of the urinary system demonstrates the collecting ducts of the kidneys by injecting a radiographic contrast medium through the ureter?
   A. Intravenous pyelogram (IVP)
   B. Hysterosalpingogram
   C. Cystogram
   D. Retrograde pyelogram

139. Which of the following represents the level of the iliac crest in the body?
    A. Second and third lumbar vertebrae
    B. Third and fourth lumbar vertebrae
    C. Fourth and fifth lumbar vertebrae
    D. Fifth lumbar and first sacral vertebrae

140. Which of the following anatomic structures articulates with the capitulum of the humerus?
    A. Styloid process of the radius
    B. Head of ulna
    C. Head of radius
    D. Styloid process of ulna

141. Which of the following radiographic methods would best demonstrate the coronoid process of the ulna?
    A. AP projection of the elbow
    B. 45° internal oblique projection of the elbow
    C. 45° external oblique projection of the elbow
    D. 90° lateral position of the elbow

142. What is the name of the bony projection that extends superiorly from the cribriform plate of the ethmoid bone?
    A. Dorsum sella
    B. Vomer
    C. Crista galli
    D. Perpendicular plate

143. What is the name of the type of skull that is considered to be of average shape and size?
    A. Brachycephalic
    B. Mesocephalic
    C. Dolichocephalic
    D. Bradycephalic

144. What radiographic projection is represented by the radiograph in Figure 1–7?
    A. AP projection in the recumbent position
    B. PA projection in the erect position
    C. Left lateral decubitus projection
    D. Right lateral decubitus projection

145. What is an anterior curvature of the vertebral column called?
    A. Lordosis
    B. Kyphosis
    C. Scoliosis
    D. Meiosis

146. How much must the patient be rotated from the horizontal position to visualize the apophyseal joints of the thoracic vertebrae?
    A. 30°
    B. 45°
    C. 70°
    D. 90°

147. The right sacroiliac (SI) joint should be *clearly* demonstrated in which of the following?
    A. AP projection
    B. PA projection
    C. RPO
    D. LPO

148. What is the rounded projection on the anterior proximal surface of the tibia called?
    A. Tibial plateau
    B. Tibial tuberosity
    C. Tibial spine
    D. Tibial condyle

149. Which of the following articulates with the medial cuneiform bone?
    A. Cuboid
    B. First metatarsus
    C. Calcaneus
    D. First phalanx

150. If the orbitomeatal line is perpendicular to the film for an AP axial (Grashey/Towne) projection of the skull, how much caudal angulation of the central ray is required?
    A. 25°
    B. 30°
    C. 37°
    D. 40°

151. Which radiographic projection of the skull should clearly demonstrate all four sets of paranasal sinuses?
    A. Submentovertex
    B. Parietoacanthial (Waters)
    C. PA (Caldwell)
    D. Lateral

152. Which of the following pathologies are well visualized by a double-contrast BE?
    A. Cirrhosis
    B. Polyps
    C. GI bleeds
    D. Hemorrhoids

153. What is the name of the process that extends superiorly from the scapula?
    A. Acromion process
    B. Coronoid process
    C. Glenoid process
    D. Coracoid process

154. Which two bones are united to form the sternoclavicular (SC) joint?
    A. Scapula and clavicle
    B. Scapula and sternum
    C. Clavicle and sternum
    D. Sternum and spine

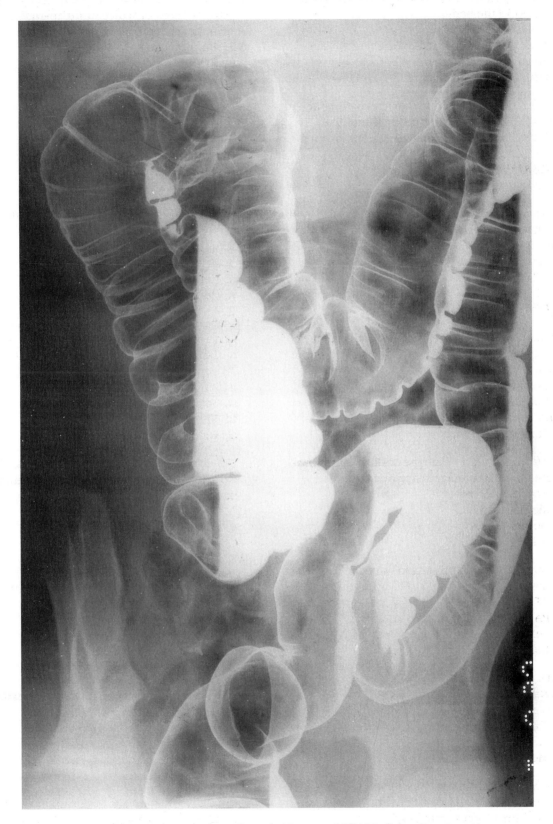

FIGURE 1–7. Air contrast colon radiograph. (Courtesy of JRMC Radiology Department.)

155. Which radiographic decubitus position is preferred for demonstrating air and fluid levels in the abdomen?
    A. Dorsal decubitus
    B. Ventral decubitus
    C. Right lateral decubitus
    D. Left lateral decubitus

156. In which of the following positions would the patient be placed during the insertion of an enema tip?
    A. Sims' position
    B. Fowler's position
    C. Trendelenburg position
    D. Prone position

157. Which of the following organs receives blood from the portal vein?
    A. Small bowel
    B. Large bowel
    C. Liver
    D. Pancreas

158. How should the patient be instructed to breathe for an AP projection of the lower ribs?
    A. Full inspiration
    B. Full expiration
    C. Normal breathing
    D. Shallow breathing

159. What is the name of the special imaging procedure or examination of the salivary ducts?
    A. Lymphangiography
    B. Sialography
    C. Hysterosalpingography
    D. TMJ arthrography

160. Which carpal bone has a characteristic hooklike process?
    A. Lunate
    B. Pisiform
    C. Scaphoid
    D. Hamate

161. What is the central ray centering point for the RAO position of the esophagus?
    A. C7–T1
    B. T5–T6
    C. T9–T10
    D. T12–L1

162. A right lateral decubitus radiograph is taken of a patient with the grid placed behind the patient. This is an example of a(an)
    A. Lateral projection
    B. Oblique projection
    C. AP projection
    D. Transaxial projection

163. During cystography, when ureteral reflux is suspected, it is often necessary to include a radiograph with the patient
    A. Voiding
    B. In the Trendelenburg position
    C. Having already voided
    D. In the erect position

164. Into which anatomic structure is the superior end of the T-tube placed for performing postoperative cholangiography?
    A. Cystic duct
    B. Hepatic duct
    C. Common bile duct
    D. Ampulla of Vater

165. What degree of central ray angulation should be used for the axial plantodorsal projection of the os calcis?
    A. 25°
    B. 35°
    C. 40°
    D. 45°

166. To better visualize the lateral thoracic spine, the patient should be instructed to:
    A. Take a full inspiration
    B. Exhale fully
    C. Breathe deeply
    D. Breathe quietly

167. Which type of pathology would be best demonstrated by a radiograph of the lower leg?
    A. Legg-Calvé-Perthes disease
    B. Monteggia's fracture
    C. Jefferson fracture
    D. Osgood-Schlatter disease

168. Where is the center of the cassette positioned for a PA projection of SC joints?
    A. Second thoracic vertebra
    B. Third thoracic vertebra
    C. Manubrial notch
    D. Body of the sternum

169. How should the patient's hands be placed for a PA projection of the ribs so that the scapulae are rotated away from the rib cage?
    A. Palm of the hands against the hips
    B. Palm of the hands against mid-thighs
    C. Back of the hands against the hips
    D. Back of the hands against mid-thighs

170. The proper medical term for a collapsed lung is:
    A. Pneumothorax
    B. Atelectasis
    C. Empyema
    D. Pleurisy

SECTION V: PATIENT CARE

171. If a radiologist instructs you to inject a patient with a radiographic contrast medium and the patient collapses from anaphylactic shock, you may be protected from a lawsuit under the doctrine of *respondeat superior*, which means:
 A. The thing speaks for itself
 B. Let the master answer
 C. Only superior authorities need to respond to legal issues
 D. Radiologists, like all physicians, are always considered liable

172. Where would a "central line" catheter be located?
 A. Stomach
 B. Trachea
 C. Subclavian vein
 D. Brachiocephalic artery

173. Which of the following methods represents a means of transmitting a disease through insect bites?
 A. Direct contact
 B. Droplet
 C. Vector
 D. Vehicle

174. Which of the following is an accepted method of sterilization?
 A. Hand washing
 B. Dry heat
 C. Antiseptic wash
 D. Bleach bath

175. What steps are necessary when performing radiographs on a patient with a head injury?
 1. Suction as necessary any nasal drainage.
 2. Check the patient's vital signs frequently.
 3. Do not remove sandbags, collars, or dressings.
 A. 1 and 2 only
 B. 2 and 3 only
 C. 1 and 3 only
 D. 1, 2, and 3

176. The proper medical term for a patient who suddenly turns pale and feels cold and clammy is:
 A. Apprehensive
 B. Febrile
 C. Hypertensive
 D. Diaphoretic

177. "Touching a patient without permission" is the legal definition of:
 A. Assault
 B. Malpractice
 C. Battery

 D. Negligence

178. Which of the following imaging procedures would require an informed consent form?
 A. Upper gastrointestinal (UGI) series
 B. Cardiac catheterization
 C. Oral cholecystogram (OCG)
 D. BE

179. Which of the following situations may cause a patient to go through the grieving process?
 1. Having a fractured clavicle
 2. Losing a spouse
 3. Being diagnosed with cancer
 A. 1 and 2 only
 B. 1 and 3 only
 C. 2 and 3 only
 D. 1, 2, and 3

180. If a patient scheduled for an arthrogram states that he or she has an allergy to an iodinated contrast medium, what other imaging method could demonstrate the anatomy without putting the patient at risk?
 A. Ultrasound
 B. Nuclear medicine
 C. Angiography
 D. Magnetic resonance imaging (MRI)

181. Which of the following pathological conditions would allow the x-ray beam to easily penetrate the patient?
 A. Edema
 B. Rheumatoid arthritis
 C. Paget's disease
 D. Pneumonia

182. What can happen if a diabetic patient has taken his or her normal dose of insulin but has been NPO since midnight?
 A. The patient can go into diabetic coma.
 B. The patient can go into insulin shock.
 C. The patient can develop difficulty breathing.
 D. The patient can become dehydrated.

183. What is the most common cause of injury to a health-care worker in the radiology department?
 A. Needle sticks
 B. Slipping and falling
 C. Lifting heavy objects
 D. Overexposure to radiation

184. Medical asepsis can be defined as the _____ of pathogenic microorganisms in the environment.
 A. Complete destruction and removal
 B. Method of encouraging growth
 C. Method of creating new types
 D. Reduction in number

185. You are called to the trauma center to perform a bedside radiographic procedure on a patient, and you suspect the patient may have hepatitis B. What are safe practices to follow to protect yourself?
    1. Always put on gloves.
    2. Always put on a mask.
    3. Always wash hands after the procedure.

    A. 1 and 2 only
    B. 1 and 3 only
    C. 2 and 3 only
    D. 1, 2, and 3

186. Which of the following is a reason why lidocaine (Xylocaine) is often used in the radiology department?
    A. To relax the colon
    B. To counteract the effects of histamine reaction
    C. To provide a topical anesthetic for invasive procedures
    D. To provide medical asepsis for invasive procedures

187. What is the normal range of diastolic pressure for an adult?
    A. 40–60 mm Hg
    B. 60–90 mm Hg
    C. 90–120 mm Hg
    D. 120–140 mm Hg

188. If a patient is scheduled for a UGI and small bowel radiological procedures, which type of radiographic contrast medium is contraindicated for the procedures if the patient is suspected of having a perforated colon?
    A. Barium
    B. Water-soluble iodine
    C. Gastroview
    D. Diatrizoate meglumine

189. A radiographic contrast medium that absorbs more radiation than the organ in which it is placed is termed a(an)
    A. Negative agent
    B. Positive agent
    C. Suspension agent
    D. Osmolality agent

190. What type of contrast medium is acceptable for use with infants who have swallowing disorders and with adults who have suspected broncho-esophageal fistulae?
    A. Water-soluble iodine
    B. Water-based barium
    C. Oil-based iodine
    D. Ethiodol

191. A patient is to be scheduled for a BE, OCG, and UGI. The proper sequence for performing these procedures is:
    A. OCG, BE, UGI
    B. BE, OCG, UGI
    C. UGI, BE, OCG
    D. OCG, UGI, BE

192. Intentional or unintentional acts performed by an individual and based on unreasonable conduct are known as:
    A. Assault and battery
    B. Misdemeanors
    C. Torts
    D. Felonies

193. The radiologist requires 60 percent more than the normal 50-cc dose of radiographic contrast medium to be used for a urologic procedure. The amount to be prepared is:
    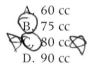
    A. 60 cc
    B. 75 cc
    C. 80 cc
    D. 90 cc

194. Destruction or alterations of medical records, such as a radiology report, by an unauthorized person is referred to as:
    A. Spoliation
    B. Negligence
    C. Consequentialism
    D. Vicarious liability

195. A common group of drugs that are used to promote defecation are termed:
    A. Emetics
    B. Cathartics
    C. Diuretics
    D. Stimulants

196. During cardiopulmonary resuscitation (CPR) of an adult, the cardiac compression rate should be about:
    A. 20 to 30 compressions per minute
    B. 40 to 60 compressions per minute
    C. 60 to 80 compressions per minute
    D. 80 to 100 compressions per minute

197. Which of the following blood pressure readings would indicate shock?
    A. Systolic pressure lower than 120 mm Hg
    B. Systolic pressure higher than 140 mm Hg
    C. Diastolic pressure higher than 140 mm Hg
    D. Diastolic pressure lower than 50 mm Hg

198. What is the average pulse rate of an infant?
    A. 40 to 60 beats per minute
    B. 70 to 80 beats per minute
    C. 80 to 100 beats per minute
    D. 115 to 130 beats per minute

199. Which method for measuring body temperature may be contraindicated for patients with cardiac conditions?
 A. The rectal method
 B. The oral method
 C. The axillary method
 D. The forehead method

200. A patient develops hives several minutes after a radiographic contrast medium is injected. Which type of drug may the patient be given to counteract this reaction?
 A. Analgesic
 B. Antihistamine
 C. Anti-inflammatory
 D. Antibiotic

Answers and Explanations

Each rationale is followed by a reference to a text listed in the bibliography at the end of this chapter.

SECTION I: RADIATION PROTECTION AND RADIOBIOLOGY

1. **(C)** Temporary sterility occurs in the adult male patient only after an acute threshold dose of approximately 2.5 Gy (250 rad). Cataractogenesis occurs only after either an acute or a chronic cumulative dose of at least 2 Gy (200 rad). Skin erythema will not typically occur at doses below 2 Gy (200 rad). A decrease in the blood count may be seen after a dose as low as 0.25 Gy (25 rad) and is the earliest response seen.
 Bushong, "Early Effects of Radiation," 1997, pp 468–470; Travis, "Radiation Pathology," pp 123–126.

2. **(B)** It is important for the pregnant radiographer to practice all of the cardinal rules of protection: *time, distance, and shielding.* It also may be advisable to avoid high-radiation areas such as fluoroscopy, and to *never* hold patients during an exposure. A radiographer has legal rights concerning any suggestion of reassignment of duty. To assess an accurate fetal dose, care must be taken to *never* get the collar badge and waist badge confused.
 Bushong, "Health Physics," 1997, p 503; Dowd, "Protecting the Radiographer and Other Workers," 1999, p 206; Statkiewicz-Sherer et al., "Protecting Occupationally Exposed Personnel during Diagnostic Radiologic Procedures," p 192.

3. **(B)** When radiographing a 3-year-old child, a grid is not necessary and should be avoided because it greatly increases radiation dose. The only

positions that demonstrate free air are upright or decubitus.
 Bontrager, "Terminology," p 19; Bushong, "The Grid," 1997, pp 225–227; Dowd, "Protecting the Patient."

4. **(D)** According to NCRP Report No. 116, the monthly dosimetry report is based on occupational exposures, both internal and external, and *excludes* any natural or background sources.

5. **(C)** An increase in kilovolts (peak) will decrease exposure to the patient *only* if a comparable decrease in milliamperage-seconds accompanies the change. In the diagnostic range, to maintain radiographic density, an increase in milliamperage-seconds will always cause an increase in patient dose even with a comparable decrease in kilovolts (peaks).
 Bushong, "Radiation Protection Procedures," 1997, pp 537–538; Statkiewicz-Sherer, "Protection of the Patient," pp 161–163.

6. **(B)** Shadow shields *cannot* be used in fluoroscopy. Tower drapes are used to protect the operator, *not* the patient. Placing the intensification tower closer to the patient (with the patient supine and the x-ray tube beneath the patient in PA fluoroscopy) will reduce excess scatter to the patient's head, neck, and extremities as compared with AP fluoroscopy, where the x-ray tube is above and situated closer to the patient.
 Statkiewicz-Sherer et al., "Protecting the Patient during Diagnostic Radiologic Procedures," p 169.

7. **(A)** The recommended monthly dose-equivalent limit for the fetus in the third trimester is 0.5 mSv (0.05 rem), according to the latest NCRP Report (No. 16.) *There is no longer a dose limit for the entire gestation period as stated in* NCRP Report No. 91.

8. **(B)** The "in air" dose, in roentgens (R), measures the charge created through the process of ionization. Scintillation and biologic and chemical changes (film badge) are more appropriate methods for stating absorbed dose or dose equivalent (occupational dose).
 Bushong, "Designing for Radiation Protection," 1997, p 515, and "Radiation Protection Procedures," p 524; Dowd, "Ionizing Radiation," pp 43–45; Statkiewicz-Sherer et al., "Radiation Monitoring," pp 226–228.

9. **(A)** According to the standards set forth in NCRP Report No. 102, 30 cm (12 in.) must be the minimum SSD in mobile fluoroscopy units (C-arm).

10. **(D)** Proper collimation of the x-ray beam has the primary effect of reducing patient dose by restricting the volume of tissue irradiated. It also reduces scatter production and improves image contrast.

Bushong, "Scatter Radiation and Beam-Restricting Devices," 1997, pp 205–206; Dowd, "Protecting the Patient in Radiography," pp 231–232; Statkiewicz-Sherer et al., "Protection of the Patient during Diagnostic Radiologic Procedures," p 150.

11. **(A)** Inverse-square law:

$$\frac{I_1}{I_2} = \frac{D_2^2}{D_1^2}; \frac{68}{x} = \frac{60^2}{40^2}$$

$$68 = \frac{(3)^2}{26} x ; 68 = \frac{9}{4} x ; \frac{4}{9} 68 = x ; x = 30.3 \text{ mR}$$

Bushong, "X-Ray Emission," 1997, p 142; Dowd, "Protecting the Radiographer."

12. **(A)** The TLD operates through the process of luminescence—no chemical reaction has occurred. Both the pocket dosimeter and the "cutie pie" operate on the principle of electric current and measure the "charge" created by ionizing radiation, although the cutie pie is *not* a personnel monitoring device. The film badge operates on the principle of the Gurney-Mott theory, which describes how x-ray photons change silver halide into atomic silver in a film emulsion—a definite chemical change.

Bushong, "Radiographic Film," 1997, pp 167–169; Carlton and Mckenaa-Adler, "Radiographic Film," p 285; Dowd, "Ionizing Radiation," pp 55–57.

13. **(B)** According to NCRP Report No. 102, the leakage radiation should be limited to 0.1 rad (100 mR) per hour at a distance of 1 m from the source.

14. **(B)** Bushong states that the tabletop intensity of a fluoroscope should not exceed 2.1 R/min for each milliampere operating at 80 kVp. Never should it exceed 10 R/min in normal modes of operation.

5 minutes × 2 R ×3 mA = 30 R (30 cGy)

Bushong, "Designing for Radiation Protection," 1997, p 512; NCRP Report No. 102.

15. **(B)** The acronym GSD stands for genetic significant dose. GSD is defined as the average gonadal dose received by an exposed population and is used to estimate the genetic impact of medical radiation doses on an entire population. In other words, protecting the gonads of *every* potentially reproductive individual in a population is absolutely essential. If only a very small fraction of the population is irradiated, this exposure may still cause a detrimental effect in terms of genetic defects in future generations. The NCRP states that the current GSD to the gonads should be limited to 20 mrad averaged over the entire population.

Dowd, "Late Effects of Radiation," p 158; Selman, "Late Effects of Ionizing Radiation," p 517; Statkiewicz-Sherer et al., "Protection of the Patient during Diagnostic Radiologic Procedures," p 172.

16. **(D)** Aplastic anemia induced by radiation would occur at doses routinely exceeding 0.25 Gy (25 rad). Cataractogenesis would occur only at an acute or cumulative dose in excess of 2 Gy (200 rad). These doses are contrary to the current dose-equivalent limits and the philosophy of ALARA. Skin erythema would be seen only in individuals who receive an acute dose of several hundred radiation absorbed doses. Because the current dose-equivalent limits keep the upper boundary of exposure at or below 50 mSv/y (5 rem/y), carcinogenesis, along with possible genetic effects, would be a potential hazard because these effects may occur at any dose (stochastic or nonthreshold effects).

Bushong, "Early Effects of Radiation," 1997, pp 467–471, and "Late Effects of Radiation," pp 478, 482–488; Dowd, "Early Effects of Radiation," pp 130–135, and "Late Effects of Radiation," pp 141–152; Travis, "Radiation Pathology," pp 112–116, 117, 127, and "Late Effects of Radiation," p 165.

17. **(D)** All equipment operating above 70 kVp should be supplied with a total filtration of at least 2.5-mm Al equivalent. For general radiographic equipment, the use of 3-mm total filtration will sometimes necessitate an increase in technical factors and therefore defeats the purpose of filtration. However, in fluoroscopy, 3 mm of Al is considered optimal.

Dowd, "Protecting the Patient in Radiography," p 251; Statkiewicz-Sherer, et al., "Protection of the Patient during Diagnostic Radiologic Procedures," p 167.

18. **(C)** Ionization leads to a chain reaction in the human body that may eventually cause biologic damage. X rays are a form of electromagnetic radiation. Only electromagnetic radiation in the very highest energy range (x, gamma, and cosmic rays) is considered to be ionizing or potentially damaging.

Bushong, 1997, "Electromagnetic Radiation," p 50, and "Molecular and Cellular Radiobiology," pp 452–453.

19. **(A)** Kilovolts (peak) and milliamperage-seconds are the *only* factors in this question that affect patient dose. Screen speed and grids would be factors only if there were a comparable change in milliamperage-seconds to offset the change in screen speed, grids, and so forth. Because the beam (kilovolts [peak] and milliamperage-seconds) exposes the patient, *not* what is placed behind the patient, you only have to concentrate on these first two factors. If distance, filtration, and beam size had been listed in this question, these factors would also affect patient dose. Steps to solve this problem are as follows:

1. Solve for milliamperage-seconds. 2. The lowest kilovolts (peak) and the lowest milliamperage-seconds would cause the lowest patient dose, because dose increases directly with the milliamperage-seconds and exponentially with the kilovolts (peak). In other words, doubling the milliamperage-seconds would double the dose to the patient. Doubling the kilovolts (peak) would result in a four times greater dose to the patient.

Bushong, "X-ray Emission," 1997, pp 140–141; Dowd, "Protecting the Patient in Radiography, pp 219–221."

20. **(D)** To calculate the cumulative dose over a radiographer's lifetime, multiply the person's age by 10 mSv (1 rem).

NCRP Report No. 116.

21. **(A)** Photoelectric interaction usually involves the ejection of an inner, or K-shell, electron. Compton scattering usually involves the ejection of an outer-shell electron. Both result in ionization of the irradiated matter. Pair production only occurs at very high energy levels and involves the interaction of the incident photon with the atom's nuclear force field, *not* the electron cloud. Pair production results in the loss of the incident photon and the creation of two new particles of matter: a positron and an electron. These particles are created by the energy of the incident photon and not from the already existing matter in the irradiated atom.

Bushong, "Interactions of X-Rays with Matter," 1997, pp 150–155; Dowd, "Interactions of Radiation with Matter," pp 67–74; Statkiewicz-Sherer et al., "Basic Interactions of X-Radiation with Matter," pp 24–31.

22. **(C)** Cesium iodide is used as the input phosphor in the image intensifier. Zinc cadmium sulfide is the material contained in the output phosphor of some image intensifiers. Sodium iodide is sometimes used as a scintillation detector in nuclear medicine gamma cameras and/or computed tomography (CT) scanners. Lithium fluoride is the phosphor used in a TLD badge.

Bushong, "Designing for Radiation Protection," 1997, p 520; Statkiewicz-Sherer et al., "Personnel Monitoring," p 223.

23. **(A)** Ion chambers operate on the principle of an electric current being generated by a charge created in air. This charge is created by an ionizing event. Either x or gamma radiation can cause this phenomenon. The coulomb per kilogram (C/kg) or the roentgen (R) is usually the unit that is used to measure a charge in air. The sievert (rad), gray (rem), and curie (becquerel) units are more appropriate for measuring absorbed doses of radiation or occupational dose.

Bushong, "Radiographic Definitions and Mathematics Review," 1997, p 13; Dowd, "Ionizing Radiation," pp 48–49; Statkiewicz-Sherer et al., "Radiation Quantities and Units," pp 40–44.

24. **(B)** Neuroblasts and spermatogonia are the stem cells, or immature cells, and therefore considered to be very sensitive to radiation. The lymphocyte is arguably *the most radiosensitive cell* in the human body, because a dose as low as 0.1 Gy (10 rad) can cause a decrease in the lymphocyte count. Erythrocytes are end cells, or mature cells, and have no nucleus, making them very resistant to radiation. Erythrocytes, like mature nerve cells, are practically immune to any damage by irradiation, and they also have a very long life span (about 4 months), as compared with several days for most other cells. It is for this reason that the depletion of red blood cells (RBCs) is not suspected of being a primary cause of death from the hemopoietic syndrome.

Bushong, "Early Effects of Radiation," 1997, pp 470–471; Dowd, "Early Effects of Radiation," p 134; Statkiewicz-Sherer et al., "Radiation Biology," p 110; Travis, "Radiation Pathology," pp 115–116.

25. **(B)** According to the latest NCRP Report (No. 116), deterministic effects are those typically associated with a threshold dose. The old term associated with these types of effects was "nonstochastic." Cataracts to the lens of the eye may be induced by a threshold dose of 2 Gy (200 rad). Genetic defects, leukemia, and thyroid cancer are considered to be stochastic effects. These effects may occur at any dose. Stochastic effects are nonthreshold effects and are the basis for total body dose-equivalent limits and the ALARA philosophy.

26. **(C)** The whole-body dose limit is based on stochastic effects that may occur at very low doses, such as cancer and genetic effects. It is set at the lowest limit (50 mSv [5 rem]) because whole-body doses are potentially more harmful than local tissue exposures. Some local tissues are allowed higher dose-equivalent limits based on deterministic effects. Examples are the lens of the eye, which is limited to an annual dose equivalent of 150 mSv (15 rem), and the extremities, which are allowed an equivalent of 500 mSv (50 rem).

NCRP Report No. 116.

27. **(C)** Using a slower speed screen would require an increase in milliamperage-seconds to maintain radiographic density and thus would increase patient dose. A decrease in kilovolts (peak) would also require an increase in milliamperage-seconds to maintain radiographic density. An increase in milliamperage-seconds would require a comparable decrease in kilovolts (peak), thus in-

creasing the dose. Using a rare earth screen would require a decrease in milliamperage-seconds and therefore would decrease dose.

Bushong, "X-Ray Emission," 1997, pp 140–142, and "Intensifying Screens," pp 196–198; Dowd, "Protecting the Patient in Radiography," pp 230–231; Statkiewicz-Sherer et al., "Protection of the Patient during Diagnostic Radiologic Procedures," p 163.

28. **(C)** Filtration serves to remove lower-energy photons and therefore increases the average energy of the x-ray beam, making the beam more penetrating. The lower-energy photons removed through filtration will protect the patient from skin exposure more than from internal organ exposure. This effect occurs because lower-energy photons are much less penetrating. Low-energy photons would not add any diagnostic quality to the image receptor.

Dowd, "Protecting the Patient in Radiography," p 222.

29. **(A)** Pocket dosimeters may only be worn for 1 day at a time and must be reset every day. Their upper limit reading is approximately 200 to 300 mR. The film badge should never be worn for longer than 1 month because of its extreme sensitivity to heat and humidity and its susceptibility to fog. A cutie pie is a radiation field survey instrument and *not* a personnel monitor. The TLD may be worn for a period up to 3 months.

Bushong, "Radiation Protection Procedures," 1997, p 534; Statkiewicz-Sherer et al., "Radiation Monitoring," p 224.

30. **(D)** The ALARA philosophy was developed by the NCRP in the 1950s to try to minimize exposure to patients, the public, and occupational personnel working in and around the radiation industry. ALARA basically states that radiation workers should try to limit their own and the public's exposure (which in diagnostic radiology includes patient exposure) to "as low as reasonably achievable." It is for this reason that the NCRP has constantly tried to lower the dose-equivalent limits to make radiology a safe occupation in which to work.

NCRP Report No. 105.

SECTION II: EQUIPMENT OPERATION AND MAINTENANCE

31. **(B)** Off-focus radiation is produced by stray electrons that bombard the anode away from the focal spot. It can diminish contrast but has little effect on resolution. The line focus principle is associated with reducing the anode angle to increase resolu-

tion. It has nothing to do with tube current. Characteristic radiation is influenced by the energy (kiloelectron volts) of the electrons, *not* the tube current. Blooming occurs with single-focus tubes (x-ray tubes with only one filament). Increasing milliamperage-seconds will increase the size of the actual focal spot even though there has not been a change in filament size. An increase in FSS will result in a decrease in resolution.

Carroll, "Quality Control," 1998, pp 400–401; Curry et al., "Geometry of the Radiographic Image," p 233; Wolbarst, "X-Ray Tubes," p 88.

32. **(B)** The input phosphor in an image intensifier is first struck by exit (remnant) radiation from the patient. This radiation stimulates light-photon emission. These light photons then strike the photocathode, which stimulates the production of electrons. These electrons are then drawn toward the output phosphor and are focused by electrostatic lenses. At the output phosphor, these electrons stimulate the screen to produce light, which is imaged by the photospot camera, camera tube, and so forth.

Bushong, "Fluoroscopy," 1997, p 324; Curry et al., "Fluoroscopic Imaging," p 168; Thompson et al., "Fluoroscopy," p 364.

33 and 34. **(C) and (B)** In Figure 1–1, 1 is the cathode block, 2 the focusing cup, 3 the filament, 4 the actual focal spot or target, 5 the rotor, 6 the stator, 7 the anode disk, and 8 the glass envelope.

Bushong, "The X-Ray Tube," 1997, pp 110, 116; Curry et al., "Production of X-Rays," p 16; Wolbarst, "X-Ray Tubes," p 89.

35. **(D)** Single-phase rectified x-ray equipment uses a one-current waveform that operates on a standard 60-Hz frequency, or 60 cycles per second. Half-wave equipment uses only half of the cycle and therefore results in 60 impulses per second. Full-wave equipment uses both halves of each cycle, resulting in 120 impulses per second. Three-phase equipment incorporates three separate circuits, each having a frequency of 60 Hz. Through different processes, 3-phase, 6-pulse machines rectify all three circuits, which results in 6 × 60 or 360 impulses per second. Three-phase, 12-pulse machines, using a different process of rectification, result in 12 impulses per cycle × 60 = 720 impulses per second. Three-phase, 12-pulse machines used to be considered the most efficient x-ray generators, possessing a voltage ripple of between 3 and 5 percent. The modern high-frequency generator uses a similar circuit as the single-phase machine and is also full-wave rectified but incorporates an additional device called a "DC chopper." High-frequency

generators greatly increase the normal frequency of 60 Hz to several thousand hertz or kilohertz. The result of this extreme high frequency is that the voltage rarely drops to zero (some texts say less than 1 percent), thus making high-frequency generators very efficient.

Curry et al., "X-Ray Generators," pp 52–53; Thompson et al., "Magnetism and Its Relation to Electricity," p 123.

36. **(C)** A farad is the unit for *capacitance* (charge per voltage). The ampere is the unit for *current* or number of electrons flowing per second. The watt is the unit of *power* (joules per second). The ohm is the unit that is used to measure *resistance*.

Carlton and McKenna-Adler, "Electricity," pp 76–77; Thompson et al., "Electricity," p 101; Wolbarst, "Resistors, Transistors and All That: The Components of an X-Ray Tube Circuit," p 72.

37. **(A)** In a typical x-ray circuit, the timer is located on the primary side of the step-up trans-

former, or between the autotransformer and the step-up transformer. In this location it is easier to control the electric current in a low-voltage circuit than in a high-voltage circuit. The only exception to this is the milliamperage-seconds timer, which is located on the secondary side of the step-up transformer. Refer to the diagram in Figure 1–8.

Bushong, "The X-Ray Unit," 1997, p 105; Carlton and McKenna-Adler "X-Ray Equipment," pp 97–98; Selman, "X-Ray Circuits," pp 237–251; Thompson et. al., "X-Ray Machine Operation: The X-Ray Circuit," pp 182–188.

38. **(B)** Brightness gain is calculated by multiplying the minification gain by the flux gain. The flux gain is the ratio of the *output screen light intensity* to the *input screen light intensity*. The minification gain is the ratio of the *area of the input screen* to the *area of the output screen*. The intensification factor is typically used to compare various screen speeds

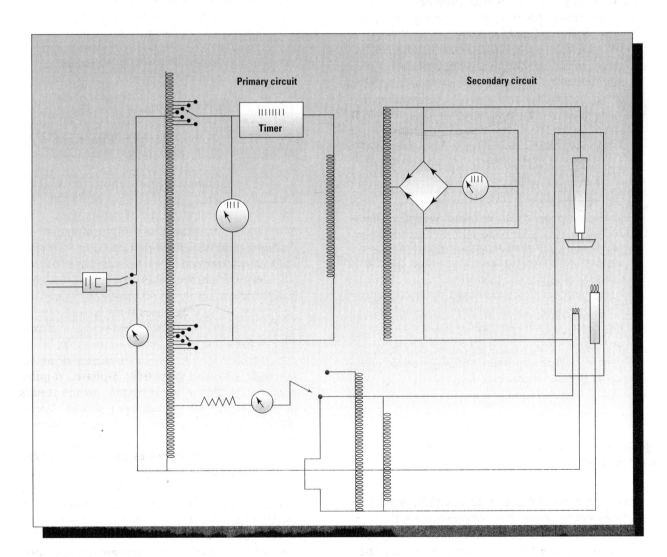

FIGURE 1–8. X-ray circuit.

or to compare the exposure needed without screens versus the exposure needed with screens.

Bushong, "Fluoroscopy," 1997, p 325; Carlton and McKenna-Adler, "Fluoroscopy," p 539; Curry et al., "Luminescent Screens," p 171; Thompson et al., "Fluoroscopy," p 366.

39. **(C)** Cine cameras have a typical frame size of 16 or 35 mm. Most photospot cameras either are 70 mm or 105 mm. The 105-mm camera is typically supplied as roll film.

Bushong, "Fluoroscopy," 1997, p 331; Carlton and McKenna-Adler, "Fluoroscopy," p 547; Curry et al., "Viewing and Recording the Fluoroscopic Image," pp 186–191; Thompson et al., "Fluoroscopy," pp 372–373.

40. **(C)** An ionization chamber is one of the more common AEC devices. To be used effectively, it must be placed between the patient and the image receptor. Another type of AEC device, the photomultiplier tube, is placed behind the x-ray cassette or image receptor. Newer units incorporate a solid-state detector.

Bushong, "The X-Ray Unit," 1997, p 98; Thompson et al. "The X-Ray Circuit," pp 183–186.

41. **(C)** The rare earth phosphors consist of lanthanum, gadolinium, and yttrium, which may be mixed with various other chemicals to produce an intensifying screen active layer. Examples of these compounds include lanthanum oxybromide, and gadolinium oxysulfide. These phosphors are capable of giving off light in the green and yellow range as well as in the blue-violet range. For x-ray film sensitivity to be properly matched with these rare earth screen phosphors, a light-absorbing dye (usually magenta) needs to be added to the emulsion to take advantage of these additional emissions. This type of film is referred to as "orthochromatic" because it is sensitive to both blue and green light.

Bushong, "Radiographic Film," 1997, p 169; Curry et al., "Photographic Characteristics of X-Ray Film," p 161; Papp, "Film Darkrooms," p 16.

42. **(B)** Luminescence is the process of giving off light as the result of some outside stimulation. There are two kinds of luminescence: (1) fluorescence, whereby the phosphor only emits light when the stimulus is present, and (2) phosphorescence, when the phosphor continues to emit light even after the stimulus is taken away. Phosphorescence may cause a problem in intensifying screens known as "afterglow" or "screen lag." Incandescence is the process of heating something to the point where it glows or gives off visible light. The filament must be heated sufficiently until it glows red for electrons to be boiled off the surface.

Hiss, "Milliamperage," p 112; Thompson et al., "In-troduction to Radiography: Principles, Equipment and Departmental Operation," p 2; Selman, "X-Rays (Roentgen Rays)," p 155.

43. **(B)** To ensure proper light field to x-ray field alignment, the mirror should be at a 45° angle to the x-ray beam. If shifts in the light field and x-ray field occur, the mirror angle should be checked. These two fields should not vary by more than 2 percent of the SID.

Carlton and McKenna-Adler, "Beam Restriction," p 242; Carroll, "Quality Control," p 396; Curry et al., "X-Ray Beam Restrictors," pp 94–95.

44. **(C)** It is not necessary to set an exact time when using an AEC device. A backup time should be set fairly high to ensure an adequate exposure. The exact time of exposure is decided by the AEC, either a photomultiplier tube or an ionization chamber. For the device to work properly, it is always important to set the photocell for field sensitivity to determine proper exposure for a specific body part. Setting the density level is also important, because the standard setting may vary from wall stand to table Bucky device.

Carlton and McKenna-Adler, "Automatic Exposure Controls," pp 504–511; Carroll, "Automatic Exposure Controls," pp 350–358; Thompson et al., "Equipment and Accessory Malfunctions or Misapplications," pp 382–384.

45. **(A)** The major and minor kilovolts (peak) selection is accomplished by the autotransformer. The actual upgrade from incoming line voltage to kilovoltage happens at the step-up transformer. The step-down transformer supplies the electrons to the filament. The rectifiers change AC supplied by the transformer to pulsating DC.

Bushong, "The X-Ray Unit," 1997, pp 94–96; Selman, "Production and Control of High Voltage," pp 130–132; Thompson et. al., "The X-Ray Circuit," pp 172–173.

46. **(B)** There is one impulse per cycle in a single-phase, half-wave rectified machine because when the current is rectified, only the crest, not the trough, of the cycle is used. A full-wave rectified machine uses both the crest and the trough of the current wave and therefore has 2 impulses per cycle. A 60-Hz incoming current consists of 120 pulses per second. In 3-phase, 6-pulse equipment, there are three transformers that are fully rectified, resulting in 6 impulses per cycle. In 3-phase, 12-pulse equipment, there are also three transformers, but its rectification system is much more complex. Suffice to say that 3-phase, 6-pulse and 3-phase, 12-pulse machines are exactly as they say—6 impulses per cycle and 12 impulses per cycle, respectively.

Curry et al., "X-Ray Generators," p 47; Tortorici, "Rectification," 1992, pp 43–53; Wolbarst, "The Nuts and Bolts of Generators," pp 80–81.

47. **(D)** The voltage ripple in single-phase equipment is 100 percent because the voltage drops to zero with each wave. A 3-phase, 6-pulse machine is much more efficient; the voltage never drops to zero but fluctuates or "ripples" about 13.5 percent of the maximum voltage. A 3-phase, 12-pulse machine is even more efficient and has a fluctuation of about 4 to 5 percent from the maximum voltage with each impulse. A high-frequency generator is more efficient than all of these because it produces a much more stable wave that fluctuates less than 4 percent of the maximum value.

Bushong, "The X-Ray Unit," 1997, p 104; Carlton and McKenna-Adler, "X-Ray Equipment," p 101.

48. **(C)** Brightness can be controlled by adjusting fluoroscopic milliamperage-seconds or kilovolts (peak). The primary factor affecting the brightness of the fluoroscopic image is the size or composition of the anatomic part.

Carlton and McKenna-Adler, "Fluoroscopy," p 540; Thompson et al., "Fluoroscopy: Viewing Motion with X-Ray," pp 366–367.

49. **(D)** According to NCRP Report No. 102, lead aprons and gloves should be tested annually to check for any defects in the lead lining.

50 and 51. **(B) and (A)** Refer to Figure 1–9. In these two graphs, the technical factor of exposure time is represented by the horizontal axis, the technical factor of milliamperage-seconds is represented by the vertical axis, and the technical factor of kilovolt (peak) is represented by the curved lines. Any combination of milliamperage-seconds and time that intersects on this graph below the level of the desired kilovolt (peak) curve is considered a "safe" technique for this particular x-ray tube. There are two graphs for this x-ray tube: one for a combination of technical factors using a large focal spot and one for a small focal spot. The graph for the large focal spot (1.2 mm) is located on the top, and the graph for the small focal spot (0.6 mm) is located on the bottom. To determine the maximum exposure time that may be safely used in combination with 90 kVp, 500 mA at a small focal spot, use the graph on the bottom and draw a line over from the 500 mA station until it intersects with the curved 90-kVp line. Next, draw a line from this point down to the horizontal axis. The intersection occurs at the 0.05-second mark, or 50 milliseconds (see Fig. 1–9[A]). To determine the maximum milliampere station that may safely be used in combi-

nation with 70 kVp at 0.5 second (500 milliseconds) at a large focal spot, use the graph on the top and draw a line from the 0.5-second mark on the horizontal axis up to the curved 70-kVp line. Next, draw a line from this point over to the vertical axis. The line falls somewhere between the 200- and 300-mA station (see Fig. 1–9[A]). Because 300 mA falls above the intersection, this would exceed the safe limit for the x-ray tube (see Fig. 1–9[B]).

Bushong, "The X-Ray Tube," 1997, pp 121–123; Carlton and McKenna-Adler, "The X-Ray Tube," pp 125–126; Thompson et al., "X-Ray Tube Components and Design," p 156.

52. **(B)** A pinhole camera checks the size of the actual focal spot. A star test pattern also checks the size of the focal spot, and it is much easier to use than the pinhole camera. An oscilloscope, or a synchronous spinning top, checks the accuracy of a timer in 3-phase equipment. A wire-mesh test device is used to determine the status of film-screen contact that would affect resolution of sharpness of detail, usually at the periphery of the image.

Carlton and McKenna-Adler, "Quality Control," p 449; Carroll, "Quality Control," p 404; Thompson et al., "Quality Control," pp 408–409.

53. **(A)** The radiograph demonstrates a synchronous spinning top that would be used to evaluate the accuracy of the timer. A quality control technologist would need either a solid-state detector attached to a computer to check the milliampere output or a penetrometer (aluminum step wedge). Kilovolt (peak) accuracy may be checked by using a Wisconsin test cassette or a solid-state detector. To check for light and x-ray field alignment, the quality control technologist could use the standard ruler test cassette or measure the light field with radiopaque objects such as pennies or paper clips.

Carroll, "Quality Control," pp 388–389; Papp, "Quality Control of Radiographic Equipment," pp 76–78.

54. **(A)** The focusing cup is a component found in the x-ray tube, not in the image intensifier. The electron gun is a component of the vidicon or plumbicon of a video monitor, not the image intensifier. The photocathode is the source of the electrons, but it does not accelerate them toward the output screen. The electrostatic lenses accomplish acceleration of the electrons.

Bushong, "Fluoroscopy," 1997, p 324; Thompson et al., "Fluoroscopy: Viewing Motion with X-Ray," p 365–366.

55. **(B)** Dirt or any foreign object on an intensifying screen will block, or attenuate, the light from the

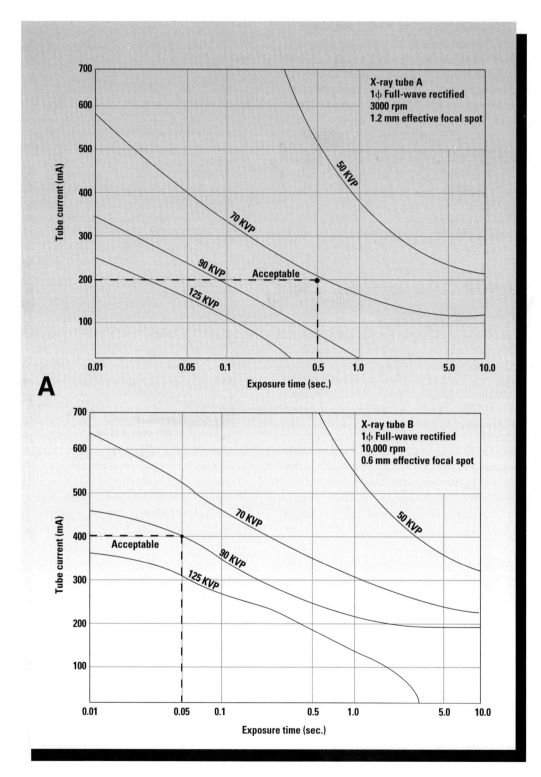

FIGURE 1–9. X-ray tube rating charts. (*A*) Acceptable maximum exposure time (bottom) and milliampere station (top). (*B*) Unacceptable maximum exposure time (bottom) and milliampere station (top).

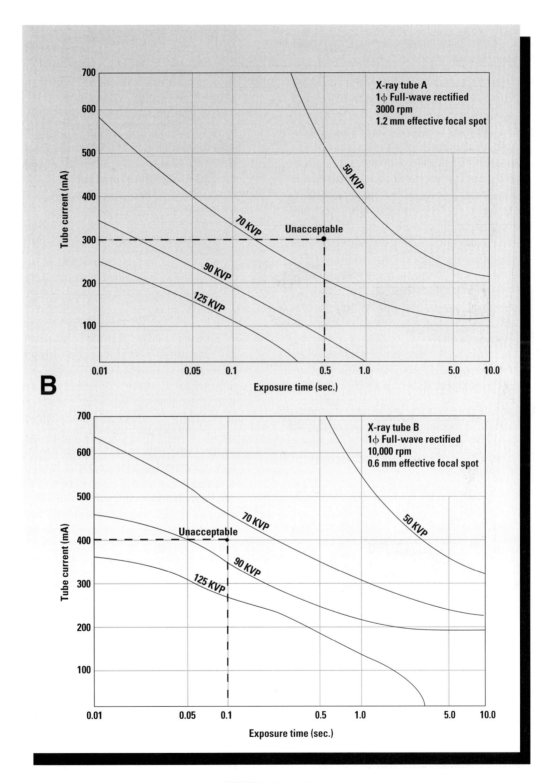

FIGURE 1–9. (*Continued*)

screen and therefore will cause an area of decreased density on the film. The area of decreased density will usually not be sufficiently large enough to cause blurring or have any effect on contrast.

Carroll, "Intensifying Screens," p 218; Cullinan, "Conventional Recording Media: Cassette," p 101.

56. **(C)** Using fast rare earth screens when the x-ray machine has been calibrated for slow speed or medium speed screens will cause an increase in radiographic density. Setting the table Bucky chamber while attempting to produce an AEC-timed radiograph of the chest of an erect patient will cause a massive increase in exposure. The reason is that the photocell in the table Bucky chamber will not receive any exposure and will therefore continue to expose until the backup timer has been activated. Using a positive density setting, as compared with the standard zero or normal setting, will increase the exposure. If a body part required at least a 2-second exposure for the proper density and if the backup time was only set for 1 second, the result would be an underexposed radiograph.

Carroll, "Automatic Exposure Controls," pp 352–353; Thompson et al., "Equipment and Accessory Malfunctions or Misapplications," p 383.

57. **(C)** Tungsten deposited on an x-ray tube window will result in decreased tube output due to an increase in the HVL and also may cause arcing of the current to the tungsten on the window instead of the anode.

Bushong, "The X-Ray Tube," 1997, p 121, and "X-Ray Emission," p 143.

58. **(D)** The formula for calculating maximum number of electrons in a shell is $2n^2$. The "n" designates the position of the shell from the nucleus. The K shell is closest, so n =1. The L shell is next, so n = 2, and so on. Thus, $2(2)^2 = 2(4) = 8$.

Bushong, "The Atom," 1997, p 35; Carlton and McKenna-Adler, "Radiation Concepts," p 27; Selman, "Structure of Matter."

59. **(C)** Grenz rays are very low-energy x rays usually not found in the diagnostic range. These low-energy rays used to be used to treat acne and psoriasis until it was discovered that they contributed to skin cancer. *Bremsstrahlung* radiation is the majority of the radiation in the beam and is created in the x-ray tube target with tungsten as the target element. Characteristic radiation is the other type of radiation that is formed at the target and can only be created at energy levels exceeding 69 keV because the binding energy of the tungsten K-shell electron is 69.5 keV. Photoelectric effect is not the formation of x rays in the tube, but rather is one of the many ways that x rays may interact with tissue.

Bushong, "X-Ray Production," 1997, p 129; Carlton and McKenna-Adler, "X-Ray Production," p 137; Hendee, "Structure of Matter," p 6, and "Special Purpose X-Ray Tubes," p 67.

60. **(C)** Heat units may be calculated by using the following formula: kVp × mA × time × 1 for single-phase generators; kVp × mA × time × 1.35 for 3-phase, 6-pulse generators; kVp × mA × time × 1.41 for 3-phase, 12-pulse generators. Thus, 75 × 400 × 0.25 × 1.41 = 10,575 HU. Also, the generator constant for a high-frequency x-ray tube that is used to calculate heat units is 1.45.

Bushong, "The X-Ray Tube," 1997, pp 122–123; Carlton and McKenna-Adler, "The X-Ray Tube," p 127; Thompson et al., "X-Ray Tube Components and Design," p 155; Tortorici, "Production of X-Rays," p 76.

SECTION III: IMAGE PRODUCTION AND EVALUATION

61. **(C)** Steps to solve this problem are as follows: 1. Rate milliamperage-seconds from 1 to 3, with 3 being the greatest density (highest milliampere-seconds). 2. Rate kilovolts from 1 to 4, with 4 being the highest kilovolts. 3. Rate the screen speed from 1 to 3, with 1 being the slowest and 3 being the fastest. 4. Rate the grid ratio. The highest grid ratio would create the least film density, so give the 12:1 grid a 1, both 8:1 grids a 2, and the 6:1 grid a 3. 5. Rate the SIDs with the farthest distance a 1, and the closest a 2. The highest total would yield the greatest radiographic density, as demonstrated in the example that follows:

mAs	kVp	Screen Speed	Grid Ratio	SID
A. 40^1	70^2	200^1	$12{:}1^1$	$100 \text{ cm}^2 = 7$
B. 80^3	75^3	400^2	$6{:}1^3$	$200 \text{ cm}^1 = 12$
C. 60^2	80^4	800^3	$8{:}1^2$	$100 \text{ cm}^2 = 13$
D. 80^3	65^1	200^1	$8{:}1^2$	$200 \text{ cm}^1 = 8$

62. **(B)** Compensating filters are used in radiography of irregularly shaped anatomic parts. The thicker portion of the filter should be placed over the thinnest or least dense anatomy. Two of the more common types are the *wedge filter,* which may be used for anatomy of graduating thickness, such as the foot or the thoracic vertebrae, and the *trough filter,* which is used to obtain balanced density in both the mediastinum and the lung fields.

Bushong, "X-Ray Emission," 1997, pp 145–146; Carlton and McKenna-Adler, "Filtration," p 173; Carroll, "Beam Filtration," pp 131–132; Thompson et al., "Factors Affecting the X-Ray Spectrum," p 230.

63. **(B)** The magnification of an object may be calculated by taking the SID/SOD ratio, or the SID/(SID − OID) ratio. In this question, the SID was 40 inches and the OID was 6 inches. So find 40/(40 − 6), or 40/34 = 1.18. The object would be magnified ×1.18.
Carlton and McKenna-Adler, "Distortion," p 420; Carroll, "Distance Ratios," pp 271–272; Tortorici, "Geometric Image Quality," pp 310–312.

64. **(D)** Size distortion or magnification is affected by the SID and the OID. However, shape distortion is *only* affected by the tube-part-film alignment: tube angulation, rotation of the anatomic part, or cassette angulation.
Carlton and McKenna-Adler, "Distortion," pp 421–422; Carroll, "Beam-Part-Film Alignment," p 278.

65. **(A)** Required filtration, as set up by the NCRP, is meant to protect the patient's skin by filtering only those x rays with insufficient energy to penetrate the anatomy. Varying normal amounts of filtration will *not* have a noticeable effect on any of the radiographic qualities (density or contrast). However, *excessive* filtration (less than 3 mm) will begin to filter out the higher energies and will decrease density and contrast.
Carlton and McKenna-Adler, "Filtration," p 175; Carroll, "Beam Filtration," p 130; NCRP Report No. 102, p 17.

66. **(A)** To answer this question, it is important to know the grid conversion factors. When changing from a nongrid technique to an exposure with a grid, the conversions are as follows:

Grid Ratio   Change in mAs (GCF)

5:1	2×
6:1	3×
8:1	4×
10:1, 12:1	5×
16:1	6×

One can then make the change in milliamperage-seconds from one grid to another by using this formula:

$$\frac{\text{New grid (GCF)}}{\text{Old grid (GCF)}} \times \text{Old mAs} = \text{New mAs}$$

$$\frac{4}{5} \times 5 \text{ mAs} = 4 \text{ mAs}$$

You could also have found the answer through process of elimination. It is not necessary to alter the kilovolts (peak) with a change in grid ratio. Therefore, you can eliminate C and D. Because the grid ratio has decreased, the technical factors would also have to decrease. This makes A the only possible choice.

Cullinan, "Technical Formulas and Related Data," p 292; Dennis and Eisenberg, "Radiographic Calculations," p 99; Wallace, "Grids and the Bucky," pp 112–113.

67. **(D)** Osteomyelitis is a destructive disease of the bone marrow and would require a decrease of 8 percent kilovolts (peak). Pneumothorax is a condition that adds excessive air into the chest cavity and would require a decrease of about 8 percent kilovolts (peak). Bowel obstruction is a pathological disorder that also results in excessive air in the small or large intestines, making them fairly easy to penetrate. Ascites is a condition in which excessive fluid collects in the peritoneal cavity and is usually a result of cirrhosis or some other liver disorder. Ascites is considered an additive pathology and requires an approximate 50 to 75 percent *increase* in milliamperage-seconds from a normal abdominal technique.
Carlton and McKenna-Adler, "The Pathology Problem," p 257; Carroll, "Pathology and Casts," pp 166–167.

68. **(B)** The anode heel effect is defined as the variation in x-ray intensity resulting from the angle at which the x rays emerge from the tungsten target. The intensity of the beam is greater at the cathode end of the tube. In some instances, this may be used to the radiographer's advantage, such as when radiographing anatomy of graduating thickness (e.g., AP projections of the thoracic vertebrae or femur). The heel effect becomes more pronounced with a steeper anode angle, which is the basis of the line focus principle meant to produce a smaller effective focal spot for better resolution. Large film sizes and short SIDs also enhance the heel effect. Shape and size distortion are unaffected by the angle of the target or line focus principle. The parallax effect has to do with tube angulation and the thickness of dual-emulsion radiographic film and is thus also unaffected by the line focus principle.
Carroll, "The Anode Bevel," pp 241–242; Thompson et al., "Geometrical Factors Affecting Image Quality," pp 292–294, and "Radiographic Film," p 238.

69. **(B)** It is not necessary to set an exact time when using an AEC device because the device automatically shuts off at the appropriate time. It is very important that one choose the correct chambers or photocells to assure an accurate density. Positioning skills are also essential when using an AEC device.
Carlton and McKenna-Adler, "Automatic Exposure Controls," pp 505–510; Carroll, "Automatic Exposure Controls," pp 350–369.

70. **(C)** Proper use of a safelight should be stressed to all darkroom personnel. The illumination will be considered safe only if the proper wattage of bulb and correct safelight filters are used. The standard of safety for all safelights is such that unexposed x-ray film may be safely handled in the light at a distance of 3 feet for 1 minute.

     Carroll, "Film Handling and Duplication Procedures," pp 515–516; Papp, "Film Darkrooms," p 15.

71. **(C)** The *only* factors that affect sharpness in this question are the SID, the OID, and the FSS. You can find the *least unsharpness* by using the formula for geometric unsharpness: OID/SOD × FSS = GU.

SID	OID	FSS	
100 cm	20 cm	1 mm	20/80 × 1 = 0.25
200 cm	60 cm	2 mm	60/140 × 2 = 0.86
150 cm	25 cm	1 mm	25/125 × 1 = 0.2
			(least unsharpness)
180 cm	30 cm	2 mm	30/150 × 2 = 0.4

     Carlton and McKenna-Adler, "Recorded Detail," p 407; Cullinan, "Radiographic Quality: Total Unsharpness," p 130; Dennis and Eisenberg, "Radiographic Calculations," p 103.

72. **(D)** The answer to this question is found by taking the formula mAs = mA × time, or one of its variations, such as mAs/time = mA. Thus, 40/0.05 seconds = 800 mA.

     Carlton and McKenna-Adler, "Exposure Conversion Problems," p 514.

73. **(D)** The tangent is the difference between least and greatest values or D-max minus D-min on a characteristic curve. This is found on the straight-line portion of the curve. The difference between the greatest useful density minus the least useful density of a radiographic film is referred to as the contrast.

     Carlton and McKenna-Adler, "Sensitometry," p 324.

74. **(A)** It is necessary to increase kilovolts (peak) to decrease contrast or to produce a longer scale. The proper adjustment would be found by using the 15 percent rule. An increase of 15 percent in kilovolts (peak) would necessitate a 50 percent reduction in milliamperage-seconds. Thus, 60 kVp × 0.15 = 9. 9 + 60 = 69 kVp; 300 mA × $^1/_{10}$ second = 30 mAs as the original technique. Letter A: 300 mA × $^1/_{20}$ = 15 mAs at 70 kVp, which is very close to the correct adjustment needed. Letter B: 400 mA × $^1/_{10}$ = 40 mAs; this represents an increase in milliamperage-seconds and would therefore be incorrect. Letter C: 600 mA × $^1/_{20}$ = 30 mAs; this would result in a film with too much density if it were accompanied by an increase in kVp to 70. Letter D: 100 mA × $^1/_{10}$ = 10 mAs with 66 kVp; both of these adjustments would fall short of the original density and would thus result in an underexposed film.

     Carlton and McKenna-Adler, "Density," pp 372–373; Carroll, "Kilovoltage-Peak," pp 107–111.

75. **(B)** All skeletal radiography, such as extremities, vertebrae, and skull require a short scale of contrast, or high contrast. Also, all studies involving an addition of a contrast medium require high contrast, or a narrow scale of density differences. Radiography of the chest requires a long scale of contrast, or many shades of gray. Because the anatomy of the chest has such naturally high subject contrast (i.e., air in lungs against dense heart and bony thorax), it becomes necessary to use high kilovolts (peak) to narrow the abrupt differences between image densities among the structures of interest.

     Bushong, "Radiographic Quality," 1997, p 248; Carlton and McKenna-Adler, "Contrast," p 390; Carroll, "Image Receptor Systems," p 228.

76. **(B)** A hypersthenic or obese patient will have the same effect as a disease process that increases water content (e.g., ascites, cancer, etc.) and thus will decrease contrast on the radiograph. Likewise, an asthenic or very small patient will have the same effect as a disease process that decreases water content (e.g., atrophy, dehydration, degenerative arthritis, etc.) and thus will increase, or shorten, the scale of radiographic contrast.

     Burns, "Radiographic Contrast," p 109; Carlton and McKenna-Adler, "Contrast," p 398; Carroll, "Interactions of X-Rays within the Patient," pp 56–60.

77. **(A)** There are three main kinds of static artifacts that are caused from low humidity in the darkroom environment. The two most common are "tree" and "crown" static, both of which can be caused by friction or rubbing the film against a surface such as the film bin or countertop. The third type, called "smudge" static, is usually caused by charged particles such as dirt or lint striking the film.

     Cullinan, "Other Recording Media," p 133; Hiss, "Intensifying Screens," p 99; Papp, "Additional Quality Management Procedures," pp 161–162.

78. **(A)** The photosensitive agents contained within the radiographic film's emulsion are made of silver halide crystals. The silver halides used in radiographic film are silver bromide, silver iodide, and silver chloride. Although the exact combination of these three halides varies greatly among film manufacturers according to the unique brand's formula, it is accepted throughout the industry that modern silver halides consist of 95 to 98 percent silver bromide.

Carlton and McKenna-Adler, "Radiographic Film," p 282; Curry et al., "Physical Characteristics of X-Ray Film and Film Processing," p 139.

79. **(D)** When using intensifying screens, as much as 99 percent of the recorded optical density (blackening) in a film is attributed to the "photographic effect." The photographic effect is the ability of the radiographic film to absorb the specific color of light emitted by the intensifying screen. Only about 2 percent of the recorded density on a radiograph is due to direct x-ray exposure.

Carlton and McKenna-Adler, "Intensifying Screens," p 330; Selman, "X-Ray Film, Film Holders and Intensifying Screens," p 279.

80. **(C)** The principal factors measured in sensitometry are the exposure to the film and the light transmitted through the film after processing. The plotting of the relationship between measurements of exposure and density is represented graphically by the characteristic curve, as shown in Figure 1–4. There are three portions to the characteristic curve: the toe, the shoulder, and the straight-line portion. The straight-line portion represents the useful range of densities for a given film; it is also referred to as the "average gradient." The average gradient represents film contrast numerically, as the rise per run or:

$$AG = \frac{D_2 - D_1}{\text{Log relative exposure}_2 - \text{Log relative exposure}_1}$$

It is not necessary to know the exact equation when comparing several films on the same graph. A sharp change in the rise per run will demonstrate a steep slope, and the film will exhibit high contrast. A slow change in the rise per run will *not* demonstrate a steep slope, and this film will exhibit low contrast, or long scale contrast, as seen in film C.

Carlton and McKenna-Adler, "Sensitometry," pp 322–324; Malott and Fodor, "Sensitometry," p 108.

81. **(A)** As explained in the previous question, characteristic curves graphically represent a film's response to exposure. *Contrast,* as mentioned, can be represented on this graph by the average gradient or difference in least and most useful densities on the film. *Speed,* or sensitivity of a film, may be represented by how quickly a film reaches a density of 1 on the characteristic curve. When visually comparing films on the same graph, it is easy to find the fastest film by locating on the graph which film is farthest to the left at a density reading of 1. On this particular graph, film A is farthest to the left at the 1 density point and is therefore the film with the greatest speed.

Carlton and McKenna-Adler, "Sensitometry," p 321; Carroll, "Sensitometry and Darkroom Quality Control," p 531; Malott and Fodor, "Sensitometry."

82. **(C)** Before attempting to answer this question, it is necessary to know which factors affect radiographic contrast. The factors of milliamperage-seconds, screen speed, SID, and FSS are irrelevant and generally need not be considered. Contrast and kilovolts (peak) are inversely proportional, which means that as kilovolts (peak) increases, contrast decreases. The factors of screen speed, grid ratio, and OID are directly proportional; as these factors increase, so does contrast. An answer to this question may be found as with other comparisons of multiple technical factors—by assigning them numbers from least to greatest contrast as follows:

kVp	Screen Speed	Grid Ratio	OID	Total
A. 75^2	200	$8:1^2$	$25\ cm^3$	= 7
B. 80^1	400	$12:1^3$	$40\ cm^4$	= 8
C. 70^3	400	$16:1^4$	$20\ cm^2$	= 9
D. 66^4	100	$6:1^1$	$15\ cm^1$	= 6

Carlton and McKenna-Adler, "Contrast," pp 395–399; Carroll, "Analyzing the Radiographic Image," pp 299–301; Wallace, "The Relationship of the Four Radiographic Qualities," pp 177–178.

83. **(D)** Some of the most common artifacts associated with automatic processors are related to the transport system. *Pi* lines are artifacts that run perpendicular to the direction of film travel at regular intervals and are caused by chemical or dirt deposits on processor rollers. Scratches that are straight and run parallel to the travel of the film indicate misaligned guide shoes seated in the processor. Failure of the film to transport may result from overlapping films; broken drive gears; or improperly seated, warped, or dirty roller racks, guide shoes, or tubes.

Carroll, "Automatic Processors," p 505; Papp, "Additional Quality Management Procedures," p 154.

84. **(A)** Hydroquinone and phenidone are the two reducing agents used in modern automatic processors. Hydroquinone helps to provide upper-scale density (blackness) on the film, represented graphically as the shoulder portion of the characteristic curve. Phenidone helps to provide intermediate or lower-scale densities (shades of gray), represented graphically as the toe portion of the characteristic curve.

Bushong, "Processing the Latent Image," 1997, p 180; Carlton and McKenna-Adler, "Radiographic Processing," pp 296–298.

85. **(C)** It is important when performing quality control checks on the automatic processor to manu-

ally check the developer temperature with a probe that is immersed directly into the solutions. Typically, external digital indicators do not directly make contact with the solution itself, but rather the outer container. The dryer thermostat controls the temperature of the dryer and has nothing to do with the developer. When performing a manual check, glass should be avoided because of its potential to break. Mercury and iodine thermometers must never be used. Bimetallic (stem or dial) thermometers are the better choice for automatic processors. Stainless steel probes are probably the best and safest design.

McKinney, "Maintenance Schedule," p 137; Papp, "Processor Quality Control," p 44.

86. **(D)** Find the answer to these technical comparisons by rating the factors affecting density from the least to the greatest radiographic density. Remember to eliminate any extraneous factors. In this case, FSS has no effect on density.

		Screen				
mAs	kVp	Speed	Grid	SID	OID	Total
A. 10^3	70^1	200^2	$8{:}1^3$	200 cm^1	20 cm^1	= 11
B. 2^2	80^2	400^3	$5{:}1^4$	100 cm^3	10 cm^2	= 16
C. 200^4	90^3	200^2	$16{:}1^1$	200 cm^1	5 cm^3	= 14
D. $.8^1$	80^2	100^1	$12{:}1^2$	150 cm^2	10 cm^2	= 10

Carlton and McKenna-Adler, "Density," pp 368–381.

87. **(D)** Increasing the OID would increase size distortion. Decreasing the SID would also increase size distortion. Tube angulation has no effect on size distortion, only shape distortion, and therefore would not correct the problem. An increase in the SID or a decrease in the OID would decrease size distortion.

Carlton and McKenna-Adler, "Distortion," pp 417–421; Wallace, "Size Distortion," pp 25–31.

88. **(C)** *Res ipsa loquitur* is a Latin term that is used in legal cases of malpractice in which the negligence is obvious, such as leaving a pair of hemostats in the abdomen of a patient during surgery. Such obvious forms of negligence do not need to be proved because "the thing speaks for itself."

Obergfell, "Civil Liability." p 52

89. **(B)** Compensating filters are used in radiography of irregularly shaped anatomic parts. The thicker portion of the filter should be placed over the thinnest or least dense anatomy. Two of the more common types are the *wedge filter*, which may be used to evaluate anatomy of graduating thickness, such as the foot or the thoracic vertebrae, and the *trough filter*, which is used to obtain balanced density in both the mediastinum and the lung fields on one PA projection.

Carlton and McKenna-Adler, "Filtration," pp 173–174; Carroll, "Beam Filtration," pp 131–132; Thompson et al., "Factors Affecting the X-Ray Spectrum," p 230.

90. **(D)** The wire mesh is a quality control device used to measure the film-screen contact of cassettes or film holders. A spinning top is used to check the accuracy of the timer and also may be used to check for rectifier failures. The Wisconsin test cassette is used to check the accuracy of the kilovolts (peak) control on the x-ray machine. The star test is one of many devices that may be used to check the FSS. Other FSS devices include the pinhole camera and the resolution bar pattern.

Carlton and McKenna-Adler, "Quality Control," pp 444–445; Carroll, "Quality Control," pp 400–403; Thompson et al., "Quality Control," pp 407–408.

91. **(B)** When an improper focal film range (SID) is used, there is a loss of peripheral density. A more severe form of bilateral grid cutoff can occur with a grid in the reverse position. The higher the grid ratio is, the more obvious the grid cutoff will be.

Carroll, "Grids," pp 189–193; Cullinan, "Grids," p 81.

92. **(C)** Oxidation is a normal chemical reaction in the development process. When the silver halide crystals in the emulsion are reduced to metallic silver on the film, the reducing agents hydroquinone and phenidone have been "oxidized." Excessive oxidation can occur from exposure to air and is termed "aerial oxidation". This is why it is essential to have close-fitting lids on replenishment tanks. Aerial oxidation can deplete these reducing agents to the point that they will no longer develop the film properly. Hydroquinone is especially sensitive to aerial oxidation. Because hydroquinone is responsible for the blackest areas, excessive oxidation will lead to a reduction in the darker regions of the film.

Bushong, "Processing the Latent Image," 1997, p 181; McKinney, "Processing: Developer Consumption," pp 44–45.

93. **(D)** The grid ratio is simply a ratio and proportion formula that is the comparison of the height of the lead strips to the distance between them. This can be represented mathematically as: R = h/d. The thickness of the lead strips is irrelevant and should not be used to calculate grid ratio. Comparing *1.6:0.1* is the same ratio as 16:1.

Curry et al., "Grids," p 100; Dennis and Eisenberg, "Radiographic Calculations," p 97.

94. **(A)** If the hardener, glutaraldehyde, becomes depleted, "any or all of the following problems can occur: plus density (wet pressure sensitiza-

tion, scratches, pressure lines, fog, scuff marks), minus density (scratches, pick-off, scuff marks), uncleared film (milky green), failure to transport (jams) or maltransport (slipping, cocking), poorly washed films (high hyporetention), and wet films."

McKinney, "Chemistry System: Development," p 62.

95. **(C)** Sensitometry is a way to measure a film's response to exposure and processing plotted as density versus log relative exposure on a characteristic curve. It is required on a daily basis and is critical to a quality assurance program.

Carlton and McKenna-Adler, "Sensitometry," pp 319–320; Carroll, "Sensitometry and Darkroom Quality Control," pp 530–531.

96. **(A)** A thick body part will produce more scatter radiation than a thin body part. An example of this is performing a PA projection of the abdomen with the patient prone rather than AP projection with the patient supine. In effect, the patient's weight will reduce the thickness of the anatomy and will increase contrast due to less scatter radiation being produced. The same result will occur with the use of a compression band stretched tight over the abdomen. Not only will this decrease scatter production and increase contrast in a thick body part, but it will also result in less patient motion when used as a restraining device.

Cullinan, "Permanent Installation: Dedicated Radiographic Units," p 44; Eisenberg and Dennis, "The Special Patient." p 337; Wallace, "Methods to Control Scatter," p 125.

97. **(C)** To be fully effective, an intensifying screen must be used only in conjunction with a film emulsion that has absorption characteristics matched to the light emitted from the screen. In other words, if the screen emits blue light, the film must be capable of absorbing light in the blue region of the electromagnetic spectrum. This is termed "spectral matching." Conversion efficiency refers to the rate at which x-ray energy is transformed into light by an intensifying screen. Intensification factor is the ratio of exposure without screens versus the exposure with screens that will produce the same optical density on the film. The line focus principle refers to the angle of the anode in an x-ray tube.

Bushong, "Intensifying Screens," 1997, p 197; Carlton and McKenna-Adler, "Intensifying Screens," pp 331–332; Wallace, "Intensifying Screens," p 165.

98. **(B)** During the photoelectric effect, the incident photon is completely absorbed, and no primary radiation will be left to expose the film. The photoelectric effect is more prevalent in tissues with high atomic numbers and with low-energy x-ray photons. There will be higher subject contrast in tissues with high atomic numbers (e.g., bone, teeth) and when using low kilovolts (peak) because of the photoelectric effect. There will be lower subject contrast when scatter is produced through Compton interactions. Compton scattering is more likely with low atomic numbers (e.g., fat, water) and high-energy x-ray photons. This is why radiographs of the abdomen result in low subject contrast and why higher-kilovolt (peak) techniques result in reduced contrast in the image. Photodisintegration does not occur in the diagnostic range, and *bremsstrahlung* radiation is produced only in the x-ray tube.

Bushong, "X-Ray Interaction with Matter," 1997, p 156; Carroll, "Interactions of X-Rays with Matter," p 53.

99. **(C)** Phosphorescence is an undesirable characteristic of a screen phosphor that sometimes may occur with older intensifying screens. Phosphorescence causes the phosphors to continue to emit light after the x-ray exposure has ceased. This can cause an increased density on the film. This increased speed of the older intensifying screen is unacceptable because it will decrease the recorded detail of the image (increased image blur).

Burns, "Imaging System," p 36; Bushong, "Intensifying Screens," 1997, p 192.

100. **(B)** An increase or decrease in the field size, which is determined by the collimator, changes the amount of scatter radiation produced. Scatter radiation affects contrast and density on the radiograph. If the field size increases, the production of scatter radiation also increases and will result in a decrease in contrast.

Carroll, "Field Size Limitation," p 138; Wallace, "Methods to Control Scatter," p 118.

101. **(C)** An important point to remember about most table Bucky devices is that they rely on the reciprocating motion of the device to blur out the grid lines. It takes a finite time for a reciprocating grid to move. If an exposure is made that is shorter than the time it takes the grid to move, the effect will be to create stop-motion, and grid lines will appear in the radiograph.

Bushong, "The Grid," 1997, pp 222–223; Hendee, "Radiographic Grids," pp 311–312.

102. **(D)** Use of a grid has nothing to do with the *production* of scatter radiation but reduces scatter from the patient before reaching the film. An increase in SID will decrease scatter because fewer photons will hit the patient. An increase in milliamperage-seconds will directly affect the number of x-ray photons produced and may indirectly affect the amount of scattering events produced but will *not* decrease scatter radiation.

The production of scatter radiation is most affected by changes in the energy of the x-ray photons, which is determined by the kilovolts (peak) A decrease in kilovolts (peak) will result in a decrease in scatter because lower-energy photons are more likely to be absorbed through the photoelectric effect.

Bushong, "X-Ray Interaction with Matter," 1997, pp 150–151; Carroll, "Kilovoltage-Peak," pp 95–96.

103. **(C)** One explanation of the formation of the latent image is referred to as the Gurney-Mott theory.

Bushong, "Radiographic Film," 1997, p 168; Carlton and McKenna-Adler, "Radiographic Film," p 285.

104. **(D)** The optical density readings recorded by a densitometer concerning how much light is transmitted can be interpreted in two ways. Either the percent transmitted or the fraction that is transmitted through the film may be used.

Percent Light Transmitted	Fraction of Light Transmitted	Density
100	1	0
10	1/10	1
1	1/100	2.0
0.1	1/1000	3.0
0.01	1/10,000	4.0

Notice that when the optical density reads 1 with the densitometer, only $1/10$ of the light from a viewbox will be transmitted through the film. The numeral 10 in $1/10$ has one zero, thus resulting in a reading of 1. When the optical density reads 2, only $1/100$ of the light from a viewbox will be transmitted through the film. The numeral 100 in $1/100$ has two zeroes, resulting in a reading of 2. When the optical density reads 3, only $1/1000$ of the light from a viewbox will be transmitted. Again, there are three zeroes in the numeral 1000, and so on. Translating the fraction $1/1000$ into a percentage, the answer is 0.1%. This memory tip may work for some. The actual formula for optical density may be found by using the calculation: log to base 10 of incident, or original light, divided by the transmitted light through the film.

$$OD = \log_{10} \frac{I_o}{I_t}$$

Bushong, "Radiographic Quality," 1997, p 233; Hendee, "X-Ray Film," p 292.

105. **(C)** Usually, 8:1 grids will provide adequate scatter reduction at tube potentials below 90 kVp. When kilovolts (peak) exceeds 90 kVp, 12:1 grids are preferred.

Bushong, "The Grid," 1997, p 225; Curry et al., "Grids," p 112.

106. **(B)** The anode heel effect results in greater radiation intensity being produced at the cathode side of the tube due to radiation absorption by the anode heel. The heel effect is more pronounced with steeper anode angles, decreased SIDs, and increased film sizes. The heel effect may be used to advantage when radiographing anatomic parts with greater subject thickness at one end than at the other. The advantage is to place the thicker body part below the cathode end of the tube. All of the anatomy listed in this question has varying part thickness at either end. Because the effect is seen to a greater degree with a large film and a short SID, the radiograph that would benefit most would be the AP projection of the femur because it requires the largest film size at the shortest distance.

Carlton and McKenna-Adler, "Density," p 369.

107. **(C)** To control the action of the reducing agents, an antifoggant, or restrainer, is added to the developer solution. The restrainer keeps the reducing agents from developing unexposed silver halide. If unexposed crystals are chemically reduced, the resulting density is termed chemical or development fog. The standard antifogging agent is potassium bromide.

Burns, "Processing the Radiograph," p 52; Carlton and McKenna-Adler, "Radiographic Processing," p 298; McKinney, "Chemistry System: Development," p 61.

108. **(B)** Rare earth screens are made of rare earth phosphors of which there are three primary types: *gadolinium, lanthanum,* and *yttrium.* The chemical with which the rare earth phosphor is mixed varies with different film manufacturers and will determine the color light emitted by the screen. There are four principal combinations: (1) *Gadolinium oxysulfide,* (2) *lanthanum oxybromide,* (3) *lanthanum oxysulfide,* and (4) *yttrium oxysulfide.* Lanthanum oxybromide emits light primarily in the blue region of the spectrum. The others typically emit in the green to blue-green to ultraviolet regions.

Bushong, "Intensifying Screens," 1997, p 197; Curry et al., "Luminescent Screens," p 129.

109. **(C)** The grid focusing distance is the range of SIDs that may be acceptable for focused grids. The grid ratio compares the height of the lead strips in a grid to the distance between them. Conversion efficiency has to do with the intensifying screen's ability to convert x-rays into light. The grid frequency is the number of grid lines per unit length, represented either in inches or centimeters. Generally, the more lead strips there are, the more efficient the grid is.

Carlton and McKenna-Adler, "The Grid," p 268; Carroll, "Grids," p 185.

110. **(C)** Chemicals in an automatic processor should be changed completely at least once every month. All tanks including developer, fixer, and wash should be completely drained and cleaned and filled with fresh chemicals at this time.

McKinney, "Maintenance: Economics," p 143; Papp, "Processor Quality Control," p 46.

SECTION IV: RADIOGRAPHIC PROCEDURES AND RELATED ANATOMY

111. **(B)** There are three accepted methods of obtaining a radiograph of the intercondylar fossa. One is referred to as the *Holmblad* method. Some refer to this position as the "humble" method because the patient is resting on all four extremities on the x-ray table, leaning slightly forward so that the femur forms a 70° angle with the table. The second method sometimes uses a curved cassette and is referred to as the *Beclere* method. The third method has the patient in the prone position with the affected leg slightly elevated to form a 30° to 40° angle to the plane of the film. This is called the *Camp-Coventry* method. The *Danelius-Miller* method (axiolateral projection) is a view of the immobile hip.

Ballinger, "Intercondylar Fossa," Vol 1, pp 250–255.

112. **(D)** When performing a lateral projection of the humerus, it is important to rotate the forearm medially to place the epicondyles perpendicular to the plane of the film. This places the back of the patient's hand against the patient's side.

Ballinger, "Humerus," Vol I, pp 116–117.

113. **(B)** When attempting to demonstrate the apophyseal joints on an oblique projection of the lumbar vertebrae, it is essential to rotate the patient's body 45° toward the side being examined. The 45° angle should demonstrate the upper four lumbar articular facets *closer* to the film. If the fifth articular facet is in question, an additional view with a 30° rotation should be obtained.

Eisenberg, "Lumbar Spine," p 188; Ballinger, "Lumbar Spine," Vol I, p 372.

114. **(A)** Refer to the radiograph in Figure 1–5. The number 1 represents the greater wing of the sphenoid bone, 2 corresponds to the lesser wing, 3 refers to the superior orbital fissure, 4 represents the crista galli of the ethmoid bone, and 5 refers to the maxillary sinus.

Bontrager, "Cranial Bones," pp 324, 328; Cornuelle and Gronefeld, "Skull," pp 324–326.

115. **(B)** In the RAO view of the upper GI tract, the entire opacified stomach and duodenum should be demonstrated. The duodenal bulb and loop should be visualized in profile.

Ballinger, "Stomach and Duodenum," Vol II, p 105–106.

116. **(A)** Anterior oblique projections are used in thoracic radiography to demonstrate the heart and great vessels and are referred to as a "cardiac series." A barium swallow is usually helpful in delineating the area of interest, especially the posterior heart and aorta. It is also ideal for demonstrating the size of the heart and thus accurately diagnosing cardiomegaly or cardiac hypertrophy.

Ballinger, "Chest: Lungs and Heart," Vol I, pp 460–463; Bontrager, "Esophagram," p 430.

117. **(D)** The hypersthenic body habitus literally means above average. About 5% of the U.S. population is considered to have a hypersthenic body habitus, which is classified as a massive build with a broad and deep thorax, short lungs that are broad at the bases, and a high diaphragm. The abdominal organs in a hypersthenic person are typically higher than the average body habitus and are more horizontal than vertical.

Ballinger, "General Anatomy and Radiographic Positioning Terminology," Vol I, p 41; Eisenberg, p 19.

118. **(C)** With the ambulatory patient radiographed in the upright position, the arms should be placed behind the back with the hands clasped together. If the patient is nonambulatory and needs to be radiographed in the recumbent position, it is advisable to place the patient's arms over the head.

Ballinger, "Sternum," Vol I, p 410; Eisenberg, p 152.

119. **(A)** The AP oblique projection of the shoulder, known as the Grashey method, is used to demonstrate the glenoid cavity in profile. The Lawrence method (transthoracic lateral projection) is used for suspected fractures of the upper third of the humerus. Both the superoinferior and inferosuperior projections are taken to demonstrate the scapulohumeral joint.

Ballinger, "Shoulder Girdle," Vol I, p 130–145; Eisenberg, "Shoulder," p 86.

120. **(C)** There are three protective layers that cover the brain and spinal cord, collectively referred to as the meninges. The outer layer, called the dura mater, which literally means "tough mother," is followed by the middle layer, called the arachnoid, which means "cobweblike" or "spiderlike."

The deepest layer that lies closest to the spinal cord is called the pia mater, or "little mother." There are spaces between each layer of the meninges where fluids form and where various drugs or other substances may be injected. Above the top layer of meninges is the epidural space where many anesthetics are placed to anesthetize the body for surgery. Between the dura mater and the arachnoid is the subdural space, which is a common site of traumatic hemorrhage. Between the arachnoid and the pia mater is the subarachnoid space. This space is bathed in spinal fluid and terminates at the level of the second sacral segment. Because the spinal cord ends at approximately the level of the first lumbar vertebra, the subarachnoid space at approximately the L3–L4 interspace is an ideal location for spinal fluid withdrawal and contrast medium injection.

Ballinger, "Myelography," Vol II, p 500; Bontrager, "Myelography," p 621; Tortorici and Apfel, "Myelography," pp 78–79.

121. **(B)** Both the inferior and superior venae cavae deliver deoxygenated blood from all parts of the body back to the heart via the right atrium, where it then passes into the right ventricle. The right ventricle pumps this deoxygenated blood to the lungs via the pulmonary arteries, the only arteries in the body which carry deoxygenated blood. The oxygenated blood from the lungs is transported back to the heart through the pulmonary veins, the only veins in the body that carry oxygenated blood. This blood is dumped into the left atrium and passes through to the left ventricle. During systolic contraction, the left ventricle pushes the oxygenated blood to the aorta, where it is circulated throughout the entire body.

Tortora and Grabowski, "The Cardiovascular System: The Heart." pp 595–597.

122. **(B)** To demonstrate the mastoid process in an axiolateral projection using the modified Law method, it is necessary to first place the patient in the true lateral position with the median sagittal plane and the infraorbitomeatal line parallel with the plane of the film. Rotate the affected side of the patient's chin toward the film until the median sagittal plane is adjusted to an angle of 15°. Finally, a central ray angulation of 15° caudal is also necessary in the modified method. The central ray should enter 2 inches posterior and superior to the uppermost external auditory meatus.

Ballinger, "Petromastoid Portion," Vol II, p 400; Eisenberg, "Mastoid Portion of the Temporal Bone," p 322.

123. **(B)** The kidneys are supported in a fairly fixed position. They may move as much as 1 inch during various respiratory phases. They typically do not drop more than 2 inches from the supine to the upright position.

Ballinger, "Urinary System." Vol I, p 152.

124. **(D)** Beneath the laryngopharynx in the throat is a structure called the larynx, otherwise known as the "voice box." This structure is responsible for sound production or phonation.

Gylys and Wedding, "Respiratory System," p 122.

125. **(B)** The Chassard-Lapine method of radiographing the hip is performed with the patient seated at the edge of the table while leaning over and grasping the lower extremities. This would be ill advised if a hip fracture were suspected. Both the Cleaves and the Lauenstein-Hickey methods are sometimes referred to as the "frog-leg" lateral projections and would also be contraindicated if a fracture were suspected. There are three methods of obtaining lateral projections of the hip that would be considered acceptable. They are all termed "axiolateral projections" or "shoot-through" methods. The first is the Danelius-Miller method or inferosuperior projection and is considered the most common. The second is the superoinferior projection or Leonard-George method and uses a curved cassette. Both of the first two projections depend a great deal on the cooperation and the ability of the patient to shift the unaffected leg out of the way. If both hips were fractured, this would not be possible. The third axiolateral projection, called the Clements-Nakayama method, is performed on patients with bilateral hip fractures.

Ballinger, "Pelvis and Upper Femora." Vol I, pp 280–295; Bontrager, "Hip and Proximal Femur: Trauma," p 239.

126. **(C)** A tangential projection of the patella known as the "sunrise" or Settegast method should demonstrate vertical or longitudinal fractures of the patella and the patellofemoral articulation.

Ballinger, "Lower Limb (Extremity)," Vol I, pp 264–265.

127. **(D)** With the patient in the prone position for the AP projection of the sacrum, the central ray should be directed to enter 2 inches superior to the symphysis pubis at an angle of 15° cephalad.

Ballinger, "Sacrum and Coccyx," Vol I, p 386.

128. **(B)** Refer to Figure 1–6.

Ballinger, "Lower Limb (Extremity)," Vol I, p 185; Bontrager, "Ankle," p 199.

129. **(D)** The wrist joint, the TMJ, and the shoulder joint may all be examined through contrast arthrography. The contrast medium of choice is usually a water-based iodinated agent sometimes mixed with air for a double-contrast effect.

Ballinger, "Contrast Arthrography," Vol I, pp 488–499.

130. **(B)** The most commonly used assessment technique to determine bone age was developed by Greulich and Pyle and compares an AP projection of the left hand and wrist to industry standards developed in the 1930s and 1940s. This method is considered extremely useful for most ages because these bones change very little in the first 2 years of life in comparison with the knee and foot bones, which develop rapidly during this time. Oftentimes, bone age protocols for the very young (younger than 2 years old) will also include an AP projection of the left knee. However, this is usually at the request of the physician and is not considered routine.

Ballinger, "Pediatric Imaging." Vol III, p 38.

131. **(D)** The transthoracic is not a plane, but rather a lateral projection in which the central ray enters on one side of the thorax and exits on the opposite side. The midsagittal or median sagittal plane divides the body into equal right and left halves. The median coronal plane divides the body into equal anterior and posterior halves and is useful in positioning for many lateral projections of the torso.

Ballinger, "Radiographic Positioning Terminology," Vol I, pp 49–50.

132. **(C)** The ampulla of Vater, also known as the hepatopancreatic ampulla, is controlled by a circular muscle known as the sphincter of the hepatopancreatic ampulla or sphincter of Oddi. Between digestive periods, the sphincter remains in a contracted state, thus routing most of the bile into the gallbladder for concentration and storage. During digestion, the sphincter relaxes to permit the bile to flow from the liver and gallbladder into the duodenum.

Ballinger, "Digestive System," Vol II, p 33.

133. **(C)** The head of the rib articulates with the vertebral body of the thoracic vertebra. The tubercle articulates with the transverse process of the thoracic vertebra. The neck of the rib is located between the head and the tubercle. The shaft extends from the tubercle on the posterior side and extends to its anterior portion, where it articulates with the sternum or the sternal cartilage.

Ballinger, "Bony Thorax," Vol I, p 402; Eisenberg et al., "Bony Thorax," p 150.

134. **(C)** In the trauma patient, it is often not feasible to obtain routine AP and lateral projections of the requested anatomy. It is critical in trauma that any injured body part must be radiographed by this rule of thumb: "two projections, 90° apart." Splints should never be removed unless a fracture has been ruled out on the radiograph. Patients are usually never moved from the trauma stretcher (and likely may need to be examined with a portable unit) until all radiographs have been "cleared" by the trauma physician or radiologist. Oblique projections are often not necessary in the proper diagnosis of traumatic injury and, in fact, can be excessively time consuming.

Ballinger, "Trauma Radiography Guidelines," Vol I, p 519; Bontrager, "Trauma and Mobile Radiography," p 551.

135. **(B)** It is important when obtaining a lateral projection of the sacrum to center the central ray 3 inches posterior to the median coronal plane. If the coccyx is of primary interest, the central ray should enter 5 inches posterior to the median coronal plane.

Ballinger, "Sacrum and Coccyx," Vol I, pp 388–389.

136. **(B)** The pedicles of each vertebra extend posteriorly from the vertebral body and exhibit superior and inferior notches. When they are stacked on top of one another, there is an opening between the vertebrae on each side of the column. Each opening, called an intervertebral foramen, permits the passage of a single spinal nerve.

Ballinger, "Vertebral Column," Vol I, p 314; Tortora and Grabowski, "The Axial Skeleton," p 186.

137. **(B)** An optimal SMV projection of the sinuses depends on (1) placing the infraorbitomeatal line as parallel with the plane of the film as possible and (2) directing the central ray perpendicular to the infraorbitomeatal line.

Ballinger, "Paranasal Sinuses," Vol II, p 384.

138. **(D)** To visualize the collecting ducts of the kidneys through the urethra, it is necessary to have the patient catheterized. A retrograde pyelogram is considered an invasive surgical procedure. Collecting ducts may be visualized nonsurgically through an intravenous injection known as an IVP or intravenous pyelogram. A cystogram also requires catheterization but is usually considered nonsurgical because the contrast medium and instrumentation devices do not extend past the bladder, which is the main area of interest. A hysterosalpingogram is an imaging procedure performed to evaluate the female reproductive system.

Ballinger, "Urinary System," Vol II, pp 179–181.

139. **(C)** The umbilicus is said to lie between the L3–L4 intervertebral disk space. The iliac crests can be palpated at approximately the L4–L5 intervertebral disk space, even though the most superior aspect of the iliac crest is closer to L4. The anterosuperior iliac spine lies at approximately the S2 segment of the sacrum.

Eisenberg et al., "Radiographic Anatomy and Positioning Terminology." p 18.

140. **(C)** The capitulum is one of the distal articulations of the humerus located on the lateral aspect of the elbow joint. The trochlea is the other and articulates with the trochlear notch of the ulna on the medial side of the elbow joint. The styloid processes of both the ulna and radius, as well as the head of the ulna, are all located at the distal end of the forearm (the wrist joint).

   Ballinger, "Upper Limb (Extremity)," Vol I, p 64; Tortora and Grabowski, "The Appendicular Skeleton." p 203.

141. **(B)** The coronoid process should be clearly demonstrated in profile in a 45° medial oblique projection (internal rotation) of the elbow. The 45° lateral oblique projection (external rotation) of the elbow is used to demonstrate the radial head.

   Ballinger, "Upper Limb (Extremity)," Vol I, pp 104–105; Eisenberg, "Elbow," pp 68–69.

142. **(C)** The crista galli is a bony projection of the ethmoid bone that extends superiorly from the cribriform plate. The perpendicular plate extends inferiorly from the cribriform. The vomer is a bone that articulates with the perpendicular plate of the ethmoid and, along with this bone, forms the inferior part of the bony nasal septum. The dorsum sella is part of the sphenoid bone.

   Eisenberg et al., "Skull," pp 265–268; Ballinger, "Skull," Vol II, p 220.

143. **(B)** There are three classifications of skull types and it is important for radiographers to become familiar with all three so that proper positioning adjustments can be made for each type compared with the average or mesocephalic shape. The mesocephalic skull has a temporal base that forms an angle of 45° to 47° to the MSP and measures approximately 15 cm (6 in.) between the parietal eminences. The brachycephalic head is short from front to back, broad from side to side, and shallow from vertex to base; its temporal base forms an angle of 54° to the MSP. The dolichocephalic head is long from front to back, narrow from side to side, and deep from vertex to base; its temporal base forms an angle of 40° to the MSP.

   Bontrager, "Skull," p 343; Eisenberg et al., "Cranium." p 271.

144. **(C)** Notice where the barium lies in this image and where the air rises. If the air had risen to the transverse colon and barium was in the cecum, rectum, and sigmoid, the patient would have been in the erect position. If the barium is filling the lateral side of the ascending colon and the medial side of the descending colon, the patient is lying on the right side. If, however, the lateral border of the descending colon and the medial border of the ascending colon are filled with barium, the patient is lying on the left side. Whatever aspect of the colon is filled with air on the decubitus projections is the aspect that will best demonstrate pathology, such as polyps.

   Ballinger, "Large Intestine," Vol II, pp 143–144; Eisenberg et al., "Colon," pp 250–251.

145. **(A)** *Lordosis* is an exaggeration of the lumbar curve of the vertebral column and is also known as "swayback." It may result from increased weight in the abdomen as in pregnancy, obesity, poor posture, rickets, and tuberculosis of the vertebrae. *Kyphosis* is an abnormal posterior convexity of the vertebral column common in older women with osteoporosis and is sometimes referred to as "hunchback" or "dowager's hump." *Scoliosis* is an abnormal lateral curvature of the vertebral column, usually in the thoracic region. It may be either congenital or due to paralysis of muscles on one side of the vertebral column, poor posture, or one leg being shorter than the other. *Meiosis* is the process by which germ cells divide.

   Tortora and Grabowski, "The Axial Skeleton," p 195.

146. **(C)** It is easiest to position the patient in the lateral recumbent position first. Then the patient may be rotated either anteriorly or posteriorly from the lateral position about 20° or about 70° from the horizontal (supine position). When the posterior oblique projection is taken, the apophyseal joints farther from the film are demonstrated. When the anterior oblique projection is taken, the apophyseal joints closer to the film are demonstrated.

   Ballinger, "Vertebral Column," Vol I, pp 362–363.

147. **(D)** The SI joints are clearly demonstrated only with the patient in the oblique position because this is the only projection that will open up the joint spaces. When the patient is in the supine position (AP oblique projection), the joints farther from the film are demonstrated.

   Ballinger, "Vertebral Column," Vol I, pp 380–381.

148. **(B)** On the anterior surface of the tibia just below the condyles is a prominent process called the "tibial tuberosity," to which the ligament patellae attaches.

   Ballinger, "Lower Limb (Extremity)," Vol I, p 182.

149. **(B)** The first or medial cuneiform articulates with the navicular, or scaphoid, at the proximal end and the first metatarsus at the distal end.

   Ballinger, "Lower Limb (Extremity)," Vol I, p 180; Eisenberg et al., "Lower Extremity et al.," p 95.

150. **(B)** If the orbitomeatal line is perpendicular to the film for an AP (Towne) projection of the skull, only a 30° caudal angle is required. If the patient is not able to sufficiently tuck the chin or is traumatized and if the infraorbitomeatal line is perpendicular to the film, a 37° central ray angle is required to demonstrate the basilar portion of the skull.

    Ballinger, "Skull," Vol II, pp 246–248; Eisenberg et al., "Skull," p 284.

151. **(D)** The SMV projection is sufficient for the demonstration of the sphenoid and ethmoid sinuses. The Waters method is the preferred view for the maxillary sinuses, and the Caldwell method is considered the best for demonstrating the frontal and ethmoid sinuses. However, only the lateral projection of the sinuses is able to clearly demonstrate all four sets. If the patient is unable to stand erect for a sinus series, a cross-table lateral projection with a horizontal beam is considered the most important projection.

    Ballinger, "Paranasal Sinuses.," Vol II, p 378; Eisenberg et al., "Paranasal Sinuses," p 285.

152. **(B)** Cirrhosis of the liver is usually diagnosed only through bloodwork, but symptoms such as hepatomegaly and ascites may be demonstrated on an abdominal radiograph or a CT scan. The introduction of a contrast medium into the colon would add little diagnostic information. GI bleeding is a symptom of many types of disease processes and is usually indicative of a perforation, in which case the use of BE with air would not be the radiological examination of choice. Internal hemorrhoids are not easily diagnosed with a BE enema examination and, in fact, may simulate other types of pathology, such as polyps. A clear diagnosis of internal hemorrhoids requires a colonoscopy.

    Ballinger, "Large Intestine," Vol II, p 131; Eisenberg and Dennis, "Gastrointestinal System"; Laudicina, "Alimentary Tract," p 78.

153. **(A)** The scapular spine arises at the superior third of the medial border of the scapula and runs obliquely superior to end in a flattened, ovoid projection called the acromion process. The coracoid process projects anteriorly and can be palpated below the clavicle. The glenoid of the scapula is not a process, but a depression that articulates with the humeral head. The coronoid process is not found on the scapula.

    Ballinger, "Shoulder Girdle," Vol I, pp 122–123.

154. **(C)** The SC joint, or sternoclavicular joint, is the articulation of the medial end of each clavicle and the lateral aspects of the manubrium of the sternum. The lateral aspect of the clavicles articulates with each scapulae at the acromion processes at the AC joints. The sternum does not articulate with either the scapula or the vertebral column.

    Ballinger, "Bony Thorax," Vol I, pp 414–415.

155. **(D)** In addition to showing the size and shape of the liver, spleen, and kidneys, the AP projection of the abdomen with the patient in the left lateral decubitus position is the most valuable for demonstrating air-fluid levels when the upright projection is unobtainable.

    Ballinger, "Digestive System," Vol II, pp 40–41; Eisenberg et al., "Abdomen," p 214.

156. **(A)** The most comfortable and the most efficient way of inserting an enema tip is with the patient in the Sims' position. For the Sims' position, the patient lies on the left side with the forward arm flexed and the posterior arm extended behind the body. The body is leaned slightly forward with the right knee bent sharply and the left knee slightly bent. This position is frequently used for diagnostic imaging of the large intestine.

    Bontrager, "Barium Enema," p 462; Torres, "Basic Patient Care and Safety in Radiographic Imaging," pp 85–86.

157. **(C)** The liver receives deoxygenated blood from the portal vein, which contains newly absorbed nutrients. These nutrients and certain toxins are extracted by the hepatic cells. In some cases of liver disease, such as cirrhosis, intrahepatic pressure may build up and cause excessive pressure in the portal vein. This is known as portal venous hypertension and can be life threatening if it leads to esophageal varices (varicose veins in the esophagus) and hemorrhaging.

    Tortora and Grabowski, "The Digestive System," p 791; Laudicina, "The Hepatobiliary System," p 92.

158. **(B)** When the lower ribs—those located below the diaphragm—are of primary interest, it is essential to instruct the patient to fully exhale before attempting the exposure. The ribs will be best demonstrated on full exhalation.

    Ballinger, "Bony Thorax," Vol I, p 426.

159. **(B)** Sialography is a special imaging procedure during which a contrast medium is injected into the salivary ducts, usually Stensen's duct of the parotid gland or Wharton's duct of the submandibular glands. To best visualize the duct for cannulization, a secretory stimulant, such as lemon juice, is squirted into the patient's mouth to dilate the salivary ducts.

    Ballinger, "Sialography," Vol II, pp 2–10.

160. **(D)** The hamate bone has a characteristic hook-like process associated with it. The lunate is shaped like a half moon (semilunar). The pisi-

form is a tiny pea-shaped bone and is the smallest carpal bone. The scaphoid, or navicular, is boat-shaped.

Tortora and Grabowski, "The Appendicular Skeleton," p 204.

161. **(B)** The central ray centering point for a radiograph of the esophagus is midthorax, which would be at approximately the level of T5–T6.

Ballinger, "Digestive System," Vol II, p 95.

162. **(C)** The term *projection* simply denotes the travel of the central ray. If the film is behind the patient and the patient is lying on the side in a decubitus position, the central ray must enter the patient's anterior surface and exit the posterior surface.

Ballinger, "General Anatomy and Radiographic Positioning Terminology," Vol I, p 50–56.

163. **(A)** When ureteral reflux is suspected, radiographs produced during both filling of the bladder and voiding through the urethra are often requested by the physician.

Ballinger, "Urinary System," Vol II, p 183.

164. **(C)** Postoperative T-tube cholangiography is performed by way of the T-shaped tube left in the *common bile duct* for postoperative drainage. It is performed to demonstrate the patency of the bile ducts, the ampulla of Vater, and the sphincter of Oddi and to detect the presence of stones or other pathological conditions that may have been missed during surgery.

Ballinger, "Digestive System," Vol II, p 78.

165. **(C)** With the patient's foot placed perpendicular to the film and the film centered to the os calcis, the central ray should be directed to enter at the level of the base of the fifth metatarsus at an angle of 40° cephalad to the long axis of the foot.

Ballinger, "Lower Limb (Extremity)," Vol I, p 215.

166. **(D)** To best obliterate the image of the ribs and the vascular markings of the lungs, it is often necessary to make the exposure during quiet breathing.

Ballinger, "Vertebral Column," Vol I, p 359.

167. **(D)** Legg-Calvé-Perthes disease is a type of avascular necrosis that affects the femoral head. This condition largely affects boys between the ages of 4 and 10. A Monteggia's fracture is a displaced fracture of the ulnar shaft associated with anterior dislocation of the radial head. A Jefferson fracture is a comminuted fracture of the ring of the atlas that involves both the anterior and posterior arches and causes displacement of bony fragments. Osgood-Schlatter disease is a painful, incomplete separation of the tibial tuberosity that primarily affects male adolescents.

Eisenberg and Dennis, "Skeletal System," pp 105–108; Laudicina, "Osseous System and Joints," pp 158–159.

168. **(B)** The central ray should be directed perpendicularly to the center of the cassette at the level of T3.

Ballinger, "Bony Thorax," Vol I, p 414.

169. **(C)** For a PA projection of the ribs with the patient in the erect position, instruct the patient to place the hands against the hips with the palms turned outward (back of hands against hips) to properly rotate the scapulae away from the rib cage.

Ballinger, "Bony Thorax," Vol I, p 424.

170. **(B)** The term *atelectasis* literally means insufficient or incomplete dilation. It is a collapse of all or part of the lung due to failure of lung expansion. If caused by trauma (punctured lung), a pneumothorax or hemothorax may accompany it.

Laudicina, "Respiratory System," p 26.

SECTION V: PATIENT CARE

171. **(B)** The legal term *respondeat superior* is a Latin term that literally means "let the master answer." It is a type of vicarious liability in which it is possible for someone to be liable for negligence they did not commit. Sometimes the negligence of one person can be attributed to another even if the other is not present. In the case of *respondeat superior*, the master may be liable for the actions of the servant. The basic premise is that one who orders some directive to be done by another is acting as if he did it himself.

Obergfell, "Civil Liability," pp 50–51.

172. **(C)** A central line may be a single-lumen or multilumen catheter that is inserted into a peripheral or central vein. Its main purposes are for monitoring pressure; for administering medications, total parenteral nutrition, or chemotherapy; or for establishing long-term venous access. The catheter may be inserted into the subclavian, jugular, or femoral vein for short-term use or the superior vena cava at the junction of the right atrium for long-term use. Some common central line catheters include Hickman, Groshong, or Raff.

Kowalczyk, "Tubes, Catheters and Vascular Access Lines," pp 141–142.

173. **(C)** A vector is a disease-carrying insect or animal that transmits germs to humans. A vector bites or stings an infected person and transmits the infection by biting or stinging another person.

Ehrlich and McCloskey, "Infection Control," p 146; Kowalczyk, "Infection Control and Aseptic Technique," pp 81–82.

174. **(B)** Although hand washing is good aseptic technique and should be practiced frequently in the medical environment to prevent the spread of infection, it is not considered a sterile technique, nor is washing with an antiseptic. Soaking instruments in a bleach or chemical solution is good for disinfecting, but it is also not considered a reliable sterilization procedure. Acceptable methods of sterilization include boiling, dry heat such as an oven, gas sterilization using freon and ethylene oxide, and autoclaving (steam).

Ehrlich and McCloskey, "Infection Control," p 166; Torres, "Surgical Asepsis," pp 106–107.

175. **(B)** Patients with head trauma should always be monitored very closely. Never remove sandbags, collars, or dressings until the radiographs have been "cleared" by a trauma physician. Keep the patient's head and neck mobilized. Check vital signs frequently. Wear sterile gloves in case any cerebrospinal fluid or blood begins to leak from the ears, mouth, or nose. *Never* perform suction on a patient with a head injury.

Torres, "Caring for Patients Needing Alternative Medical Treatments," p 226.

176. **(D)** *Diaphoresis* is defined as a condition in which the patient is pale, cold and clammy, and sweating profusely. A diaphoretic patient may be in shock, have diabetes, or be an acutely ill patient who is experiencing extreme pain. Hypertension usually does not produce a diaphoretic reaction, or "cold sweat." A febrile patient is someone with an extremely high fever.

Ehrlich and McCloskey, "Patient Care and Assessment," p 120.

177. **(C)** Threatening someone, such as verbally arguing with a patient about having a procedure performed, is the legal definition of assault. Actually carrying out the threat, such as touching someone without permission, is the legal definition of battery. Touching patients is a necessary part of performing radiological procedures, but before attempting to position patients, you should obtain permission from the patient and carefully explain what you are about to do and why.

Ehrlich and McCloskey, "The Radiographer as a Member of the Health Care Team," pp 56–57; Kowalczyk, "Medical Ethics and Legalities," pp 68–69.

178. **(B)** Before performing any invasive, interventional, or potentially hazardous procedure such as a cardiac catheterization, the patient must sign a consent form. The ordering physician usually completes this responsibility, but it is a radiographer's responsibility to confirm that an informed consent form was signed for all invasive procedures.

Ehrlich and McCloskey, "The Radiographer as a Member of the Health Care Team," pp 54, 56; Kowalczyk, "Medical Ethics and Legalities," p 71; Torres, "Professional Issues in Radiologic Technology," p 13.

179. **(C)** An individual may experience the grieving process when suffering a loss. Losses may include a loss of a loved one, social status, a beloved material possession or loss or changes in the body as a result of the aging process, disease, or physical injury that leaves the person *disabled* in some way. All of these changes are extreme and *permanent* and can alter a person's self-concept. Elisabeth Kübler-Ross states that the grieving process occurs in five stages: (1) denial, (2) anger, (3) bargaining, (4) depression, and (5) acceptance. It is highly unlikely that a person would grieve over a fractured clavicle, which would not be a permanent disability.

Ehrlich and McCloskey, "Professional Communications," p 77; Torres, "Patient Rights Related to Death, Dying and Medical Treatment," pp 32–33.

180. **(D)** With the development of MRI, the number of contrast arthrograms performed in imaging centers has been significantly reduced. MRI offers a noninvasive technique because no contrast material is injected. The main advantage of MRI is its superior low-contrast resolution. It also uses no ionizing radiation. For these reasons, contrast arthrography is now almost nonexistent in many radiology departments and is reserved for only specialized functions.

Ballinger, "Contrast Arthrography," Vol I, p 488; Bushong, "Physical Principles of Magnetic Resonance Imaging," 1993, pp 450–451.

181. **(B)** Any pathology that causes destructive damage to tissue is considered *easy to penetrate*—usually requiring the radiographer to decrease kilovolts (peak). Arthritis is a destructive process that destroys bone and connective tissue, whereas edema, Paget's disease, and pneumonia are additive disease processes because they increase tissue density and therefore require an increase in technical factors, usually kilovolts (peak).

Carroll, "Pathology and Casts," pp 166–167; Wallace, "Radiographic Technique Charts," pp 212–213.

182. **(B)** When a diabetic patient has been without food for a given period of time, the patient may suffer from hypoglycemia, or low blood sugar. If hypoglycemia is also accompanied by hyperinsulinism (too much insulin in the blood), it may

quickly lead to insulin shock. This may result from a diabetic patient who has been both NPO and receives a normal dose of insulin. This is usually why it is best to schedule diabetic patients early in the morning for any procedures that require them to be NPO. The opposite effect is diabetic coma, or ketoacidosis, in which the patient is suffering from hyperglycemia (too much blood sugar and a lack of insulin). It is important to closely monitor diabetic patients who have been without food for a time to prevent them from going into insulin shock. When the patient is hypoglycemic, a simple treatment, such as giving the patient fruit juice or a candy bar, may curtail the onset of shock. For the patient in insulin shock, glucose administered intravenously is usually required.

Gylys and Wedding, "The Endocrine System," pp 305–306; Kowalczyk, "Patient Care in Critical Situations," pp 213–216.

183. **(C)** The most common *types* of injuries found in the imaging department are back injuries caused from lifting heavy objects, such as patients, cases of film, heavy cassettes, and so forth. The use of proper body mechanics is essential for the safety of the patient and the health-care worker.

Ehrlich and McCloskey, "Safety, Transfer and Positioning," p 91; Kowalczyk, "Patient Assessment and Assistance," p 122; Torres, "Basic Patient Care and Safety in Radiographic Imaging: Body Mechanics," p 73.

184. **(D)** Medical asepsis, such as practicing good hand-washing techniques and using alcohol wipes to prepare a site for IV injection, serves to reduce the number of pathogenic microorganisms in the immediate environment. Only surgical asepsis (autoclave, dry heat, etc.) involves the complete destruction and removal of pathogens.

Ehrlich and McCloskey, "Infection Control," p 153; Kowalczyk, "Infection Control and Aseptic Technique," p 79.

185. **(D)** Universal precautions should always be used whenever contact with blood or body fluids is likely. According to the Occupational Safety and Health Administration, the following guidelines should be practiced on all patients as universal, now called standard, precautions against blood-borne pathogens such as hepatitis B:
1. Gloves should be worn when handling patients.   2. Gloves should be changed after each patient.   3. Masks and protective eye shields should be worn, especially during procedures, such as trauma, in which droplets of blood may be generated.   4. Protective gowns should be worn.   5. Hands should be thoroughly washed immediately following the procedure.

Ehrlich and McCloskey, "Infection Control," pp 152–153; Kowalczyk, "Infection Control and Aseptic Technique," p 86; Torres, "Techniques of Infection Control," p 52.

186. **(C)** *Glucagon* is a drug that is often used in radiology departments during barium enema examinations to relax the colon and to prevent spasms. *Diphenhydramine (Benadryl)*, an antihistamine, is used to counteract allergic reactions that release histamines into the body. Examples of common medical aseptics used in skin preparation are *alcohol* or *povidone-iodine (Betadine)*. *Lidocaine (Xylocaine)* is used as a local anesthetic for limited invasive procedures such as arthrography, myelography, and needle biopsy.

Ehrlich and McCloskey, "Medications and Their Administration," p 191; Torres, "Pharmacology for Radiographers," p 258.

187. **(B)** The normal range of blood pressure for both adult men and women ranges from 110–140 mm Hg for systolic pressure and 60–90 mm Hg for diastolic pressure.

Ehrlich and McCloskey, "Patient Care and Assessment," p 127; Torres, "Vital Signs and Oxygen Administration: Blood Pressure," p 138.

188. **(A)** When perforation of the GI tract is suspected, a water-soluble iodinated contrast medium such as diatrizoate meglumine (Gastrografin) must be used instead. Barium sulfate suspension can be toxic if it leaks through a perforation in the digestive tract and therefore is contraindicated with suspected bowel perforation.

Kowalczyk, "Medication Administration," p 190; Laudicina, "Alimentary Tract," p 51; Torres, "Care of Patients during Imaging Examinations of the Gastrointestinal System," p 200.

189. **(B)** There are two broad categories of contrast media: negative and positive. Positive agents absorb more radiation than their surrounding tissue and increase subject contrast. Examples include BE and iodine. Negative agents decrease organ density by the addition of materials into the organ that are very easy to penetrate, such as air or carbon dioxide. These also tend to increase subject contrast because the surrounding soft tissue is now more difficult to penetrate than the negative contrast agent. Typically, lower-kilovolt (peak) techniques are used with the addition of negative agents.

Kowalczyk, "Medication Administration," pp 189–190; Torres, "Care of Patients during Imaging Examinations of the Gastrointestinal System," p 200.

190. **(A)** Swallowing disorders in infants can indicate a congenital disorder known as tracheo-

esophageal fistula. Usually barium is the contrast medium of choice in infants because iodine can cause dehydration very quickly in small children. However, in the instance of any perforation, or opening of the GI tract, barium is always contraindicated and should be replaced by a water-soluble agent such as diatrizoate meglumine.

Laudicina, "Alimentary Tract," pp 53–55.

191. **(A)** Ehrlich and McCloskey suggested the following guidelines for scheduling multiple examinations:
1. All radiographic examinations *not* requiring an injection of a contrast medium 2. Laboratory studies for iodine uptake (nuclear medicine) 3. Radiographic examinations of the urinary tract 4. Radiographic examinations of the biliary tract 5. Lower GI series (BE enema) 6. UGI series.
Sequence: 4, 5, and 6 (OCG, BE, UGI).

Ehrlich and McCloskey, "Preparation and Examination of the Gastrointestinal Tract," p 243.

192. **(C)** The most probable type of legal action that may be brought against a radiographer is a tort. A tort involves personal injury or damage resulting in civil action or litigation to obtain reparation for damages incurred. It may be either intentional or unintentional and is based on *unreasonable* conduct. An example would be a patient injured by falling off a stretcher after a radiographer had completed a bedside examination. The negligence in this case would be clearly unintentional because the radiographer had completed the examination and ensured the patient's safety to the best of his knowledge before leaving. However, the patient could still bring a civil suit against him for an unintentional tort. It is for this reason that a prudent radiographer will become educated in the law as it affects the health-care environment.

Obergfell, "Civil Liability," p 41; Torres, "Professional Issues in Radiologic Technology," p 12.

193. **(C)** Many times in the imaging department, routine protocols may be altered for various reasons. It is important for the radiographer to have a working knowledge of basic mathematics, including percentages, ratios, and proportions. To find the percentage of something, simply multiply the original amount by the percentage in decimal form; for example, 60 percent in decimal form is 0.60. If the question is asking for an increase in the original amount, the percentage will be added to the original to obtain the answer: 50 cc × 0.6 = 30; 50 + 30 = 80. 80 cc is the desired amount needed for injection.

Dennis and Eisenberg, "Percentages," p 13

194. **(A)** An alteration of a medical record by an unauthorized person, or spoliation, may be avoided by the radiographer by following two simple rules:
1. If corrections are needed on a medical record, draw a single line through the original entry and initial and date the entry. Attempts to obliterate the original record by scribbling or whiting out the original entry send up a "red flag" to a lawyer searching for negligence or inappropriate care. 2. Entries in a medical record, such as the patient's chart, should be made on every single available line. Skipping lines leaves room for tampering with records. Also, be sure to put the exact time of the procedure clearly designated in military time or AM and PM.

Obergfell, "Documentation and Record Keeping," pp 73–74.

195. **(B)** Cathartics, or laxatives, are often prescribed for cleansing the bowel. Drinking fluids along with the medication usually enhances the effects of these drugs. Often the orders include a prescription for cathartics along with increased fluid intake.

Ehrlich and McCloskey, "Preparation and Examination of the Gastrointestinal Tract," pp 244–245; Torres, "Pharmacology for Radiographers," p 262.

196. **(D)** According to the latest recommendations published by the American Heart Association, the average rate of compressions when performing CPR on an adult should be between 80 to 100 compressions per minute.

American Heart Association (AHA), "Adult Basic Life Support," pp 4–12; Kowalczyk, "Patient Care in Critical Situations," p 206.

197. **(D)** When you take blood pressure, the lower number is the diastolic reading. A normal range of diastolic pressure is between 60–90 mm Hg. Consistent diastolic pressure below 50 mm Hg may indicate shock.

Ehrlich and McCloskey, "Patient Care and Assessment," p 127; Torres, "Vital Signs and Oxygen Administration: Blood Pressure," p 138.

198. **(D)** Torres stated that the average pulse rate for an infant is approximately 120 beats per minute. Kowalczyk stated it may range anywhere from 100 to 180 beats per minute.

Kowalczyk, "Patient Assessment and Assistance," p 112; Torres, "Vital Signs and Oxygen Administration: Pulse," p 133.

199. **(A)** Monitoring a patient's temperature rectally is arguably the most accurate indication of a person's true core body temperature. However, this method may be contraindicated in some patients

with cardiac conditions because it may stimulate the vagus nerve.

Ehrlich and McCloskey, "Patient Care and Assessment," pp 120–121.

200. **(B)** An allergic reaction to any outside substance typically involves the release of histamines in the body, which results in symptoms such as redness of the skin, hives (urticaria), and itching. The best medication to administer to the patient with a mild histamine reaction is an antihistamine such as diphenhydramine.

Ehrlich and McCloskey, "Medications and Their Administration," pp 186–187; Kowalczyk, "Medication Administration," p 173.

BIBLIOGRAPHY

Adler, AM, and Carlton, RR: Introduction to Radiography and Patient Care. WB Saunders, Philadelphia, 1993.

American Heart Association (AHA): Basic Life Support for Healthcare Providers. AHA, Dallas, TX, 1997.

Ballinger, PW: Merrill's Atlas of Radiographic Positions and Radiologic Procedures, ed 8, 3 vols. Mosby–Year Book, St Louis, 1995.

Bontrager, KL: Textbook of Radiographic Positioning and Related Anatomy, ed 4. Mosby–Year Book, St Louis, 1997.

Burns, EF: Radiographic Imaging: A Guide for Producing Quality Radiographs. WB Saunders, Philadelphia, 1992.

Bushong, S: Radiologic Science for Technologists: Physics, Biology and Protection, ed 6. Mosby–Year Book, St Louis, 1997.

Bushong, S: Radiologic Science for Technologists: Physics, Biology and Protection, ed 5. Mosby–Year Book, St Louis, 1993.

Carlton R, and McKenna-Adler A: Principles of Radiographic Imaging: An Art and a Science, ed 2. Delmar, Albany, NY, 1996.

Carroll, QB: Fuchs's Radiographic Exposure, Processing and Quality Control, ed 6. Charles C Thomas, Springfield, IL, 1998.

Carroll, QB: Evaluating Radiographs. Charles C Thomas, Springfield, IL, 1993.

Centers for Disease Control and Prevention: Infection Control Standards and Guidelines for Healthcare Workers. Author, Atlanta, GA, 1997.

Cornuelle, AG, and Gronefeld, DH: Radiographic Anatomy and Positioning: An Integrated Approach. Appleton & Lange, Stamford, CT, 1998.

Cullinan, AM: Producing Quality Radiographs, ed 2. Lippincott, Philadelphia, 1994.

Curry, TS, et al: Christensen's Physics of Diagnostic Radiology, ed 4. Lea & Febiger, Philadelphia, 1990.

Dennis, CA, and Eisenberg, RL: Applied Radiographic Calculations, WB Saunders, Philadelphia, 1993.

Dowd, SB: Practical Radiation Protection and Applied Radiobiology. WB Saunders, Philadelphia, 1994.

Ehrlich, RA, and McCloskey, ED: Patient Care in Radiography, ed 5. Mosby, St Louis, 1999.

Eisenberg, RL, and Dennis, CA: Comprehensive Radiographic Pathology, ed 2. Mosby, St. Louis, 1995.

Eisenberg, RL, et al: Radiographic Positioning. Little, Brown & Co, Boston, 1989.

Garza, D, and Becan-McBride, K: Phlebotomy Handbook, ed 3. Appleton & Lange, Norwalk, CT, 1993.

Gould, BE: Pathophysiology for the Health Related Professions. WB Saunders, Philadelphia,1997.

Gray, JE, et al: Quality Control in Diagnostic Imaging. University Park Press, Baltimore, 1983.

Greathouse, JS: Radiographic Positioning and Procedures, 3 vols. Delmar, Albany, NY, 1998.

Gurley, LT, and Callaway, WJ: Introduction to Radiologic Technology, ed 4. Mosby, St Louis, 1996.

Gylys, BA, and Wedding, ME: Medical Terminology: A Systems Approach, ed 4. FA Davis, 1999.

Hendee, WR: Medical Radiation Physics: Roentgenology, Nuclear Medicine and Ultrasound, ed 2. Year Book Medical Publishers, Chicago, 1979.

Hiss, SS: Understanding Radiography, ed 3. CC Thomas, Springfield, IL, 1993.

Ireland, SJ: Integrated Mathematics of Radiographic Exposure. Mosby, St Louis, 1994.

Kowalczyk, N: Integrated Patient Care for the Imaging Professional. Mosby, St Louis, 1996.

Laudicina, P: Applied Pathology for Radiographers. Saunders, Philadelphia, 1989.

Linn-Watson, TA: Radiographic Pathology. Saunders, Philadelphia, 1996.

Mace, JD, and Kowalczyk, N: Radiographic Pathology, ed 2. St. Mosby–Year Book, St Louis, 1994.

Mallett, M: Anatomy and Physiology for Students of Medical Radiation Technology. Burnell, Mankato, MN, 1981.

Malott, JC, and Fodor, J: The Art and Science of Medical Radiography, ed 7. Mosby, St. Louis, 1993.

McKinney, WEJ: Radiographic Processing and Quality Control. Lippincott, Philadelphia, 1988.

Memmler, RL, and Wood, DL: The Human Body in Health and Disease, ed 5. JB Lippincott, Philadelphia, 1983.

Mosby's Medical, Nursing and Allied Health Dictionary. Mosby, St Louis, 1993.

National Council on Radiation Protection and Measurements (NCRP): Limitation of Exposure to Ionizing Radiation, Report No. 116. Author, Bethesda, MD, 1993.

NCRP: Medical X-Ray Electron Beam and Gamma-Ray Protection for Energies up to 50 MeV (Equipment Design, Performance and Use), Report No. 102. Author, Bethesda, MD, 1989.

NCRP: Quality Assurance for Diagnostic Imaging, Report No. 99. Author, Bethesda, MD, 1988.

NCRP: Radiation Protection for Medical and Allied Health Personnel. Report, No.105. Author, Bethesda, MD, 1989.

Obergfell, AM: Law and Ethics in Diagnostic Imaging and Therapeutic Radiology. Saunders, Philadelphia, 1995.

Papp, J: Quality Management in the Radiologic Sciences. Mosby, St Louis, 1998.

Scanlon, VC, and Sanders, T: Essentials of Anatomy and Physiology, ed 3. FA Davis, Philadelphia, 1999.

Selman, J: The Fundamentals of X-Ray and Radium Physics, ed 8. Charles C Thomas, Springfield, IL, 1994.

Sheldon, H: Boyd's Introduction to the Study of Disease, ed 10. Lea & Febiger, Philadelphia, 1988.

Snopek, AM: Fundamentals of Special Radiographic Procedures, ed 3. WB Saunders, Philadelphia, 1992.

Springhouse: Medication Administration and I.V. Therapy Manual: Process and Procedures. Springhouse Corporation, Springhouse, PA, 1988.

Statkiewicz-Sherer, MA, et al: Radiation Protection in Medical Radiography, ed 3. Mosby, St Louis, 1998.

Sweeney, RJ: Radiographic Artifacts: Their Cause and Control. Lippincott, Philadelphia, 1983.

Taber's Cyclopedic Medical Dictionary, ed 18. FA Davis, Philadelphia, 1996.

Tamparo, CD, and Lewis, MA: Diseases of the Human Body, ed 2. FA Davis, Philadelphia, 1995.

Thompson, MA, et al: Principles of Imaging Science and Protection. Saunders, Philadelphia, 1994.

Torres, LS: Basic Medical Techniques and Patient Care in Imaging Technology, ed 5. Lippincott, Philadelphia, 1997.

Tortora, GJ, and Grabowski, SR: Principles of Anatomy and Physiology, ed 7. HarperCollins, New York, 1993.

Tortorici, MR: Concepts in Medical Radiographic Imaging: Circuitry, Exposure and Quality Control. WB Saunders, Philadelphia, 1992.

Tortorici, MR, and Apfel, PJ: Advanced Radiographic and Angiographic Procedures. FA Davis, Philadelphia, 1995.

Travis, EL: Primer of Medical Radiobiology, ed 2. Year Book, Chicago, 1989.

Wallace, JE: Radiographic Exposure: Principles and Practice. FA Davis, Philadelphia, 1995.

Wilson, BG: Ethics and Basic Law for Medical Imaging Professionals. FA Davis, Philadelphia, 1997.

Wolbarst AB: Physics of Radiology. Appleton & Lange, Norwalk, CT, 1993.

SIMULATION TEST #1

NAME_____

           Last   First   Middle

ADDRESS _____

           Street

           _____

           City   State   Zip

· ·

MAKE
ERASURES
COMPLETE

PLEASE USE NO. 2 PENCIL ONLY.

↓ BEGIN HERE

**Radiation Protection
and Radiobiology**

01 Ⓐ Ⓑ Ⓒ Ⓓ   21 Ⓐ Ⓑ Ⓒ Ⓓ   41 Ⓐ Ⓑ Ⓒ Ⓓ **Image Production and Evaluation** 61 Ⓐ Ⓑ Ⓒ Ⓓ

02 Ⓐ Ⓑ Ⓒ Ⓓ   22 Ⓐ Ⓑ Ⓒ Ⓓ   42 Ⓐ Ⓑ Ⓒ Ⓓ   62 Ⓐ Ⓑ Ⓒ Ⓓ

03 Ⓐ Ⓑ Ⓒ Ⓓ   23 Ⓐ Ⓑ Ⓒ Ⓓ   43 Ⓐ Ⓑ Ⓒ Ⓓ   63 Ⓐ Ⓑ Ⓒ Ⓓ

04 Ⓐ Ⓑ Ⓒ Ⓓ   24 Ⓐ Ⓑ Ⓒ Ⓓ   44 Ⓐ Ⓑ Ⓒ Ⓓ   64 Ⓐ Ⓑ Ⓒ Ⓓ

05 Ⓐ Ⓑ Ⓒ Ⓓ   25 Ⓐ Ⓑ Ⓒ Ⓓ   45 Ⓐ Ⓑ Ⓒ Ⓓ   65 Ⓐ Ⓑ Ⓒ Ⓓ

06 Ⓐ Ⓑ Ⓒ Ⓓ   26 Ⓐ Ⓑ Ⓒ Ⓓ   46 Ⓐ Ⓑ Ⓒ Ⓓ   66 Ⓐ Ⓑ Ⓒ Ⓓ

07 Ⓐ Ⓑ Ⓒ Ⓓ   27 Ⓐ Ⓑ Ⓒ Ⓓ   47 Ⓐ Ⓑ Ⓒ Ⓓ   67 Ⓐ Ⓑ Ⓒ Ⓓ

08 Ⓐ Ⓑ Ⓒ Ⓓ   28 Ⓐ Ⓑ Ⓒ Ⓓ   48 Ⓐ Ⓑ Ⓒ Ⓓ   68 Ⓐ Ⓑ Ⓒ Ⓓ

09 Ⓐ Ⓑ Ⓒ Ⓓ   29 Ⓐ Ⓑ Ⓒ Ⓓ   49 Ⓐ Ⓑ Ⓒ Ⓓ   69 Ⓐ Ⓑ Ⓒ Ⓓ

10 Ⓐ Ⓑ Ⓒ Ⓓ   30 Ⓐ Ⓑ Ⓒ Ⓓ   50 Ⓐ Ⓑ Ⓒ Ⓓ   70 Ⓐ Ⓑ Ⓒ Ⓓ

11 Ⓐ Ⓑ Ⓒ Ⓓ **Equipment Operation and Maintenance** 31 Ⓐ Ⓑ Ⓒ Ⓓ   51 Ⓐ Ⓑ Ⓒ Ⓓ   71 Ⓐ Ⓑ Ⓒ Ⓓ

12 Ⓐ Ⓑ Ⓒ Ⓓ   32 Ⓐ Ⓑ Ⓒ Ⓓ   52 Ⓐ Ⓑ Ⓒ Ⓓ   72 Ⓐ Ⓑ Ⓒ Ⓓ

13 Ⓐ Ⓑ Ⓒ Ⓓ   33 Ⓐ Ⓑ Ⓒ Ⓓ   53 Ⓐ Ⓑ Ⓒ Ⓓ   73 Ⓐ Ⓑ Ⓒ Ⓓ

14 Ⓐ Ⓑ Ⓒ Ⓓ   34 Ⓐ Ⓑ Ⓒ Ⓓ   54 Ⓐ Ⓑ Ⓒ Ⓓ   74 Ⓐ Ⓑ Ⓒ Ⓓ

15 Ⓐ Ⓑ Ⓒ Ⓓ   35 Ⓐ Ⓑ Ⓒ Ⓓ   55 Ⓐ Ⓑ Ⓒ Ⓓ   75 Ⓐ Ⓑ Ⓒ Ⓓ

16 Ⓐ Ⓑ Ⓒ Ⓓ   36 Ⓐ Ⓑ Ⓒ Ⓓ   56 Ⓐ Ⓑ Ⓒ Ⓓ   76 Ⓐ Ⓑ Ⓒ Ⓓ

17 Ⓐ Ⓑ Ⓒ Ⓓ   37 Ⓐ Ⓑ Ⓒ Ⓓ   57 Ⓐ Ⓑ Ⓒ Ⓓ   77 Ⓐ Ⓑ Ⓒ Ⓓ

18 Ⓐ Ⓑ Ⓒ Ⓓ   38 Ⓐ Ⓑ Ⓒ Ⓓ   58 Ⓐ Ⓑ Ⓒ Ⓓ   78 Ⓐ Ⓑ Ⓒ Ⓓ

19 Ⓐ Ⓑ Ⓒ Ⓓ   39 Ⓐ Ⓑ Ⓒ Ⓓ   59 Ⓐ Ⓑ Ⓒ Ⓓ   79 Ⓐ Ⓑ Ⓒ Ⓓ

20 Ⓐ Ⓑ Ⓒ Ⓓ   40 Ⓐ Ⓑ Ⓒ Ⓓ   60 Ⓐ Ⓑ Ⓒ Ⓓ   80 Ⓐ Ⓑ Ⓒ Ⓓ

081 Ⓐ Ⓑ Ⓒ Ⓓ

Radiographic Procedures and Related Anatomy

111 Ⓐ Ⓑ Ⓒ Ⓓ

141 Ⓐ Ⓑ Ⓒ Ⓓ

Patient Care

171 Ⓐ Ⓑ Ⓒ Ⓓ

082 Ⓐ Ⓑ Ⓒ Ⓓ   112 Ⓐ Ⓑ Ⓒ Ⓓ   142 Ⓐ Ⓑ Ⓒ Ⓓ   172 Ⓐ Ⓑ Ⓒ Ⓓ

083 Ⓐ Ⓑ Ⓒ Ⓓ   113 Ⓐ Ⓑ Ⓒ Ⓓ   143 Ⓐ Ⓑ Ⓒ Ⓓ   173 Ⓐ Ⓑ Ⓒ Ⓓ

084 Ⓐ Ⓑ Ⓒ Ⓓ   114 Ⓐ Ⓑ Ⓒ Ⓓ   144 Ⓐ Ⓑ Ⓒ Ⓓ   174 Ⓐ Ⓑ Ⓒ Ⓓ

085 Ⓐ Ⓑ Ⓒ Ⓓ   115 Ⓐ Ⓑ Ⓒ Ⓓ   145 Ⓐ Ⓑ Ⓒ Ⓓ   175 Ⓐ Ⓑ Ⓒ Ⓓ

086 Ⓐ Ⓑ Ⓒ Ⓓ   116 Ⓐ Ⓑ Ⓒ Ⓓ   146 Ⓐ Ⓑ Ⓒ Ⓓ   176 Ⓐ Ⓑ Ⓒ Ⓓ

087 Ⓐ Ⓑ Ⓒ Ⓓ   117 Ⓐ Ⓑ Ⓒ Ⓓ   147 Ⓐ Ⓑ Ⓒ Ⓓ   177 Ⓐ Ⓑ Ⓒ Ⓓ

088 Ⓐ Ⓑ Ⓒ Ⓓ   118 Ⓐ Ⓑ Ⓒ Ⓓ   148 Ⓐ Ⓑ Ⓒ Ⓓ   178 Ⓐ Ⓑ Ⓒ Ⓓ

089 Ⓐ Ⓑ Ⓒ Ⓓ   119 Ⓐ Ⓑ Ⓒ Ⓓ   149 Ⓐ Ⓑ Ⓒ Ⓓ   179 Ⓐ Ⓑ Ⓒ Ⓓ

090 Ⓐ Ⓑ Ⓒ Ⓓ   120 Ⓐ Ⓑ Ⓒ Ⓓ   150 Ⓐ Ⓑ Ⓒ Ⓓ   180 Ⓐ Ⓑ Ⓒ Ⓓ

091 Ⓐ Ⓑ Ⓒ Ⓓ   121 Ⓐ Ⓑ Ⓒ Ⓓ   151 Ⓐ Ⓑ Ⓒ Ⓓ   181 Ⓐ Ⓑ Ⓒ Ⓓ

092 Ⓐ Ⓑ Ⓒ Ⓓ   122 Ⓐ Ⓑ Ⓒ Ⓓ   152 Ⓐ Ⓑ Ⓒ Ⓓ   182 Ⓐ Ⓑ Ⓒ Ⓓ

093 Ⓐ Ⓑ Ⓒ Ⓓ   123 Ⓐ Ⓑ Ⓒ Ⓓ   153 Ⓐ Ⓑ Ⓒ Ⓓ   183 Ⓐ Ⓑ Ⓒ Ⓓ

094 Ⓐ Ⓑ Ⓒ Ⓓ   124 Ⓐ Ⓑ Ⓒ Ⓓ   154 Ⓐ Ⓑ Ⓒ Ⓓ   184 Ⓐ Ⓑ Ⓒ Ⓓ

095 Ⓐ Ⓑ Ⓒ Ⓓ   125 Ⓐ Ⓑ Ⓒ Ⓓ   155 Ⓐ Ⓑ Ⓒ Ⓓ   185 Ⓐ Ⓑ Ⓒ Ⓓ

096 Ⓐ Ⓑ Ⓒ Ⓓ   126 Ⓐ Ⓑ Ⓒ Ⓓ   156 Ⓐ Ⓑ Ⓒ Ⓓ   186 Ⓐ Ⓑ Ⓒ Ⓓ

097 Ⓐ Ⓑ Ⓒ Ⓓ   127 Ⓐ Ⓑ Ⓒ Ⓓ   157 Ⓐ Ⓑ Ⓒ Ⓓ   187 Ⓐ Ⓑ Ⓒ Ⓓ

098 Ⓐ Ⓑ Ⓒ Ⓓ   128 Ⓐ Ⓑ Ⓒ Ⓓ   158 Ⓐ Ⓑ Ⓒ Ⓓ   188 Ⓐ Ⓑ Ⓒ Ⓓ

099 Ⓐ Ⓑ Ⓒ Ⓓ   129 Ⓐ Ⓑ Ⓒ Ⓓ   159 Ⓐ Ⓑ Ⓒ Ⓓ   189 Ⓐ Ⓑ Ⓒ Ⓓ

100 Ⓐ Ⓑ Ⓒ Ⓓ   130 Ⓐ Ⓑ Ⓒ Ⓓ   160 Ⓐ Ⓑ Ⓒ Ⓓ   190 Ⓐ Ⓑ Ⓒ Ⓓ

101 Ⓐ Ⓑ Ⓒ Ⓓ   131 Ⓐ Ⓑ Ⓒ Ⓓ   161 Ⓐ Ⓑ Ⓒ Ⓓ   191 Ⓐ Ⓑ Ⓒ Ⓓ

102 Ⓐ Ⓑ Ⓒ Ⓓ   132 Ⓐ Ⓑ Ⓒ Ⓓ   162 Ⓐ Ⓑ Ⓒ Ⓓ   192 Ⓐ Ⓑ Ⓒ Ⓓ

103 Ⓐ Ⓑ Ⓒ Ⓓ   133 Ⓐ Ⓑ Ⓒ Ⓓ   163 Ⓐ Ⓑ Ⓒ Ⓓ   193 Ⓐ Ⓑ Ⓒ Ⓓ

104 Ⓐ Ⓑ Ⓒ Ⓓ   134 Ⓐ Ⓑ Ⓒ Ⓓ   164 Ⓐ Ⓑ Ⓒ Ⓓ   194 Ⓐ Ⓑ Ⓒ Ⓓ

105 Ⓐ Ⓑ Ⓒ Ⓓ   135 Ⓐ Ⓑ Ⓒ Ⓓ   165 Ⓐ Ⓑ Ⓒ Ⓓ   195 Ⓐ Ⓑ Ⓒ Ⓓ

106 Ⓐ Ⓑ Ⓒ Ⓓ   136 Ⓐ Ⓑ Ⓒ Ⓓ   166 Ⓐ Ⓑ Ⓒ Ⓓ   196 Ⓐ Ⓑ Ⓒ Ⓓ

107 Ⓐ Ⓑ Ⓒ Ⓓ   137 Ⓐ Ⓑ Ⓒ Ⓓ   167 Ⓐ Ⓑ Ⓒ Ⓓ   197 Ⓐ Ⓑ Ⓒ Ⓓ

108 Ⓐ Ⓑ Ⓒ Ⓓ   138 Ⓐ Ⓑ Ⓒ Ⓓ   168 Ⓐ Ⓑ Ⓒ Ⓓ   198 Ⓐ Ⓑ Ⓒ Ⓓ

109 Ⓐ Ⓑ Ⓒ Ⓓ   139 Ⓐ Ⓑ Ⓒ Ⓓ   169 Ⓐ Ⓑ Ⓒ Ⓓ   199 Ⓐ Ⓑ Ⓒ Ⓓ

110 Ⓐ Ⓑ Ⓒ Ⓓ   140 Ⓐ Ⓑ Ⓒ Ⓓ   170 Ⓐ Ⓑ Ⓒ Ⓓ   200 Ⓐ Ⓑ Ⓒ Ⓓ

SIMULATION EXAMINATION 2

Questions

Directions: (Questions 1 to 200) For each of the following items, select the best answer among the four possible choices (A, B, C, or D). For ease of scoring, it is suggested that you use the bubble sheets provided in the back of this book. Make sure to answer all questions. You should allow yourself a maximum of 3 hours to take this examination.

Refer to the scale in the back of the book to determine a passing score in each section. It is not necessary that you pass each section, but you must receive a total "scaled" score of 75 to pass the examination.

SECTION I: RADIATION PROTECTION AND RADIOBIOLOGY

1. What is the most radiosensitive part of any human cell?
   A. Cytoplasm
   B. Chromosome
   C. Centromere
   D. Golgi body

2. For occupational personnel, the annual dose equivalent limits for the skin, hands, and feet are:
   A. 150 mSv (15 rem)
   B. 250 mSv (25 rem)
   C. 500 mSv (50 rem)
   D. 750 mSv (75 rem)

3. Which type of shielding should be used while imaging a young child with a typical fixed fluoroscopic unit?
   A. Shadow shield
   B. Shaped contact shield
   C. Flat contact shield over the pelvis
   D. Lead apron placed under the pelvis

4. According to the National Council on Radiation Protection and Measurement (NCRP), how many times should the primary beam scatter before reaching the operator behind a control booth?
   A. Never
   B. Once
   C. Twice
   D. Four times

5. When the x-ray beam is projected through the patient's body, the part that receives the largest exposure is the
   A. Exit surface
   B. Bone marrow
   C. Entrance surface
   D. Gonads

6. If the exposure rate is 25 R/min at a source-skin distance (SSD) of 80 cm, what would the exposure rate be (roentgens per minute) if the SSD is changed to 90 cm?
   A. 16 R/min
   B. 20 R/min
   C. 32 R/min
   D. 42 R/min

7. What is the annual dose-equivalent limit for the lens of the eye for the general public?
   A. 15 mSv (1.5 rem)
   B. 25 mSv (2.5 rem)
   C. 50 mSv (5 rem)
   D. 150 mSv (15 rem)

8. Which radiation measuring and detection device has a wide range and is accurate in measuring radiation exposure for personnel, patients, and stationary area monitoring?
   A. Proportional counter
   B. Scintillation detector
   C. Thermoluminescent detector (TLD)
   D. Ionization chamber

9. What is the main purpose of a filter in diagnostic radiology?
   A. To remove the low-energy photons
   B. To decrease scatter radiation
   C. To increase recorded detail
   D. To increase quantity of the beam

10. Which of the following projections would be most beneficial to reduce radiation exposure to certain radiosensitive body tissues?

    1. Posteroanterior (PA) projection of the skull
    2. Anteroposterior (AP) projection—scoliosis series
    3. AP projection for intravenous urogram (IVU) (female patients)

    A. 1 and 2 only
    B. 2 and 3 only
    C. 1 and 3 only
    D. 1, 2, and 3

11. An occupational worker must wear a personnel monitoring device any time that individual receives, or is likely to receive, a whole-body dose that exceeds:
    A. 10 mrem/wk
    B. 25 mrem/wk
    C. 50 mrem/wk
    D. 100 mrem/wk

12. Most radiation survey instruments used to calibrate radiographic equipment use a(an)
    A. Scintillation crystal
    B. Piece of radiographic film
    C. Ionization chamber
    D. Spinning top

13. The biologic effects of radiation that increase in *severity* in proportion to the dose are categorized as:
    A. Long-term effects
    B. Stochastic effects
    C. Nonthreshold effects
    D. Deterministic effects

For questions 14 and 15, refer to Figure 2–1:

14. Using technical factors of 300 mA, 200 milliseconds, and 80 kilovolts (peak) (kVp) at a 100-cm source-image receptor-distance (SID), what would be the approximate skin dose to the patient?
    A. 18 mR
    B. 56 mR
    C. 118 mR
    D. 204 mR

15. What would the estimated entrance skin exposure (ESE) be if the technical factors were changed to 600 mA, 50 milliseconds, at 90 kVp?
    A. 14 mR
    B. 71 mR
    C. 126 mR
    D. 270 mR

16. What is the most likely effect that may be exhibited by a fetus irradiated during major organogenesis?
    A. Spontaneous abortion
    B. Congenital defects
    C. Childhood leukemia
    D. There would be no effect during this stage

17. Which type of interaction of x rays with matter is responsible for the majority of the dose to the patient?
    A. Classical scattering
    B. Photoelectric effect
    C. Compton scattering
    D. Pair production

mR/mAs at a 100 cm SID

KVp	60	70	80	90	100
mR/mAs	1.2	2.3	3.4	4.2	5.6

FIGURE 2–1. mR/mAs chart.

18. During juvenile scoliosis examinations, what organ should be protected from the primary beam of x-radiation?
    A. Lens of the eye
    B. Thyroid gland
    C. Breast
    D. Blood-forming organs

19. The shielding device attached to the collimator of the x-ray unit is called a
    A. Contact shield
    B. Gonadal shield
    C. Shadow shield
    D. Thyroid shield

20. An occupational worker should be monitored to determine the estimated exposure to ionizing radiation. The most common personnel monitoring device is the:
    A. Pocket dosimeter
    B. TLD badge
    C. Cutie pie
    D. Film badge

Refer to Figure 2–2 to answer questions 21 and 22:

21. According to the graph in Figure 2–2, the linear, nonthreshold-type relationship is illustrated by:
    1. Curve A
    2. Curve B
    3. Curve C

    A. 1 and 2 only
    B. 1 and 3 only
    C. 2 and 3 only
    D. 1, 2, and 3

22. The nonlinear, threshold response relationship is illustrated by:
    A. Curve A
    B. Curve B
    C. Curve C
    D. Curve D

23. The second stage of response in the acute radiation syndrome (ARS), in which the organism shows no signs or symptoms, is called:
    A. Prodromal stage
    B. Latent stage
    C. Major organogenesis stage
    D. Manifest stage

24. The maximum cumulative whole-body exposure that is allowed for a 28-year-old occupational worker is:
    A. 1.08 Sv (108 rem)
    B. 0.88 Sv (88 rem)
    C. 0.28 Sv (28 rem)
    D. 0.028 Sv (2.8 rem)

25. According to NCRP recommendations, what should be the minimum thickness of protection for the tower drape on a fluoroscopic unit?
    A. 0.15-mm lead (Pb) equivalent
    B. 0.25-mm Pb equivalent
    C. 1.5-mm aluminum (Al) equivalent
    D. 2.5-mm Al equivalent

26. Which individual should never assist in holding patients during an exposure to x-radiation?
    A. Patient transport aides
    B. Patient's relative
    C. Nurse
    D. Radiographer

27. On fluoroscopic equipment, a "dead-man" switch is incorporated in the circuitry in order to:
    A. Automatically collimate to the film size
    B. Initiate the high-dose mode
    C. Activate the x-ray exposure by the fluoroscopist
    D. Control the automatic brightness gain

28. In what unit is the radiation measured "in air" expressed?
    1. Gray
    2. Roentgen
    3. Coulomb (C) kilogram

    A. 1 and 2
    B. 1 and 3
    C. 2 and 3
    D. 1, 2, and 3

29. Radiation that possesses a high linear energy transfer (LET) also:
    A. Has a low ability to ionize
    B. Has a low relative biologic effect (RBE)
    C. Is highly penetrating
    D. Is highly ionizing

30. While using an automatic exposure control (AEC) device on a sthenic patient, what should the radiographer do to minimize patient dose during abdominal radiography?

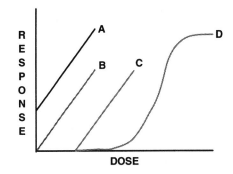

FIGURE 2–2. Dose-response curves.

A. Position the anatomy of interest over the correct photocell.
B. Use a positive density setting.
C. Use a lower kilovolt (peak) compared to that used on an asthenic patient.
D. Use a 400-mA setting with a 2-second backup time

SECTION II: EQUIPMENT OPERATION AND MAINTENANCE

31. Safe technical factors applied to the x-ray tube for a single exposure are determined by the
    A. Tube rating chart
    B. Hurter and Driffield (H & D) chart
    C. Technique chart
    D. Anode cooling chart

32. Which of these types of electromagnetic radiation will possess the shortest wavelength?
    A. X rays
    B. Cosmic rays
    C. Gamma rays
    D. Radio waves

33. In a x-ray machine, the induction motor is used to:
    A. Heat the filament of the cathode
    B. Drive the portable machine
    C. Rotate the rotor of the anode
    D. Operate the autotransformer

34. When operating a mobile unit with a capacitor discharge generator, high-speed image receptors should be used to:
    A. Take advantage of the high-kilovolt (peak) output of the generator
    B. Improve the recorded detail of the mobile image
    C. Overcome the limited output of the mobile unit's generator
    D. Reduce the screen lag often seen with slower-speed imaging receptors

35. What is the main advantage of image-intensified fluoroscopy compared with conventional radiography?
    A. Lower patient dose
    B. Real-time viewing
    C. Higher resolution
    D. Higher milliampere output

36. What type of meter is wired in a series circuit?
    A. Ammeter
    B. Voltmeter
    C. Ohmmeter
    D. Penetrometer

37. The area of the anode target that is struck by the electron beam is called the
    A. Effective focal spot
    B. Projected focal spot
    C. Actual focal spot
    D. Anode heel

38. Failure to properly warm-up the x-ray tube prior to a single large exposure may result in:
    A. A cracked anode
    B. Burned-out rectifier tubes
    C. A cracked glass envelope
    D. Overexposure to the patient

39. To avoid the hazard of electrical shock, which part of the x-ray circuit is grounded?
    A. Primary side of the step-up transformer
    B. Secondary side of the step-up transformer
    C. Primary side of the filament transformer
    D. Secondary side of the filament transformer

40. The quality of an x-ray beam may be expressed in terms of:
    A. Exposure linearity
    B. Reproducibility
    C. Half-value layer (HVL)
    D. Focal spot size (FSS)

41. In which part of the image intensifier is the electronic image created?
    A. At the input phosphor
    B. At the output phosphor
    C. At the electrostatic lenses
    D. At the photocathode

42. What type of radiation is produced when an incident electron interacts with the force field of an atomic nucleus?
    A. Characteristic radiation
    B. Annihilation radiation
    C. *Bremsstrahlung*
    D. Compton scattering

43. If the x-ray tube produces a loud grinding noise during the boost stage prior to the exposure, it is usually an indication of:
    A. "A gassy" x-ray tube
    B. A cracked glass envelope
    C. A pitted anode
    D. Damaged rotor bearings

44. The TV camera tubes most often used in intensified fluoroscopy are:
    1. Thyratron
    2. Vidicon
    3. Plumbicon

    A. 1 and 2
    B. 1 and 3
    C. 2 and 3
    D. 1, 2, and 3

45. A 3-phase, 12-pulse unit has a maximum anode heat storage capacity of 500,000 heat units (HU). How many rapid exposures of 400 mA, 300 milliseconds, and 75 kVp can be made before exceeding the storage capacity of this anode?
    A. 36
    B. 39
    C. 41
    D. 55

Refer to Figure 2–3 to answer questions 46 and 47:

46. The drawing in Figure 2–3 illustrates a sine curve of:
    A. Single-phase DC
    B. Single-phase AC
    C. Pulsating DC
    D. 3-phase AC

47. The length of time that it takes the current to travel from point C to point E is:
    A. 1 second
    B. ⅓₀ second
    C. ⅟₆₀ second
    D. ⅟₁₂₀ second

48. How many neutrons are in an isotope of barium that has an atomic number of 56 and a mass number of 138?
    A. 56
    B. 82
    C. 138
    D. 194

49. Reproducibility from one exposure to the next using identical factors of milliamperes, time, and kilovolts (peak) should not vary in intensity by more than _____percent.
    A. 2
    B. 5
    C. 10
    D. 15

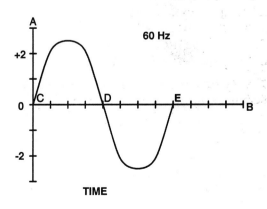

FIGURE 2–3. Sine curve of alternating current (AC).

50. If a 180-cm (72-in.) SID is used with a chest unit, the light field and x-ray beam must be accurate to within _____ on each side of the image receptor.
    A. 2 cm (0.8 in.)
    B. 3.6 cm (1.44 in.)
    C. 5.08 cm (2 in.)
    D. 9.2 cm (3.6 in.)

51. After loading a cassette with film, how long should you wait before performing a quality assurance test for screen contact?
    A. 2 minutes
    B. 5 minutes
    C. 15 minutes
    D. 30 minutes

52. When performing a noninvasive timer test on a 3-phase, 6-pulse unit, what should appear on the radiograph with a timer setting of 50 milliseconds?
    A. 3 dots or dashes
    B. 6 dots or dashes
    C. 18° arc
    D. 36° arc

53. Examples of devices that control the size and shape of the useful beam are:
    1. Cone
    2. Collimator
    3. Aperture diaphragm

    A. 1 and 2
    B. 1 and 3
    C. 2 and 3
    D. 1, 2, and 3

54. In the x-ray circuit, the terms "star," "wye," or "delta" are used to describe types of:
    A. Transformers
    B. Rectifiers
    C. Generators
    D. X-ray tubes

55. What type of quality assurance test would be used to detect the buildup of tungsten inside the glass envelope?
    A. Reproducibility
    B. Exposure linearity
    C. FSS
    D. Beam quality

56. The current needed to heat the filament in the x-ray tube ranges between:
    A. 200 to 500 A
    B. 200 to 500 mA
    C. 3 to 5 A
    D. 3 to 5 mA

57. Which of the following equipment errors may cause a failure to initiate an exposure in a machine with positive beam limitation (PBL)?
    1. The Bucky tray is not pushed in all the way.
    2. Both table Bucky and chest stand AEC controls are depressed.
    3. The tube crane is not in the correct SID position.
    A. 1 and 2
    B. 1 and 3
    C. 2 and 3
    D. 1, 2, and 3

58. The undesirable decrease in brightness at the periphery of a fluoroscopic image is called:
    A. Size distortion
    B. Vignetting
    C. Minification gain
    D. Flux gain

59. Which one of the following imaging devices that may be coupled to the output phosphor in an image intensifier delivers the greatest patient dose?
    A. Cine camera
    B. Cassette-loaded spot film
    C. Photospot camera
    D. Videotape recorder

60. What is the voltage if a circuit has a resistance of 4 ohms (Ω) and a current of 6 A?
    A. 0.67 V
    B. 1.5 V
    C. 10 V
    D. 24 V

SECTION III: IMAGE PRODUCTION AND EVALUATION

61. Which one of the following will reduce magnification?
    A. Use of a short object-image receptor-distance (OID)
    B. Use of a long OID
    C. Placing the object parallel to the film
    D. Placing the central ray perpendicular to the object

62. Which one of these would tell the radiographer what new milliamperage-seconds to use when the SID changes to maintain film density?
    A. The reciprocity law
    B. The inverse-square law
    C. Coulomb's law
    D. The direct-square law

63. When performing an IVU series on the same patient, how should the milliamperage-seconds be altered if the scout film was taken in a 3-phase machine and if the rest of the radiographs were taken on a single-phase unit?
    A. Increase by a factor of 2
    B. Increase by a factor of 1.5
    C. Decrease by a factor of 2
    D. Decrease by a factor of 1.5

64. Which set of technical factors would produce the greatest image blur?
    A. 160-cm SID, 20-cm OID, 0.3-mm FSS
    B. 100-cm SID, 15-cm OID, 2-mm FSS
    C. 80-cm SID, 25-cm OID, 1-mm FSS
    D. 100-cm SID, 25-cm OID, 0.6-mm FSS

65. When performing a portable knee radiograph on a trauma patient without a grid, how much should the radiographer alter the technical factors if the patient were to be followed up with radiographs in a routine 3-phase radiographic room with an 8:1 ratio Bucky grid?
    A. Increase kilovolts (peak) by 15 percent.
    B. Increase milliamperage-seconds by 30 percent.
    C. Increase milliamperage-seconds by a factor of 3.
    D. Increase kilovolts (peak) by 10, and double the milliamperage-seconds.

66. If it is desirable to reduce radiographic density by one-half, the radiographer may:
    A. Reduce SID by one-half
    B. Decrease kilovolts (peak) by 10
    C. Double the milliamperage-seconds
    D. Reduce kilovolts (peak) by 15 percent

67. Which of the following chemicals will reduce silver halide crystals to black metallic silver?
    A. Sodium sulfite
    B. Ammonium thiosulfate
    C. Hydroquinone
    D. Glutaraldehyde

68. In comparison to lower-energy x rays, increasing the energy of the x-ray beam will result in a radiograph that exhibits:
    A. Short scale of contrast
    B. Long scale of contrast
    C. Reduction of noise
    D. An increase in recorded detail

69. The modern rare earth intensifying screens are used primarily to:
    A. Reduce patient dose
    B. Decrease quantum mottle
    C. Decrease cost
    D. Increase exposure time

70. What effect does excessive developer temperature have on a finished radiograph?
    A. Increased contrast and decreased density
    B. Increased contrast and increased density
    C. Decreased contrast and decreased density
    D. Decreased contrast and increased density

71. In which equal volume of tissue does the least amount of absorption occur when the body is exposed to diagnostic x rays?
    A. Muscle
    B. Liver
    C. Bone
    D. Fat

72. If the technical factors remained the same when adjusting from an aperture diaphragm to an extension cylinder, the result would be:
    A. An increase in contrast
    B. A decrease in SID
    C. An increase in density
    D. An increase in patient dose

73. What radiographic technical adjustment is recommended for most advanced destructive pathological conditions?
    A. An increase in kilovolts (peak) by 10 percent
    B. An increase in milliamperage-seconds by 30 percent
    C. A decrease in kilovolts (peak) by 15 percent
    D. A decrease in milliamperage-seconds by 30 percent

74. Compared with a low-ratio grid, a high-ratio grid will:
    1. Absorb more primary radiation
    2. Absorb more secondary radiation
    3. Allow more centering latitude
    A. 1 and 2
    B. 1 and 3
    C. 2 and 3
    D. 1, 2, and 3

75. Which of the following sets of technical factors will result in a radiograph with the highest radiographic contrast?

	mA	Time	kVp	Grid Ratio	FSS
A.	800	120 ms	90	8:1	1 mm
B.	400	150 ms	85	12:1	2 mm
C.	600	200 ms	94	6:1	0.5 mm
D.	200	100 ms	88	5:1	1 mm

76. The recorded detail in an image may be enhanced by the use of:
    A. High-speed screens
    B. Rare earth screens
    C. Large FSS
    D. Small FSS

77. When comparing the two radiographs in Figure 2–4, the film on the right exhibits:
    A. Decreased radiographic contrast
    B. Increased recorded detail
    C. Decreased radiographic density
    D. Increased radiographic contrast

78. An exposure is made using 32 mAs at a SID of 100 cm (40 in.). If the SID is changed to 150 cm (60 in.), what new mAs must be used to maintain radiographic density?
    A. 14 mAs
    B. 21 mAs
    C. 48 mAs
    D. 72 mAs

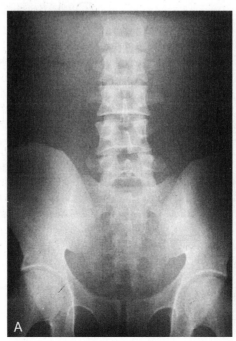
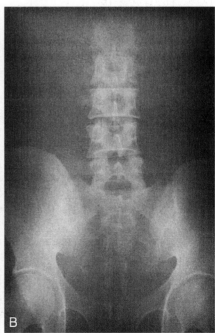

FIGURE 2–4. *(A)* Radiograph of the lumbar spine taken at 80 kVp and 12.5 mAs. *(B)* Radiograph of the same area at 92 kVp and 6.25 mAs. (From Wallace, JE: Radiographic Exposure: Principles and Practice. FA Davis, Philadelphia, 1995, p 96, with permission.)

79. The unit of measure used to express resolution in an imaging system is:
    A. Tesla
    B. Penumbra
    C. Line pairs per millimeter
    D. Hertz

80. What is the term referring to a condition in which all of the anatomic structures are on top of each other in the image?
    A. Elongation
    B. Spatial distortion
    C. Foreshortening
    D. Superimposition

81. Which of the following is a factor that controls shape distortion?
    A. Milliamperage-seconds
    B. Beam-part-film alignment
    C. SID
    D. FSS

82. Which advanced pathological condition requires a decrease in exposure factors?
    A. Ascites
    B. Bowel obstruction
    C. Paget's disease
    D. Acromegaly

83. Which one of the following sets of technical factors would result in the film with the lowest radiographic density?

	mA	Time	kVp	Screen Speed	Grid Ratio	SID
A.	400	100 ms	70	200	12:1	150 cm
B.	200	400 ms	75	400	6:1	200 cm
C.	300	200 ms	80	800	8:1	100 cm
D.	800	100 ms	65	200	8:1	200 cm

84. Which of the following must be identified on all radiographs?
    1. Patient's name or identification (ID) number
    2. Right or left marker
    3. Institutional ID

    A. 1 and 2
    B. 1 and 3
    C. 2 and 3
    D. 1, 2, and 3

85. Which of the following is a result of the anode heel effect?
    A. Radiation intensity is increased on the anode side of the tube.
    B. Effective FSS is smallest on the cathode side.
    C. Radiation intensity is increased on the cathode side of the tube.
    D. Focal spot blur is greatest on the anode side of the tube.

86. When using a fixed kilovolt (peak) technique chart, which of the following technical factors should be adjusted for variations in part thickness?
    A. Kilovolts (peak)
    B. Milliamperage-seconds
    C. SID
    D. Screen speed

87. If it is desirable to increase radiographic contrast, the radiographer might try selecting a:
    A. Smaller focal spot
    B. Shorter SID
    C. Smaller beam restrictor
    D. Lower ratio grid

88. Which of the following types of technique charts requires the most precise positioning skills?
    A. Fixed kilovoltage
    B. Variable kilovoltage
    C. High kilovoltage
    D. AEC

89. For which of the following clinical situations should the density controls on an AEC device be adjusted?
    A. When adjustments for variations in part thickness need to be made
    B. When an adjustment in kilovolts (peak) is also necessary
    C. When changing to a faster-speed screen
    D. When solving temporary problems with the sensing chamber

90. Which of the following imaging procedures would most likely require the use of a high-kilovoltage technique chart?
    A. Barium swallow
    B. Shoulder
    C. Pelvis
    D. Mammography

91. What type of quality assurance test tool is used to evaluate the kilovolt (peak) settings when performing equipment calibration on x-ray units?
    A. Sensitometer
    B. Resolution bar pattern
    C. Wisconsin test cassette
    D. Star test pattern

92. If a blue light–sensitive film is used with a green light–emitting screen, the resultant radiograph will display:
    A. Loss of contrast
    B. Loss of density
    C. Loss of recorded detail
    D. Quantum mottle

93. Which one of the following has the most dramatic effect on the production of scatter radiation?
    A. Air-gap technique
    B. X-ray beam intensity
    C. Amount of tissue exposed
    D. Type of grid used

94. Foreshortening of an object on a radiograph is a form of:
    A. Magnification
    B. Image blur
    C. Noise
    D. Distortion

95. When two linear grids are placed on top of each other with the grid lines overlapping, a _____ artifact may occur.
    A. Moiré
    B. Treelike
    C. Mottling
    D. Fogging

96. Which of the following sets of technical factors would result in the best recorded detail?

	mAs	kVp	OID	SID	FSS
A.	20	78	20 cm	100 cm	2.0 mm
B.	40	84	30 cm	180 cm	1.0 mm
C.	60	74	15 cm	170 cm	2.0 mm
D.	40	82	25 cm	200 cm	0.5 mm

97. Minimum filtration is required by federal regulations on all radiographic equipment for the primary purpose of:
    A. Improving resolution
    B. Absorbing scatter radiation
    C. Reducing patient dose
    D. Increasing beam intensity

98. Most scatter radiation is produced in the:
    A. Cassette
    B. Film
    C. X-ray tube
    D. Patient

99. If a lumbar vertebrae technique produced sufficient radiographic density using technical factors of 75 kVp and 50 mAs with a 200-speed screen, what technical factors would be necessary for a 400-speed screen?
    A. 75 kVp and 100 mAs
    B. 65 kVp and 50 mAs
    C. 75 kVp and 25 mAs
    D. 65 kVp and 100 mAs

100. When using the 15 percent rule, if the kilovolts (peak) is increased by 15 percent, the milliamperage-seconds should be:

A. Doubled
B. Reduced by half
C. Reduced by 15 percent
D. Quadrupled

101. Which of the following sets of technical factors will result in an image showing the greatest radiographic density?

	mA	Time	kVp	Screen Speed	SID	FSS
A.	400	50 ms	80	100	200 cm	1 mm
B.	200	150 ms	75	200	100 cm	2 mm
C.	500	200 ms	80	50	200 cm	0.5 mm
D.	400	150 ms	85	200	100 cm	1 mm

102. With a reduction in field size and all other technical factors remaining unchanged, the radiographic scale of contrast will:
    A. Shorten
    B. Lengthen
    C. Be unaffected
    D. Change, but not visibly

103. When there are drastic temperature differences between the developer and fixer tanks in an automatic processor, a _____ artifact may appear on the image.
    A. Crescent mark
    B. Streaking
    C. Reticulation "wrinkling"
    D. Green-tinted

104. If technical factors of 70 kVp and 40 mAs were selected and if the time setting was 50 milliseconds, the milliamperes must have been selected at:
    A. 200
    B. 400
    C. 800
    D. 1000

105. Which chemical in the developer causes the film emulsion to swell?
    A. Phenidone
    B. Potassium bromide
    C. Sodium sulfite
    D. Sodium carbonate

106. Where should the base-plus-fog be measured when performing a sensitometry test?
    A. On a high-density step
    B. On a medium-density step
    C. On a low-density step
    D. On any unexposed area of the film

107. Which one of the following would require an alteration of technical factors?
    1. Changing the relative screen speed
    2. Changing the grid ratio
    3. Increasing the collimation

A. 1 and 2 only
B. 1 and 3 only
C. 2 and 3 only
D. 1, 2, and 3

108. Which of these changes will produce a radiograph with higher contrast when using an AEC device?
A. Decreasing the milliampere station
B. Increasing the backup time
C. Decreasing the density setting
D. Decreasing the kilovolts (peak)

109. The device used to test the resolution of a film-screen imaging system is a
A. Wire-mesh test tool
B. Resolution grid
C. Penetrometer
D. Densitometer

110. When using a trough filter, it should be placed:
A. On the patient's gonads
B. Between the patient and the x-ray film
C. In the track under the x-ray tube
D. Between the focal spot and the x-ray tube window

SECTION IV: RADIOGRAPHIC PROCEDURES AND RELATED ANATOMY

111. Which of the following bones lies on the medial aspect of the foot?
A. Navicular
B. Cuboid
C. Third or external cuneiform
D. Fifth middle phalanx

112. A rotational movement of the hand starting from the anatomic position and ending with the palmar surface closest to the cassette is termed:
A. Pronation
B. Supination
C. Abduction
D. Adduction

113. Which of the following types of pathology could a radiograph of the cervical vertebrae diagnose?
A. Colles' fracture
B. Jefferson fracture
C. Pott's fracture
D. Smith's fracture

114. Which baseline should be adjusted perpendicular to the film when performing a PA projection of the skull?
A. Orbitomeatal line (OML)
B. Glabellomeatal line
C. Infraorbitomeatal line (IOML)
D. Acanthomeatal line

115. Routine chest radiography should be performed:
A. With the patient recumbent
B. At the end of full inspiration
C. At the end of full expiration
D. At the end of the second full inspiration

116. Which of the following is demonstrated by the Camp-Coventry method for knee radiography?
A. Lateral epicondyle
B. Intercondyloid fossa
C. Patellofemoral articulation
D. Medial epicondyle

117. Where should the central ray enter for a dorsoplantar projection of the foot?
A. Anterior talus
B. Third metatarsophalangeal joint
C. Base of the third metatarsal
D. First cuneiform

118. What is the bony landmark used to center the patient to the middle of the cassette for a recumbent abdominal radiograph?
A. AP iliac spine
B. Symphysis pubis
C. Third lumbar vertebra
D. Iliac crest

119. For which of the following procedures is a long exposure time (breathing technique) useful?
A. AP projection of the cervical vertebrae
B. "Swimmer's lateral" method of the cervicothoracic region
C. Right anterior oblique (RAO) position of the sternum
D. AP projection of the odontoid process

120. The joints formed by the superior and inferior articulating processes of the lumbar vertebrae can be best demonstrated with a(an)
A. AP projection
B. 25° PA oblique projection
C. 45° AP oblique projection
D. Lateral projection

121. What anatomic structures are located in the folds of the small intestine?
A. Rugae
B. Haustra
C. Villi
D. Cilia

122. How many bones are found in a normal adult skeleton?
A. 178
B. 206
C. 212
D. 256

123. Where does the capitulum lie in comparison to the trochlea?
    A. Superior
    B. Inferior
    C. Medial
    D. Lateral

124. How long should the patient remain in the upright position prior to the exposure before the radiographer attempts to perform an erect abdominal radiograph for the demonstration of free air?
    A. 2 minutes
    B. 5 minutes
    C. 10 minutes
    D. 20 minutes

125. The medical term that is defined as the act of or the position assumed when lying down is called:
    A. Decubitus
    B. Recumbent
    C. Supine
    D. Trendelenburg

126. How should the patient be positioned for an AP lordotic projection of the chest?
    1. Have patient lean backward in extreme lordosis, resting shoulders on cassette.
    2. Place the top of the cassette 3 to 4 inches above the top of the shoulders.
    3. Elbows and shoulders should be rolled forward.
    A. 1 and 2
    B. 1 and 3
    C. 2 and 3
    D. 1, 2, and 3

127. Which projection would you use to demonstrate the space between the first and second metatarsal joints and the intertarsal joints between the first and second cuneiforms?
    A. Tangential projection of the instep
    B. Lateral oblique projection of the foot
    C. Medial oblique projection of the foot
    D. Mediolateral projection of the foot

128. Which of the following examinations may be used to image the colon?
    1. Diatrizoate meglumine (Gastrografin) enema
    2. Enteroclysis —small bowel
    3. Barium with air
    A. 1 and 2
    B. 1 and 3
    C. 2 and 3
    D. 1, 2, and 3

129. The part of the pelvis that forms the cavity between the pelvic inlet and the pelvic outlet is the
    A. Filum terminale
    B. False pelvis

    C. Fovea capitis
    D. True pelvis

130. One characteristic of the brachycephalic skull is that the petrous ridges form an angle with the midsagittal plane (MSP) of:
    A. 35°
    B. 47°
    C. 54°
    D. 62°

131. The sutures of the skull are classified as:
    A. Diarthrodial joints
    B. Synarthrodial joints
    C. Ambiarthrodial joints
    D. Amphiarthrodial joints

132. A special projection of the wrist may be requested if the scaphoid bone is of primary interest. How should the part be positioned?
    A. In radial flexion
    B. In ulnar flexion
    C. With the wrist pronated
    D. With the wrist supinated

133. In which projection of the ankle should the malleoli be equidistant to the film?
    A. Mediolateral
    B. 15° to 20° medial oblique
    C. 30° to 45° lateral oblique
    D. AP

134. A radiographic examination of the upper gastrointestinal tract with the patient in the Trendelenburg position is taken primarily to demonstrate:
    A. Esophageal varices
    B. Diverticula of the esophagus
    C. Gastric polyps
    D. Hiatal hernia

135. What radiographic examination uses the positioning terms "craniocaudal," "mediolateral," and "axillary"?
    A. Shoulder arthrogram
    B. Nephrotomogram
    C. Mammogram
    D. Dental radiography

136. Which projection would best demonstrate the intervertebral foramina of the thoracic vertebrae?
    A. AP
    B. Lateral
    C. 45° oblique
    D. 70° oblique apophyseal joints profile

137. With what other bony structure does the auricular surface of the sacrum articulate?
    A. The inferior articulating process of L5
    B. The intervertebral disk of L5
    C. The auricular surface of the ilium
    D. The superior articulating process of the coccyx

138. Filtration of the organic salts, fluids, and nitrogenous compounds from the circulating blood occurs across a membrane called the
    A. Renal pelvis
    B. Hypothalamus
    C. Glomerulus
    D. Major calyx

For questions 139 and 140, refer to Figure 2–5:

139. In Figure 2–5, 4 represents the _____ bone.
    A. Sacral
    B. Iliac
    C. Ischial
    D. Pubic

140. In Figure 2–5, 7 represents the:
    A. Ischial tuberosity
    B. Ischial spine
    C. Coccyx
    D. Symphysis pubis

141. To prevent the joint space from being obscured by the magnified shadow of the medial femoral condyle in the lateral projection of the knee, the radiographer should:
    A. Angle the central ray 5° cephalad
    B. Place the knee joint in 90° flexion
    C. Rotate the knee so that the patella forms a 45° angle to the film
    D. Fully extend the patient's lower leg

142. Which of the following ducts transfers saliva from the parotid glands to the oral cavity?
    A. Stensen's
    B. Santorini's
    C. Bartholin's
    D. Wharton's

143. For positioning purposes, in the average adult skull, the difference between the OML and the IOML is approximately:

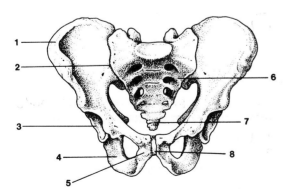

FIGURE 2–5. Innominate bone of the pelvis. (From Scanlon, VC, and Sanders, T: Student Workbook for Essentials of Anatomy and Physiology, ed 3. FA Davis, Philadelphia, 1999, p 85, with permission.)

A. 5°
B. 7°
C. 10°
D. 12°

144. Which basal skull foramen is usually projected into the maxillary sinus during a parietoacanthial (Waters) projection?
    A. Foramen ovale
    B. Foramen rotundum
    C. Foramen lacerum
    D. Foramen spinosum

145. In a typical vertebra, which of the following anatomic parts projects posteriorly from the lateral borders of the vertebral body?
    A. Lamina
    B. Spinous process
    C. Transverse process
    D. Pedicle

146. When radiographing a routine skull in the lateral position, the central ray should be directed perpendicular to the MSP to enter:
    A. 1 inch posterior and inferior to the outer canthus
    B. ¾ inch anterior and superior to the external auditory meatus (EAM)
    C. 2 inches anterior and 1 inch superior to the EAM
    D. 2 inches superior to the EAM

147. For a PA projection of the chest, crosswise placement of the cassette is recommended for:
    A. Broad-shouldered patients
    B. All male patients
    C. Obese patients
    D. Female patients with large breasts

148. On an AP abdominal radiograph, what is indicated if the left obturator foramen appears foreshortened compared with the right obturator foramen?
    A. Rotation toward the patient's right
    B. Rotation toward the patient's left
    C. Cephalic tube angulation
    D. Horizontal alignment of the body on the table

149. Which of the following would correct this view for a parietoacanthial projection (Waters method) if the patient cannot extend his chin any farther and the petrous ridges are seen in the middle of the maxillary sinuses?
    A. Tilt the cassette 15° away from the forehead
    B. Angle the beam 5° to 7° cephalad
    C. Angle the beam 10° to 12° caudal
    D. Angle the beam 15° cephalad

150. In which position is the patient placed for the radiograph of the lumbar vertebrae in Figure 2–6?

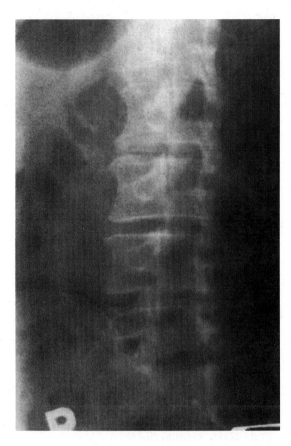

FIGURE 2–6. Radiograph of the lumbar spine. (From Wallace, JE: Radiographic Exposure: Principles and Practice. FA Davis, Philadelphia, 1995, p 84, Fig. 7–12*(A)*, with permission.)

A. Supine
B. Left posterior oblique (LPO)
C. Right posterior oblique (RPO)
D. Left lateral

151. What other examination to evaluate the heart size and great vessels may be combined with a routine radiographic examination of the chest?
 A. Cardiac catheterization
 B. Barium swallow
 C. Apical lordotic view
 D. Electrocardiogram

152. A radiograph obtained with the elbow in acute flexion and the central ray perpendicular to the forearm gives a view of the
 1. Radial head
 2. Medial epicondyle
 3. Olecranon process

 A. 1 and 2
 B. 1 and 3
 C. 2 and 3
 D. 1, 2, and 3

153. The oral contrast agent that is given to the patient for cholecystography is excreted by the
 A. Kidneys
 B. Pancreas
 C. Liver
 D. Duodenum

154. The most common radiographic finding of myelography is:
 A. Metastatic bone cancer
 B. Meningocele
 C. Herniated disk
 D. Osteomyelitis

155. What correction should be made for an AP projection of the pelvis if the greater trochanters are seen partially overlapping the femoral necks?
 A. Abduct the femurs 30°.
 B. Invert the lower extremities 15°.
 C. The patient is rotated; make sure the pelvis is horizontal.
 D. Externally rotate the lower extremities 45°.

156. A hysterosalpingogram (HSG) may be contraindicated in instances such as:
 A. Multiple abortions or miscarriages
 B. Pelvic inflammatory disease (PID)
 C. The absence of the menstrual cycle
 D. A suspected fistula

157. Which of the following anatomic landmarks is located at the interspace between the fourth and fifth thoracic vertebrae?
 A. Thyroid cartilage
 B. Jugular notch
 C. Sternal angle
 D. Xiphoid process

158. What is the general body position described when the patient is in the supine position with the knees and hips flexed and with the thighs abducted and rotated externally and supported by leg and ankle supports?
 A. Fowler's position
 B. Lithotomy position
 C. Sims' position
 D. Trendelenburg position

159. The tangential projection of the carpal bridge is recommended for the demonstration of:
 1. Lunate dislocations
 2. Foreign bodies in the wrist
 3. Navicular fractures

 A. 1 and 2
 B. 1 and 3
 C. 2 and 3
 D. 1, 2, and 3

160. In which position is the left sacroiliac joint best demonstrated?
    A. 25° left anterior oblique (LAO)
    B. 30° right anterior oblique
    C. 30° LPO
    D. 45° RPO

161. The roughened areas on bones that serve for the attachment of tendons are called:
    A. Condyles
    B. Foramen
    C. Meati
    D. Tubercles

162. The mastoid air cells are located posterior to the ear within a large, bony prominence of the
    A. Occipital bone
    B. Temporal bone
    C. Malar bone
    D. Sphenoid bone

163. The appearance of haustral folds is in large part due to the action of three flat bands of muscle fibers on the exterior of the colon called the
    A. *Escherichia coli*
    B. Teniae coli
    C. Epiploicae
    D. Gyri

164. Cirrhosis of the liver is often associated with the excessive intake of a toxic substance known as:
    A. Cholesterol
    B. Bilirubin
    C. Alcohol
    D. Renin

165. When performing a barium enema examination, which position or projection may require a second radiograph centered 2 to 4 inches above the iliac crests?
    A. Left lateral decubitus
    B. LPO
    C. Anteroposterior axial
    D. RPO

For questions 166 and 167, refer to Figure 2–7:

166. What anatomic structure is represented by the number 7 in the diagram in Figure 2–7?
    A. Cystic duct
    B. Common hepatic duct
    C. Common bile duct
    D. Ampulla of Vater

167. What anatomic structure is represented by the number 5 in the same diagram?
    A. Pancreatic duct
    B. Duct of Santorini
    C. Common bile duct
    D. Ampulla of Vater

168. Which of the following anatomic structures would be best demonstrated in the plantodorsal projection?
    A. Instep of the foot
    B. Mortise joint
    C. Os calcis
    D. Subtalar joint

169. How much should the patient be rotated for the posterior oblique position during excretory urography?
    A. 15°
    B. 25°
    C. 30°
    D. 45°

170. Which of the following positions would best demonstrate the axillary ribs of the right rib cage?
    A. Supine
    B. Right posterior oblique (RPO)
    C. Right anterior oblique (RAO)
    D. Prone

SECTION V: PATIENT CARE

171. Ninety-five percent of all contrast medium reactions occur in the first _____ minutes.
    A. 5
    B. 10
    C. 15
    D. 20

172. The burden of proof for medical negligence rests with the _____
    A. Physician
    B. Patient
    C. Radiographer
    D. Risk manager

173. In which direction should the top flap be opened when opening a wrapped sterile package?
    A. Toward the individual
    B. Away from the individual
    C. Toward the dominant hand
    D. Away from the dominant hand

174. During the Seldinger technique of vessel puncture, an anesthetic may be administered to prevent:
    A. Vasospasm
    B. Cardiac arrest
    C. High blood pressure
    D. Bronchospasm

175. What type of transmission occurs when the host inhales infectious droplets or dust particles?
    A. Fomites
    B. Inhalation
    C. Airborne
    D. Vector

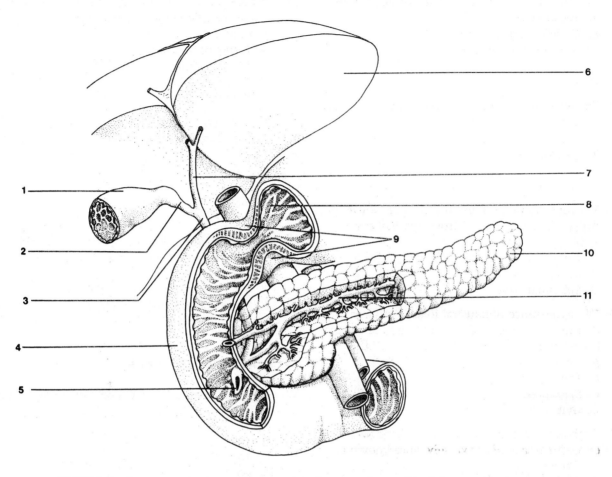

FIGURE 2–7. Biliary system. (From Scanlon, VC, and Sanders, T: Student Workbook for Essentials of Anatomy and Physiology, ed 3. FA Davis, Philadelphia, 1999, p 275, with permission.)

176. When preparing a patient for an oral cholecystogram (OCG), the patient should be instructed to avoid _____ during the 12 hours preceding the procedure.

    1. Smoking
    2. High-fat foods
    3. Laxatives

    A. 1 and 2 only
    B. 1 and 3 only
    C. 2 and 3 only
    D. 1, 2, and 3

177. The passing of a tube into the trachea to administer oxygen to aid in respiration is called:
    A. Suction
    B. Resuscitation
    C. Intubation
    D. Aspiration

178. If a patient is left unattended by the radiographer and the patient falls off the radiographic table, the radiographer could be sued for:

    A. Battery
    B. Felony
    C. Negligence
    D. Assault

179. What is the first duty the radiographer should perform when beginning a radiographic examination?
    A. Check the physician's orders in the chart.
    B. Verify the patient's identity.
    C. Place the film in the Bucky tray.
    D. Obtain an accurate medical history on the patient.

180. Which of the following conditions require protective, or "reverse," isolation technique?

    1. Leukemia
    2. Hepatitis B
    3. Third-degree burns

    A. 1 and 2
    B. 1 and 3
    C. 2 and 3
    D. 1, 2, and 3

181. What abbreviation is used in a patient's chart to assign medication as needed?
    A. PRN
    B. bid
    C. NPO
    D. qid

182. A very serious and life-threatening response to an injection of contrast medium is called:
    A. Hypoglycemia
    B. Anaphylaxis
    C. Urticaria
    D. Hypovolemic shock

183. Which of these are included among the major categories of microorganisms?

    1. Fungi
    2. Protozoa
    3. Viruses

    A. 1 and 2
    B. 1 and 3
    C. 2 and 3
    D. 1, 2, and 3

184. Care should be taken when radiographing infants with "brittle bone disease," otherwise known as:
    A. Osteomyelitis
    B. Erythrocythemia
    C. Osteochondritis dissecans
    D. Osteogenesis imperfecta

185. After completing either an oral or rectal barium examination on an elderly patient, the physician may recommend the use of cathartics to prevent:
    A. Excessive dehydration from diarrhea
    B. Absorption of barium into the bloodstream from causing septicemia
    C. Constipation or fecal impaction
    D. Electrolyte imbalance from diarrhea

186. What is the first step the radiographer should take when establishing that an adult patient is unresponsive?
    A. Open the airway and check for breathing
    B. Call for immediate assistance
    C. Check for a pulse
    D. Start mouth-to-mouth resuscitation

187. Iodine is used as a contrast medium principally because of its
    A. High atomic number
    B. High osmolality
    C. Radiolucent characteristics
    D. Low toxicity

188. It is recommended that a(an) _____ should witness an informed consent for an invasive radiographic procedure.
    A. Radiographer
    B. Disinterested health-care worker

189. C. Radiologist
    D. Radiology staff nurse

189. Which of the following imaging modalities should be used if the results of a radiographic metastatic bone survey are inconclusive?
    A. Computed tomography scan
    B. Arthrography
    C. Magnetic resonance imaging
    D. Nuclear medicine

190. It is important for a radiographer to empathize with a patient who may be going through the stages of the grieving process. The first stage of this process is usually:
    A. Anger
    B. Denial
    C. Depression
    D. Bargaining

191. When a patient's IV drip infiltrates, the radiographer's responsibility should be to:
    A. Push 50 cc of air into the IV bag
    B. Reposition the needle
    C. Slow the flow rate and call a nurse
    D. Apply mild compression with a cool cloth

192. Adding 2 tsp of salt per liter of water used in an enema preparation may prevent:
    A. Hypoxia
    B. Hypervolemia
    C. Hyponatremia
    D. Hyperpnea

193. Allergic-type reactions may occur during a barium enema procedure because of:

    1. Sensitivity to barium
    2. Preservatives added to the solution
    3. Latex used in retention catheters

    A. 1 and 2
    B. 1 and 3
    C. 2 and 3
    D. 1, 2, and 3

194. During the movement and transfer of patients, urinary catheter bags should be placed:
    A. Below the level of the radiographic table
    B. At the foot end of the radiographic table
    C. Below the level of the urinary bladder
    D. On the stretcher or the wheelchair

195. A system set up by the Centers for Disease Control and Prevention (CDC) that requires the use of barriers between individuals and makes the assumption that all patients are potentially infectious is called:
    A. Sterile technique
    B. Universal precautions
    C. Antitoxicity
    D. Medical septicemia

196. An example of a moderate allergic reaction to a contrast medium is:
    A. Metallic taste in the mouth
    B. Urticaria
    C. Bronchospasm
    D. Cyanosis

197. Radiographers should take care to use proper body mechanics when lifting patients to avoid injury to the
    A. Arms and shoulders
    B. Thighs and lower legs
    C. Lumbosacral spine
    D. Cervical spine

198. When performing one-rescuer cardiopulmonary resuscitation (CPR) on an adult, the rate of compressions to ventilations should be:
    A. 5:1
    B. 5:2
    C. 15:1
    D. 15:2

199. The safest and most desirable route of drug administration (when it can be used) is:
    A. Oral
    B. Rectal
    C. IM
    D. IV

200. Following a sudden change of posture from the recumbent to the erect position, the patient may experience syncope or fainting due to a condition known as:
    A. Orthostatic hypotension
    B. Neurogenic shock
    C. Hypovolemic shock
    D. Renal hypertension

Answers and Explanations

Each rationale is followed by references to texts listed in the bibliography at the end of this chapter.

SECTION I: RADIATION PROTECTION AND RADIOBIOLOGY

1. **(B)** The most sensitive part of any human cell to ionizing radiation is the DNA molecule that forms individual chromosomes. The DNA material may be found within the nucleus of the cell. The cytoplasm is less sensitive and contains mostly water and organelles such as mitochondria, ribosomes, Golgi bodies, t-RNA (transfer-RNA), and so forth. Although these complex organelles (called macromolecules) are more radiosensitive than the surrounding water molecules, the DNA is still far more sensitive than any other cell structure.

Selman, "Modes of Action of Ionizing Radiation on Living Matter," p 57; Thompson et al., "General Radiation Biology," p 419; Travis, "Basic Biologic Interactions of Radiation," p 33.

2. **(C)** According to the National Council on Radiation Protection and Measurement (NCRP), the only tissues and organs not included in the whole-body dose are the lens of the eye, which has an annual limit of 150 mSv (15 rcm), and the skin, hands, and feet, which are allowed an annual limit of 500 mSv (50 rem). The whole-body limit is 50 mSv (5 rem). In general, the public's exposure is limited to approximately ⅒ the occupational limit.
    NCRP, No. 116, p 56.

3. **(D)** Most fixed fluoroscopic units are installed in such a way that the x-ray tube is fixed under the radiographic table and the image intensifier is placed above the table. To limit the exposure to a child to as low as reasonably achievable, it is not only necessary to shield the gonads, but also as much of the bone marrow as possible. The only way to properly shield a child during a typical fluoroscopic examination is to place a protective lead apron underneath the child's pelvis (as long as this placement will not interfere with ability to image the structures of interest).
    Dowd and Tilson, "Protecting the Patient in Radiography," pp 232–233.

4. **(C)** Every time an x-ray beam scatters, its intensity decreases by a factor of 1000 at a distance of 1 m. To minimize operator exposure, the examination room should be designed so that no x-ray photons can enter the shielded booth unless they have been scattered at least twice. After undergoing two scattering events, the original beam would have decreased by a factor of 1 million, ensuring the least possible dose to the operator.
    Dowd and Tilson, "Protecting the Radiographer," p 202; NCRP Report No. 105, "Shielded Booths," p 48.

5. **(C)** The largest dose of radiation in the diagnostic range received by the patient is the skin dose. The entrance skin exposure (ESE) is the measurement most often used to represent radiation dose to the patient because the tissue absorbs the majority of the x-ray beam.
    Carlton and McKenna-Adler, "Minimizing Patient Dose," p 205; Dowd and Tilson, "Interactions of X-Rays with Matter," p 62.

6. **(B)** Using the inverse-square law, set up the problem as follows:

$$\frac{25}{x} = \frac{90^2}{80^2}; \frac{25}{x} = \frac{8100}{6400}; \frac{25}{x} = 1.265;$$

$$\frac{25}{1.265} = x; x = 19.76$$

Thompson et al., "Factors Affecting the X-Ray Spectrum," pp 231–233.

7. **(A)** A rule of thumb when determining the dose-equivalent limit for the public is that it is usually ¹⁄₁₀ of the occupational limit. The dose equivalent for occupational workers for the lens of the eye is 150 mSv (15 rem). Therefore, the public is allowed 15 mSv (1.5 rem) annually.
NCRP Report No. 116.

8. **(C)** The TLD badge is the most accurate dosimetry device because it absorbs radiation similarly to human tissue. It cannot measure doses below 5 mR, as the pocket dosimeter can, but it is still very sensitive. It also has a very wide range and is accurate to doses as high as 1000 R. It also has limited function as a stationary area monitor.
Bushong, "Designing for Radiation Protection," 1997, p 643; Selman, "Protection in Radiology: Health Physics," p 513.

9. **(A)** The main purpose of filtration in a diagnostic x-ray tube is to "harden" the beam by removing the low-energy photons. The photons that are removed by the aluminum filter are diagnostically useless and ultimately are absorbed into the patient's skin because they do not have sufficient energy to penetrate human tissue. Filtration not only reduces the patient's skin dose, but it also increases the quality of the beam because it increases its average energy.
Statkiewicz-Sherer et al., "Protection of the Patient during Diagnostic Radiologic Procedures," p 155.

10. **(C)** Certain radiographic projections are better when considering radiation protection of specific radiosensitive organs. The PA projection of the skull, rather than the AP projection, is superior because it limits radiation dose to the lens of the eye by 95 percent. When performing an IVU on a female patient, the AP projection is better because the contrast-filled bladder may act as a shield to the gonads. When performing a scoliosis series, the PA projection offers better radiation protection because it may reduce exposure to the breast tissue by as much as 99 percent.
Dowd and Tilson, "Protecting the Patient in Radiography," pp 228–229.

11. **(B)** The NCRP recommends that personnel be considered "occupational workers" and participate in a personnel monitoring program anytime that individual has the possibility of exceeding a dose of 25 mR/wk or one-quarter the dose-equivalent limit.
Bushong, "Radiation Protection Procedures," Dowd and Tilson, "Health Physics," p 182; NCRP Report No. 105, p 19.

12. **(C)** The cutie pie and the Victoreen condenser R-meter are two of the more common types of ion chambers that may be used for area survey measurements. It is important to note that although ionization chambers are excellent in terms of estimating approximate exposure in air, they do not reveal the type of energy present. Ionization chambers should not be relied on for personnel monitoring or for estimating patient doses. Patient and personnel doses are usually estimated through the use of scintillation or solid-state detectors, not ion chambers.
Selman, "Protection in Radiology—Health Physics," p 539; Statkiewicz-Sherer et al., "Radiation Monitoring," pp 224–228.

13. **(D)** Biologic effects that increase in severity with the dose (that is, the effects are more severe with a higher dose than with a lower dose) are called deterministic effects. Deterministic effects were once termed nonstochastic effects. Examples are (1) skin erythema that becomes progressively worse as the dose increases and (2) cataracts that have a threshold of 2 Gy (200 rad). In the latter case, the entire lens can become opacified, which may lead to complete blindness at doses of 1000 rad or more.
Carlton and McKenna-Adler, "Radiation Protection Procedures for Patients and Personnel," p 156; Dowd and Tilson, "Principles of Radiobiology," pp 112–113; NCRP Report No. 116.

14. **(D)** For questions 14 and 15, three steps are required. *First,* calculate the milliamperage-seconds. *Second,* look on the chart to determine what the exposure rate would be at the kilovolts (peak) in the question. In this case, 80 kVp has a rate of 3.4 mR/mAs. The *third* step requires you to set up a ratio and proportion equation. If there are 3.4 mR for every 1 mAs, how many milliroentgens are there in 60 mAs?

$$\frac{3.4 \text{ mR}}{1 \text{ mAs}} = \frac{x}{60}; \frac{3.4 \text{ mR} \times 60 \text{ mAs}}{1 \text{ mAs}} = x; x = 204 \text{ mR}$$

Bushong, "Radiation Protection Procedures," 1997, pp 526–529.

15. **(C)** Step 1: Find the milliamperage-seconds, which is 30. Step 2: Find the exposure rate at 90 kVp, which is 4.2 mR/mAs. Step 3: Set up a ratio and proportion:

$$\frac{4.2 \text{ mR}}{1 \text{ mAs}} = \frac{x}{30 \text{ mAs}}; \frac{4.2 \text{ mR} \times 30 \text{ mAs}}{1 \text{ mAs}} = x$$

$$x = 126 \text{ mR}$$

Bushong, "Radiation Protection Procedures," 1997, pp 526–529.

16. **(B)** Radiation is a known teratogen, an agent that causes birth defects. Other types of teratogens are alcohol, lithium, rubella, and mercury. In the very early stages of fetal development, specifically the preimplantation stage, radiation may destroy enough developing cells to terminate the pregnancy. Congenital defects are highly unlikely. In the second stage of fetal development, called *major organogenesis,* which occurs between implantation through the 10th week of gestation, cells rapidly divide and differentiate (specialize). The developing fetus is especially sensitive to the effects of chemicals or ionizing radiation, which may result in congenital defects or effects seen at birth. In the third and final stage, known as the *fetal stage,* which occurs between the 10th week of gestation and birth, the fetus is fully developed and simply grows in size. The most likely effects of irradiation that may be induced during this stage are long-term late effects, such as leukemia or other childhood cancers.

   Bushong, "Late Effects of Radiation," 1997, p 490; Dowd and Tilson, "Late Effects of Radiation," p 161; Travis, "Total Body Radiation Response," pp 152–161.

17. **(B)** The patient absorbs more energy through the photoelectric effect than from Compton scattering. The entire energy of the photon is absorbed when a photoelectric effect occurs, whereas only part of the photon's energy is absorbed when Compton scattering occurs. Photoelectric effects increase with increasing atomic number of tissues (such as bone or dental enamel) and decreasing kilovolts (peak). Consequently, using lower-kilovolt (peak) techniques usually increases patient dose through photoelectric effects. Because more absorption through the photoelectric effect means a greater patient dose, the radiographer should be prudent in selecting the optimum kilovolts (peak) while being careful to provide the desired image quality coupled with patient safety.

   Bushong, "X-Ray Interaction with Matter," 1997; Dowd and Tilson, "Interactions of Radiation with Matter"; Statkiewicz-Sherer et al., "Basic Interactions of X-Radiation with Matter."

18. **(C)** There are many types of shielding available to both patients and operators who are exposed to radiation. Gonadal shielding is the most common. Thyroid shields and breast shields are also available because of the sensitivity of both of these tissues. Use of a breast shield is especially recommended for juvenile scoliosis examinations because this tissue may be exposed to the primary beam. If a breast shield is not available, it is recommended that the patient be radiographed with a PA projection instead of an AP projection to protect the breast tissue. The thyroid, although radiosensitive, is usually not in the primary beam when performing a scoliosis series. A lead shield is only effective in protecting the patient from the primary beam, not from internal patient scatter.

   Bushong, "Radiation Protection Procedures," 1997, p 538; Dowd and Tilson, "Protecting the Patient in Radiography," p 236.

19. **(C)** There are three main types of gonadal shielding: (1) contact shields, which are placed directly on top of the patient; (2) shaped contact shields, which are specifically designed for the male gonads; (3) shadow shields, which attach to the collimator and are especially useful for examinations requiring sterile technique. A special type of shadow shield is the clear lead gonadal and breast shielding, made of transparent lead-plastic material that provides shielding for scoliosis examinations. There is also clear lead shielding that may act as a compensating filter because they provide uniform density to the vertebral column during scoliosis examinations.

   Dowd and Tilson, "Protecting the Patient in Radiography," pp 232–233.

20. **(D)** There are three basic types of personnel monitors: film badges, TLD, and pocket ionization chambers. Film badges have many advantages over the other two and are therefore the most often used. They are relatively inexpensive, easy to handle, easy to process, give a permanent record of exposure, and are ideal for detecting low-energy scatter radiation that is the occupational worker's primary source of exposure.

   Bushong, "Radiation Protection Procedures," 1997, pp 532–533; Dowd and Tilson, "Ionizing Radiation," pp 50–59.

21. **(A)** Dose-response curves vary in two basic ways: (1) they are either linear, in which a proportional response is observed in relation to dose, or nonlinear, in which a proportional response is not observed in relation to dose; and (2) they are either threshold, in which a level is reached below which no effects are observed, or nonthreshold, in which theoretically even a small dose could cause an effect. Diagnostic radiology is concerned primarily with linear, nonthreshold dose-response curves because the low doses received mainly cause late effects. Curves A and B are both nonthreshold because these effects may occur at any dose reflected in the line drawn straight up from zero. Curve A starts at a higher level on the graph because it takes into account the natural occurrence of the effect in the population prior to radiation exposure. For example, a certain percentage of the population

may be expected to develop breast cancer without x-ray exposure. The x-ray exposure simply increases the already existing disease occurrence in the population.

Bushong, "Fundamental Principles of Radiobiology," 1997, pp 444–445; Dowd and Tilson, "Principles of Radiobiology," pp 109–111.

22. **(D)** Curves C and D are both threshold dose-response curves because the response is evident above a certain threshold. Notice from the graph that these lines do not begin immediately at zero but appear farther to the right on the graph. This means that there must have been a certain minimum dose that had to occur before the response, or radiation-induced effect, developed. A nonlinear graph is simply a curve that is *not* a straight line. The line may be a hyperbola, a parabola, or a sigmoidal shape. Curve D is both threshold and nonlinear, or sigmoidal.

Bushong, "Fundamental Principles of Radiobiology," 1997, p 445; Dowd and Tilson, "Principles of Radiobiology," pp 109–111.

23. **(B)** The ARS will occur only after a very high-dose total body exposure to radiation. There are four stages to the ARS: (1) the prodromal stage, also known as the "nausea-vomiting-diarrhea syndrome" because these are the symptoms in this initial stage; (2) the latent stage, which is a brief period between the initial prodromal stage and the manifest illness stage in which there are no symptoms and the patient feels better (the shorter this stage, the poorer the patient's prognosis); (3) the manifest illness stage, in which the major system that was damaged by the radiation displays its effects (hemopoietic, gastrointestinal, or central nervous system); and (4) recovery or death. Victims may only recover from damage to the hemopoietic system. If the gastrointestinal or central nervous systems display irradiation effects, life span may be as short as 24 hours to 10 days.

Bushong, "Early Effects of Radiation," 1997, pp 464–467; Dowd and Tilson, "Early Effects of Radiation," pp 128–130; Travis, "Total Body Radiation Response," p 137.

24. **(C)** According to NCRP, the formula that is now used to calculate the cumulative exposure over the course of an occupational worker's lifetime is: (N) × 10 mSv (1 rem). The letter *N* designates the person's age in years. The old formula was 5(N − 18), taking into account the fact that no one under the age of 18 would be employed in the radiation industry. The new formula limits exposure to a greater degree for those who have been employed for several years.

NCRP Report No. 116.

25. **(B)** According to the NCRP, all tower drapes are attached to the image intensifier to protect the fluoroscopist from scatter radiation and should have a minimum thickness of at least 0.25-mm Pb equivalent.

Bushong, "Designing for Radiation Protection," 1997, p 512; NCRP Report No. 102; Statkiewicz-Sherer et al., "Protecting Occupationally Exposed Personnel," p 225.

26. **(D)** The NCRP states that occupational personnel should *never* stand in the primary beam to restrain a patient during a radiographic exposure. Other nonoccupational persons wearing appropriate apparel or mechanical restraining devices should be used to perform this function when required.

NCRP Report, No. 102, p 9; Statkiewicz-Sherer et al., "Protecting Occupationally Exposed Personnel," pp 233–235.

27. **(C)** The fluoroscopic exposure switch should be the dead-man type; that is, if the operator should "drop dead," the exposure would be deactivated. Most fluoroscopic dead-man switches use a foot pedal to serve this purpose.

Bushong, "Designing for Radiation Protection," 1997, p 512; NCRP Report No. 102, p 15.

28. **(C)** The unit in the "traditional" system used to measure the in air exposure is the roentgen (R). The unit that corresponds to the roentgen in the MKS system, or *System Internationale*, is the coulomb per kilogram (C/kg).

Bushong, "Radiographic Definitions and Mathematics Review," 1997, p 13; Statkiewicz-Sherer et al., "Radiation Quantities and Units," pp 50–51.

29. **(D)** Linear energy transfer (LET) designates the amount of energy that is deposited by radiation in tissue. LET is measured in units of kiloelectron-volts per micrometer (keV/μm). Radiation that has a high LET tends to deposit all of its energy at once. This radiation is therefore not very penetrating but is highly ionizing. Types of radiation that are considered to have a high LET values are (1) alpha particles, which may deposit as much as 100 keV/μm; (2) slow neutrons, which may deposit 20 keV/μm; and (3) beta particles, which deposit approximately 12 keV/μm. Comparatively, x- and gamma radiation have very low LET values and are highly penetrating. They have an average LET of approximately 3 keV/μm. Alpha particles deposit all of their energy at once and have a half-value layer of 0.1 mm of human tissue. Beta particles are slightly more penetrating in tissue with a half-value layer (HVL) of about 1 to 2 cm of human tissue. X- and gamma

radiation, on the other hand, have an HVL of 10 cm of tissue.

Bushong, "Fundamental Principles of Radiobiology," 1997, p 442; Dowd and Tilson, "Interactions of X-rays with Matter," pp 76–78; Thompson et al., "General Radiation Biology," pp 420–421; Travis, "Basic Biologic Interactions of Radiation," p 31.

30. **(A)** One of the biggest problems with using AEC devices is correctly positioning the anatomy of interest. If the desired anatomy is not placed correctly over the photocell, the radiograph will appear either too dark or too light, resulting in a repeated examination and excessive dose to the patient. On an average-size (sthenic) patient, using a positive density setting will most likely result in an overexposed radiograph and unnecessary exposure to the patient. Using low kilovolts (peak) will result in the AEC producing higher milliamperage-seconds and unnecessary overexposure to the patient. When selecting technical factors on an AEC, it is important to use a balance between milliamperes and time that will not potentially overexpose the patient. If an adequate exposure required only 40 mAs for a sthenic patient, selecting the 200-mA setting with a 1-second backup time would be wiser. This combination would eliminate the possibility of grossly overexposing the patient in the event of a malfunction. Some authorities recommend using only 1.5 times the expected milliamperage-seconds when combining the milliampere setting and the backup time.

Dowd and Tilson, "Protecting the Patient in Radiography," pp 221–222; Thompson et al., "Equipment & Accessory Malfunctions or Misapplications," pp 388–389.

SECTION II: EQUIPMENT OPERATION AND MAINTENANCE

31. **(A)** The tube rating chart is used to determine safe exposure factors of milliamperes, time, kilovolts (peak), and FSS that may be used for a single exposure without damaging the tube. The H & D curve is used to plot radiographic exposure versus radiographic density on a radiographic film. The anode cooling chart is used to determine how many exposures may be made without exceeding the heat capacity of the anode. The heat capacity may be assessed with the heat unit formula, which is as follows: Milliamperes × Time × Kilovolts (peak) × Constant for generator type. A technique chart is used for determining correct exposure factors for various radiographic procedures.

Bushong, "The X-Ray Tube," 1997, p 121; Carlton and McKenna-Adler, "Vascular Imaging Equipment," pp 598–599.

32. **(B)** On the electromagnetic spectrum, radio waves are located at the low-energy end of the continuum. These are followed by microwaves, infrared, visible light, x and gamma rays, and cosmic rays, which are at the opposite (high-energy) end of the spectrum. Because all electromagnetic energies travel at the speed of light, the properties that differentiate them are energy, frequency, and wavelength. Frequency and wavelength are inversely proportional: as the frequency of the wave increases, the wavelength decreases. Energy and wavelength are also inversely proportional: as the energy of the wave increases, the wavelength decreases. Cosmic rays have the greatest energy and the shortest wavelength.

Carlton and McKenna-Adler, "Radiation Concepts," pp 32–33.

33. **(C)** A motor is an electrical device that converts electrical energy into mechanical energy (motion). In an induction motor, the rotating armature is an iron bar (rotor) that attempts to align itself with the induced magnetic field of the series of wire loops (stator). The electromagnets (stators) surrounding the rotor are energized in sequence when the radiographer depresses the "prep" button on the control panel. The induced current flow produced in the rotor windings generates a magnetic field. This field attempts to align itself with the magnetic field of the stator. Because these electromagnets are being energized in sequence, the rotor begins to rotate, trying to bring its magnetic north pole in alignment with the stator's south pole. In an AC circuit, the result is that the rotor can never fully catch up with the alternating magnetic field of the stator and therefore continuously rotates. The rotation of the anode should operate at a speed of at least 3000 rotations per minute (rpm) prior to the exposure. On most modern x-ray units, the preparatory stage has a minimum delay time before the x-ray exposure occurs to prevent damage to the anode.

Bushong, "Electromagnetism," 1997, pp 81–82; Carlton and McKenna-Adler, "Electromagnetism," pp 71–73; Selman, "Electric Generators and Motors," pp 118–119.

34. **(C)** A capacitor discharge generator was the most common type of generator available in older mobile units. Most mobile x-ray machines now operate with battery-powered 3-phase equipment or high-frequency generators that are much more efficient. Because the capacitor dis-

charge units are much less efficient than these modern types, it is advisable to use higher-speed screens to overcome the limited output of this type of generator. Using high-speed screens requires a lower exposure because of the efficiency of the screen. The phosphors are larger with higher-speed screens, resulting in poorer resolution compared with slower-speed screens. Screen lag is usually not a problem for any modern intensifying screens regardless of the speed.

Bushong, "The X-Ray Unit," 1997, pp 103–104, and "Intensifying Screens," p 194; Carlton and McKenna-Adler, "Mobile Radiography," pp 529–530, and "Intensifying Screens," p 333; Curry et al., "X-Ray Generators," pp 51–52.

35. **(B)** Image-intensified fluoroscopy provides real-time viewing of an image, such as imaging of a patient swallowing barium during an upper gastrointestinal tract (UGI) examination and demonstrating peristalsis during a small-bowel follow-through examination. Real-time viewing is otherwise known as "dynamic imaging." The dose to a patient during fluoroscopy greatly exceeds that of routine radiography. Typical doses during fluoroscopy range from 2 rad/min (2000 mR) to as high as 10 rad/min (10,000 mR). Compare this to doses during routine radiography, which may range from as low as 10 mR for a PA projection of the chest to approximately 800 mR for a lateral projection of the lumbar vertebrae on a sthenic patient. Resolution in a fluoroscopic imaging system is much more difficult to maintain than in static radiography because there are so many complex variables (i.e., image enhancement by the image intensifier, video camera tube, and eventually the cathode-ray tube [CRT]). The milliampere settings for fluoroscopy are much lower (0.5 to 5 milliamperes) than for conventional radiography (50 to 1200 mA).

Bushong, "Fluoroscopy," 1997, and "Radiation Protection Procedures," pp 526–529; Carlton and McKenna-Adler, "Fluoroscopy," p 536.

36. **(A)** Both voltmeters and ohmmeters are wired in parallel in the circuit. Voltmeters read potential difference when the circuit is closed. Ohmmeters read resistance when the circuit is open. Ammeters are wired in series in the circuit. In an x-ray circuit, the prereading voltmeter, or kilovolt-meter, is wired between the autotransformer and the primary side of the step-up transformer, and the milliampere meter is wired before the rectification system and the x-ray tube. A penetrometer is also known as a "step wedge" and is not used in an electrical circuit.

Carlton and McKenna-Adler, "Electromagnetism," p 73; Selman, "Electrodynamics," p 75; Thompson et

al., "Electricity," pp 96–97; Tortorici, "Measuring Volts, Amperes and Ohms," 1992, pp 30–34.

37. **(C)** The focal spot in most modern x-ray tubes is determined by selecting the size of the filament that is the source of "boiled-off" electrons. The actual focal spot is that part of the anode target that is actually struck by this supply of electrons from the filament. The larger the filament, the larger the cloud of electrons that is sent to the target during the exposure and the larger the actual focal spot. The apparent, or effective, focal spot is created by using what is known as the line focus principle. The steeper the anode bevel of the target, the smaller the effective or projected focal spot (even though the actual focal spot remains the same). The heel of the anode is the most inferior portion of the anode and is not in the target area where electrons from the filament strike. The *anode heel effect* is a phenomenon in which x rays that are produced at the target are absorbed by the heel of the anode. This effect is more prominent with larger filaments and steeper anode bevels.

Bushong, "The X-Ray Tube," 1997, pp 116–117; Thompson et al., "X-Ray Tube Components and Design," p 148.

38. **(A)** Failure to properly warm-up the anode of an x-ray tube by using low milliamperes, high kilovolts (peak), and 1- to 2-second exposures may result in cracking of the anode due to the sudden change in temperature. The rectification system is located outside of the x-ray tube and is therefore unaffected by the heat produced within the x-ray tube housing. The x-ray tube housing can withstand much more heat than the anode target and is usually not overloaded by a single exposure. It may overheat from multiple exposures such as those used in angiography and special procedures. X-ray tube rating charts should be posted in every diagnostic x-ray room to alert the radiographer to safe technical factors that may be used for a single exposure. Any damage done to a x-ray tube anode due to heat will usually result in a decrease in exposure, not an increase.

Carlton and McKenna-Adler, "The X-Ray Tube," p 117; Selman, "X-Ray Tubes and Rectifiers," pp 216–222.

39. **(B)** The midpoint of the secondary coil of the high-tension (step-up) transformer is grounded. These cables are designed to eliminate the danger of shock, provided the insulation remains intact. Very heavy insulation is required to prevent the high voltage from sparking over to the patient or other objects near the cable. The grounded wo-

ven wire sheath surrounding the cable prevents the danger of shock.

Selman, "X-Ray Circuits," p 248.

40. **(C)** Reproducibility and linearity are quality assurance assessments that are used to check the accuracy of the kilovolt (peak), milliampere, and time stations on a particular x-ray unit. Reproducibility is the ability of the machine to reproduce multiple exposures when using identical factors of kilovolt (peak), time, and milliampere. Reproducibility must be accurate to within 5 percent. Linearity is based on the "reciprocity law" whereby the milliamperage-seconds should equal the milliamperage-seconds for multiple exposures regardless of which milliampere and time stations are used. Multiple exposures of milliamperage-seconds equals milliamperage-seconds should not vary by more than 10 percent. FSS has an effect on the resolution of the image but does not affect beam "quality." Beam quality is a measure of the average energy of the beam. The higher the average energy is, the higher the quality. Beam quality is measured by the HVL and may be affected by the factors of kilovolt (peak) and filtration.

Carroll, "Quality Control," 1998, pp 390–391; Papp, "Radiographic Ancillary Equipment," pp 97–98.

41. **(D)** During fluoroscopic imaging, exit radiation leaves the patient and strikes the image intensifier at the input phosphor. The input phosphor converts x rays into light. The light photons given off by the input phosphor then strike the photocathode, which converts this light into electrons (the electronic image). The electron stream is focused toward the output phosphor by the electrostatic lenses. Finally, the electronic image is converted back into a light image by the output phosphor. This light image can then be directly observed or, as in most modern systems, may be transmitted through a complex television (TV) system where the image appears on a monitor (CRT).

Bushong, "Fluoroscopy," 1997, pp 324–325; Carlton and McKenna-Adler, "Fluoroscopy," pp 536–538; Thompson et al., "Fluoroscopy: Viewing Motion with X-Ray," pp 364–365.

42. **(C)** At the anode target of the x-ray tube, two types of radiation are produced. Characteristic radiation only occurs above 69 keV in a tungsten atom and occurs when an incident electron strikes an electron in an inner shell of a target atom, causing ionization. *Bremsstrahlung* radiation is more common and is produced when an incident electron decelerates or changes direction as it passes by the nuclear force field of a target

atom. Annihilation radiation and Compton scatter only occur when x rays strike matter, not when electrons strike matter.

Bushong, "X-Ray Production," 1997, p 132; Carlton and McKenna-Adler, "X-Ray Production," pp 134–138.

43. **(D)** A common cause of tube failure is bad bearings caused by long use at high temperatures. Although the rotating stem of the anode, which is made of molybdenum, is made to withstand a minimum amount of heat, the ball bearings eventually become imperfectly round. These irregular bearings lead to a grinding noise and wobbling of the rotor.

Bushong, "The X-Ray Tube," 1997, p 120; Carlton and McKenna-Adler, "The X-Ray Tube," p, 123.

44. **(C)** The image intensifier serves to increase the brightness of a fluoroscopic image. The TV camera tubes, such as the vidicon and the plumbicon, function to send this image to the CRT or TV monitor and are usually coupled to the output phosphor of the image intensifier via fiber optics. The TV camera tube converts the light image into an electric signal that is then sent to the TV monitor and changed back into a light image.

Bushong, "Fluoroscopy," 1997, p 327; Carlton and McKenna-Adler, "Fluoroscopy," p 543; Thompson et al., "Fluoroscopy," p 370.

45. **(B)** To calculate heat units for a 3-phase, 12-pulse generator, the formula is mA × Time × kVp × 1.41. Thus, 400 × 0.30 × 75 × 1.41 = 12,690 HU. If the maximum heat capacity of the tube is 500,000 HU, then 500,000/12,690 = 39.41. It would be possible to produce 39 rapid exposures at a technique of 400 mA, 300 milliseconds, and 75 kVp for this machine.

Bushong, "The X-Ray Tube," 1997, pp 122–123; Carlton and McKenna-Adler, "The X-Ray Tube," pp 126–127; Curry et al., "The X-Ray Tube.

For answers 46 and 47, refer to Figure 2–3:

46. **(B)** The illustrated wave is an example of a single-phase AC because it alternates between positive and negative ends of the cycle. Most power lines operate on AC, which is ideal for the operation of the transformers in a x-ray circuit. Transformers cannot operate on DC, and x-ray tubes cannot operate on AC. A rectification system, which changes AC to DC, is placed between the high-tension transformer and the x-ray tube. A half-wave rectified circuit supplies 60 impulses per second because it uses only the positive end of the cycle. A full-wave rectified circuit is twice as efficient because it uses both ends of the cycle and produces 120 impulses per second.

Bushong, "The X-Ray Unit," 1997, pp 100–102; Selman, "Electric Generators & Motors," p 109; Thompson et al., "X-Ray Machine Operation," p 170.

47. **(C)** In most hospitals, the incoming power supplied is 220 V at a frequency of 60 Hz (which means 60 cycles per second). One full cycle can be measured from peak to peak, or from zero to positive peak back to zero to negative peak and back to zero again. Because there are 60 of these cycles per second, one cycle (designated by the starting point of letter C and ending point of letter E) would take exactly $\frac{1}{60}$ of a second.

Bushong, "The X-Ray Unit," 1997, pp 100–102; Selman, "Electric Generators & Motors," p 109; Thompson et al., "X-Ray Machine Operation," p 170.

48. **(B)** The atomic number of an atom is determined by the number of protons in its nucleus. The mass number is determined by the sum of the protons and neutrons in the nucleus of an atom. Isotopes of an element are usually represented by their atomic mass number because the number of neutrons determines the stability of the element. For instance, there are several isotopes of barium (^{127}Ba, ^{128}Ba, ^{129}Ba, ^{130}Ba, etc.). All of the isotopes of barium have the same atomic number of 56 because they all have 56 protons in their nucleus. To determine the number of neutrons in an isotope of barium with a mass number of 138, simply subtract 56 from 138. There are 82 neutrons in the isotope of ^{138}Ba.

Bushong, "The Atom," 1997, p 37; Carlton and McKenna-Adler, "Radiation Concepts," pp 25–29; Selman, "The Structure of Matter," p 44.

49. **(B)** A quality assurance test for reproducibility is one of the many tests that should be performed on radiographic equipment. Reproducibility ensures that the technical factors selected by the radiographer at the control panel are those that are actually produced by the x-ray tube. Reproducibility should be checked by making repeated exposures of the same technique and observing that the average variation in radiation intensity does not exceed 5 percent. Reciprocity, or linearity, is a similar term that means as milliampere and time stations are changed to produce the same total milliamperage-seconds, the radiation intensity should not vary by more than 10 percent. It is important to distinguish between the two.

Bushong, "Designing for Radiation Protection," 1997, pp 511, 520; Carlton and McKenna-Adler, "Quality Control," p 446; Carroll, "Quality Control," 1998, p 391; Gray et al., "X-Ray Generators," p 119.

50. **(B)** The light field and x-ray field should be accurate to within 2 percent of the source SID. At a SID of 180 cm (72 in.), this would be as follows:

$180 \times 0.02 = 3.6$ cm on each side

Bushong, "Designing for Radiation Protection," 1997, pp 511, 520; Carlton and McKenna-Adler, "Quality Control," p 445; Carroll, "Quality Control," 1998, p 396; Gray et al., "X-Ray Tubes and Collimators," p 88.

51. **(C)** A freshly loaded cassette may exhibit poor contact because of entrapped air. It is recommended that the quality control technologist wait a minimum of 10 to 15 minutes after cassette loading before making screen contact tests.

Gray et al., "Basic Tests," p 56.

52. **(C)** In 3-phase equipment, there are no gaps of x-ray production during the exposure, as are seen in single-phase equipment. Single-phase circuits are pulsating and have a voltage ripple of 100 percent. For every impulse, a dot or dash will appear on the radiograph of a manual spin top. For half-wave rectified machines, the electric current will fluctuate 60 times per second. For full-wave rectified machines, the electric current fluctuates 120 times per second. For 3-phase equipment, the x-ray production is relatively constant and the exposed portion of the radiograph of a spin top will appear as a steady line or arc. When testing the equipment with a synchronous spinning top, which rotates at a speed of 1 revolution per second, the quality assurance technologist should calculate the estimated time for 3-phase equipment by measuring this arc with a protractor. By dividing the degrees of the arc degrees by the constant of 360°, or multiplying 360° by the time, the exposure time is found:

$$\frac{x}{360°} = 50 \text{ ms}; 360° \times 50 \text{ ms} = x; x = 18°$$

Carroll, "Quality Control," 1998, pp 388–390; Gray et al., "X-Ray Generators," pp 107–111; Thompson et al., "Quality Control," pp 406–407.

53. **(D)** Beam-restricting devices have two main purposes: (1) to reduce unnecessary exposure to the patient and (2) to improve image contrast. These devices include aperture diaphragms, cones, cylinders, and variable-aperture collimators. All serve to shape and limit the beam to only the area of interest.

Bushong, "Scatter Radiation and Beam-Restricting Devices," 1997, p 209; Carlton and McKenna-Adler, "Beam Restriction," p 239; Carroll, "Field Size Limitation," 1998, p 136.

54. **(A)** In a 3-phase x-ray machine, the circuitry is complicated. Instead of having one autotransformer and one high-tension transformer, there are three of each. On the primary side of the high-tension transformer, three transformers are

found that form a delta shape. On the secondary side, there are usually two sets of transformers, either two delta transformers or one delta, and one star transformer. The star formation is also called a "wye" formation because it is shaped like the letter "Y."

Carlton and McKenna-Adler, "X-Ray Equipment," p 96; Curry et al., "X-Ray Generators," pp 50–51; Selman, " X-Ray Circuits," pp 255–256; Tortorici, "Rectification," 1992, pp 48–49; Wolbarst, "The Nuts and Bolts of Generators," p 81.

55. **(D)** The consistency of the x-ray beam energy can be tested by measuring the HVL. The HVL of the x-ray beam may be used as a reference for kilovolt (peak) calibration or tube aging. Tube aging produces hardening of the beam, which results from deposits of tungsten on the inside of the glass housing.

Carlton and McKenna-Adler, "Quality Control," p 445, and "The X-Ray Tube," p 113; Thompson et al., "Quality Control," p 405.

56. **(C)** The current through the filament must be sufficiently high to cause thermionic emission, or the boiling off of electrons. This current is usually in excess of 4 A but may range from 3 to 5 A. This current heats the filament and does not represent the current across the x-ray tube. The filament circuit is supplied by a step-down transformer and has a higher current than the tube current. The filament current heats the filament and is measured in amperes. The tube current is the flow of electrons across the x-ray tube and is measured in milliamperes.

Bushong, "The X-Ray Tube," 1997, p 110; Curry et al., "X-Ray Generators," p 40; Selman, "X-Ray Circuits," p 245.

57. **(D)** If the x-ray unit is supplied with PBL, there may be several different reasons for a failure to initiate an exposure. In most instances, the interlocks do not allow the preparatory stage to engage. This interference may be the result of the Bucky tray not being pushed in all the way, the tube crane not being locked into the correct position (either horizontally or vertically), or the AEC devices for both the table and the upright Bucky having been depressed.

Thompson et al., "Equipment and Accessory Malfunctions or Misapplications," p 380.

58. **(B)** Some types of image intensifiers have the capability to magnify the image. The technique of magnification in an image intensifier varies from a static radiograph because changing the electrostatic focal point within the tube may change the image size. The magnified image may appear to have more distortion than in the minified image.

Size distortion, or magnification, may have an effect on the overall brightness of the entire image, not just at the periphery. Shape distortion may occur in intensified fluoroscopy because of the shape of the image intensification tube. Even though the input screen is concave, it does not totally eliminate edge distortion at the output screen. Electrons at the outer edges tend to flare out, causing a loss in image brightness at the periphery. This is known as vignetting or the "pincushion" effect. Both minification gain and flux gain cause an increase in brightness.

Bushong, "Fluoroscopy," 1997, p 326; Carlton and McKenna-Adler, "Fluoroscopy," p 541.

59. **(A)** Patient dose during cinefluorography is significant. The dose may be as high as 7.2 R/min. Spot film recorders vary in dose but may average 30 mR per exposure for a cassette-loaded spot film, or 10 mR per exposure for a photospot camera (70 or 105 mm). Videotape recorders record the image directly off the TV monitor. Their advantages include the following: (1) they are easy to use, (2) they do not require film processing, and (3) they can provide instant playback. More important, they do not provide additional dosage to the patient.

Bushong, "Fluoroscopy," 1997, p 331; Carlton and McKenna-Adler, "Fluoroscopy," p 548; Thompson et al., "Fluoroscopy," p 373.

60. **(D)** According to Ohm's law, voltage is equal to amperage times the resistance (V = IR). The current in this circuit measured 6 A and the resistance 4 ohms. Therefore:

$$6 \times 4 = x \text{ volts}; 6 \times 4 = 24 \text{ V}$$

Bushong, "Electricity," 1997, p 63; Carlton and McKenna-Adler, "Electricity," p 50; Selman, "Electrodynamics," p 71.

SECTION III: IMAGE PRODUCTION AND EVALUATION

61. **(A)** Magnification is also called size distortion. The four factors that affect size distortion are: (1) SID, which is inversely proportional to magnification (as SID increases, size distortion, or magnification, decreases); (2) OID, which is directly proportional to magnification (as the OID increases, the size distortion increases); (3) SOD, which is also inversely proportional to magnification (as the source-object receptor-distance [SOD] increases, the size distortion decreases); and (4) the thickness of the patient. The placement of the object and x-ray tube at various an-

gles to the image receptor has an effect on shape distortion, not size distortion.

Carlton and McKenna-Adler, "Distortion," p 429; Carroll, "Distance Ratios," 1998, pp 271–275.

62. **(D)** The reciprocity law states that when setting the same milliamperage-seconds at varying time and milliampere station, the radiation intensity should not vary by more than 10 percent for multiple exposures. This is also known as linearity and is represented by the following equation: mAs = mAs. The inverse-square law is used to determine what the radiation intensity would be at various distances from the source. It is set as an inverse proportion as follows:

$$\frac{I_1}{I_2} = \frac{(D_2)^2}{(D_1)^2}$$

Coulomb's law is simply a measure of the magnitude of an electrostatic force and does not have application to this question. The direct-square law is similar to the inverse-square law except that it is set up as a direct proportion. As distance increases, intensity decreases with the square of the distance (as stated in the inverse-square law), the milliamperage-seconds needs to be increased to compensate. This is accomplished by using the following formula:

$$\frac{mAs_1}{mAs_2} = \frac{(D_1)^2}{(D_2)^2}$$

Bushong, "Electricity," 1997, p 60; Carlton and McKenna-Adler, "Exposure Conversion Problems," p 514; Carroll, "Source-Image Receptor Distance," 1998, p 257; Ireland, "Direct, Inverse, and Inverse-Square Proportions," pp 39–71.

63. **(A)** When performing an IVP on the same patient and it is necessary to alternate from a 3-phase machine to a single-phase machine, the radiographer should increase the milliamperage-seconds by a factor of 2.

Carlton and McKenna-Adler, "Exposure Conversion Problems," p 514; Carroll, "Machine Phase and Rectification," 1998, pp 124–125.

64. **(B)** To determine image blur, use the formula to calculate geometric unsharpness (GU). GU increases with increasing OID, decreasing SOD, and increasing FSS. It can be written mathematically as follows:

$$GU = FSS \times \frac{OID}{SOD}$$

A. 20/140 X 0.3 = 0.04 mm
B. 15/85 X 2 = 0.35 mm
C. 25/75 X 1 = 0.33 mm
D. 25/75 X 0.6 = 0.19 mm

In the ideal situation, the smallest FSS, the shortest OID, and the longest SOD would result in the least image blur or best recorded detail.

Carlton and McKenna-Adler, "Recorded Detail," p 407; Cullinan, "Technical Formulas and Related Data," p 297.

65. **(C)** As a rule of thumb, when changing from tabletop nongrid techniques to the Bucky grid, it is necessary to increase the milliamperage-seconds by a factor of 3. It should not be necessary to adjust the kilovolts (peak).

Carroll, "Grids," 1998, p 187.

66. **(D)** The 15 percent rule states that an increase in kilovolts (peak) of 15 percent will result in a doubling of radiographic density (a similar effect as doubling the milliamperage-seconds). The opposite is also true. A reduction in kilovolts (peak) of 15 percent will result in a 50 percent reduction in radiographic density.

Carlton and McKenna-Adler, "The Prime Factors," p 184; Carroll, "Kilovoltage Peak," 1998, pp 107–110; Wallace, "mAs and kVp Relationship," p 93.

67. **(C)** The reducing agents in an automatic processor are hydroquinone and phenidone. They are found in the developer tank and serve to reduce the exposed silver halide crystals in the x-ray film emulsion to black metallic silver. Sodium sulfite is the preservative in both the fixer and developer tanks. Ammonium thiosulfate is found in the fixer and serves to remove the unexposed silver crystals from the film.

Carlton and McKenna-Adler, "Radiographic Processing," p 297; Cullinan, "Automatic Processing," p 109; Wallace, "Radiographic Film and Development," pp 144–145.

68. **(B)** The average energy of the x-ray beam is controlled by the kilovolts (peak) but is also affected by changes in filtration. As kilovolts (peak), or energy, increases, the scale of contrast gets longer and the noise increases because of increased scatter fog. Kilovolts (peak) affects the visibility functions of the image, as does milliamperage-seconds. Recorded detail is unaffected by changes in energy.

Carroll, "Kilovoltage Peak," 1998, pp 89–90, and "Beam Filtration," p 130; Wallace, "Radiographic Contrast," pp 81–85.

69. **(A)** Use of rare earth screens compared with conventional calcium tungstate screens will result in a reduction in exposure factors. The superior conversion efficiency of the rare earth materials makes them much "faster" than conventional screens. Rare earth screens do not require as many milliamperage-seconds; there-

fore, shorter exposure times and lower-milliampere stations may be used. Using rare earth screens reduces stress on the x-ray tube as well as exposure to the patient. Unfortunately, this increased speed does come at a price. Rare earth screens are more expensive than conventional screens, and in some cases, resolution may be decreased with rare earth screens because of quantum mottle.

Bushong, "Intensifying Screens," 1997, pp 198– 199; Carlton and McKenna-Adler, "Intensifying Screens," pp 332–333; Wallace, "Intensifying Screens," pp 164–165.

70. **(D)** The temperature of the developer is essential to film quality. A typical developer temperature will usually be between 93°F and 98°F. A visible difference may be noticed by a fluctuation of only +0.5°F in that the radiograph will be overdeveloped, have excessive density, and have reduced contrast due to chemical fog.

Bushong, "Processing the Latent Image," 1997, p 181; Carlton and McKenna-Adler, "Radiographic Processing," p 306; Wallace, "Radiographic Film and Development," p 144.

71. **(D)** Absorption of x rays is dependent on the photoelectric effect, which occurs more often with low-energy photons and tissues of high atomic number. The tissue with the greatest absorption coefficient due to the photoelectric effect is dental enamel, because of the relatively high atomic number of calcium, followed by bone, muscle, dense organs, fat, and air. Fat has the lowest effective atomic number of human tissue and will absorb the least amount of x rays.

Bushong, "X-Ray Interaction with Matter," 1997, p 154; Carroll, "Patient Status and Contrast Agents," 1998, pp 149–150.

72. **(A)** Using an extension cylinder is essentially using two apertures: one close to the source and one closer to the patient. The SID has not changed. The result of this dual collimation is a reduction in off-focus radiation and a smaller field size. Because the field size has decreased, less of the patient is exposed, resulting in a decrease in patient dose if identical technical factors have been set. This reduction in field size and off-focus radiation results in a lower radiographic density with an increase in radiographic contrast. Although the cylinder does not directly absorb scatter radiation (scatter is only produced in the patient), it does effectively expose a smaller area of tissue, which ultimately will decrease the number of scattered x rays produced in the patient.

Bushong, "Scatter Radiation and Beam-Restricting Devices," 1997, p 211; Carlton and McKenna-Adler,

"Beam Restriction," pp 240–241; Carroll, "Field Size Limitation," 1998, pp 132–138.

73. **(D)** Destructive pathology usually leads to an increase in air or fat or a decrease in normal body fluid or bone. Both air and fat are significantly less dense than fluid and absorb fewer x-ray photons. The milliamperage-seconds may need to be reduced by 30 percent to 50 percent for most destructive diseases (i.e., bowel obstruction, emphysema, osteomalacia, osteoporosis). A rule of thumb is that a destructive disease requires a 30 percent decrease in milliamperage-seconds or a 5 percent reduction in kilovolts (peak).

Carlton and McKenna-Adler, "The Pathology Problem," pp 259–260; Carroll, "Pathology & Casts," 1998, pp 166–167.

74. **(A)** A properly functioning grid should absorb very little primary radiation. An artifact will appear in the image, called "grid cutoff," if too much primary radiation is absorbed. High-ratio grids are more effective in absorbing secondary radiation; however, their major disadvantage is the lack of centering latitude. Centering must be precise with high ratio-grids to reduce the chance of grid cutoff. High-ratio grids most often used are those in which the central ray is at a fixed centering point, as in a dedicated chest unit.

Bushong, "The Grid," 1997, p 216; Carlton and McKenna-Adler, "The Grid," p 268; Carroll, "Grids," 1998, pp 189–190; Wallace, "Grids and the Bucky," p 112.

75. **(B)** The only factors in this problem that affect contrast are kilovolts (peak) and grid ratio. The lower the kilovolts (peak) and the higher the grid ratio, the higher the contrast. A kilovolt (peak) of 85 and a grid ratio of 12:1 provide the highest contrast of all of these in this question.

Bushong, "The Grid," 1997, pp 215–216; Carlton and McKenna-Adler, "The Grid," p 268, and "Contrast," p 390; Carroll, "Grids," 1998, pp 179–180.

76. **(D)** The best way to improve recorded detail or resolution in an image is to use a small FSS. The use of detail or slow-speed screens is another way to improve recorded detail. Most rare earth screens are considerably faster than conventional calcium tungstate screens. The resolution of screens can be increased by using smaller crystals and a smaller active layer.

Carroll, "Focal Spot Size," 1998, p 233, and "Intensifying Screens," pp 214–216; Wallace, "Intensifying Screens," p 162, and "Geometric Factors Affecting Recorded Detail," p 134.

77. **(A)** The radiograph on the right was exposed using 92 kVp and 6.25 mAs. The radiograph on the

left was exposed using 80 kVp and 12.5 mAs. The density and recorded detail on both films are sufficient. However, the film on the right has poor radiographic contrast because of excessively high kilovolts (peak). This ultimately affects visibility of detail but not recorded detail. The optimum kilovolts (peak) that should be used in the abdomen is 70 because of the soft-tissue structures, which contribute to Compton scattering. If technical factors need to be increased, the milliamperage-seconds should be the factor of choice to keep this scatter to a minimum.

Wallace, "mAs and kVp Relationship,"p 96.

78. **(D)** Using the direct-square law, this problem may be set up two different ways as long as the components of new and old are directly proportional:

1. $$\frac{\text{Old mAs}}{\text{New mAs}} = \frac{\text{Old Distance}^2}{\text{New Distance}^2}$$

Because the new milliamperage-seconds is the unknown, set up this problem as follows:

2. $$\frac{\text{New mAs}}{\text{Old mAs}} = \frac{\text{New Distance}^2}{\text{Old Distance}^2}$$

$$\text{New mAs} = \frac{\text{Old mAs} \times \text{New Distance}^2}{\text{Old Distance}^2}$$

$$x = \frac{32 \times (60)^2}{(40)^2}$$

$$x = \frac{32 \times 3600}{1600}$$

$$x = \frac{115{,}200}{1600}$$

$$x = 72 \text{ mAs}$$

Carlton and McKenna-Adler, "Exposure Conversion Problems," p 514; Carroll, "Source-Image Receptor Distance," 1998, p 257; Cullinan, "Technical Formulas and Related Data," p 294; Ireland, "Direct, Inverse, and Inverse-Square Proportions," p 41.

79. **(C)** Image resolution may be measured by the unit line-pairs per millimeter using a special quality assurance test tool. The smaller the line resolution, the more lines that would fit into 1 mm. This measurement is also called *spatial frequency*. *Spatial resolution* is defined as the number of details that fit into a given space of 1 mm and are still visibly distinct. Tesla is a measure of magnetism, hertz is a measure of frequency, and penumbra is image blur at the edge of a radiographic image.

Bushong, "Intensifying Screens," 1997, pp 194–195; Carlton and McKenna-Adler, "Film/Screen Combinations," p 346; Carroll, "Analyzing the Radiographic Image," 1998, p 307.

80. **(D)** Superimposition occurs when structures lie directly on top of one another. Sometimes it is necessary to angle the x-ray tube or the anatomic part to overcome superimposition. With angulation techniques, structures may become either elongated or foreshortened but are visible because the overlying structure has moved in position. For example, during radiography of the colon, it is necessary to angle the x-ray tube and sometimes rotate the patient to properly demonstrate the rectosigmoid colon.

Bontrager, "Positioning Principles," p 50; Carroll, "Beam-Part-Film Alignment," 1998, pp 277; Wallace, "Shape Distortion," pp 42–44.

81. **(B)** There are four major factors that affect shape distortion: (1) the shape and thickness of the object being radiographed, (2) the centering of the central ray with respect to the object, (3) the angle formed between the central ray and the long axis of the object, and (4) the angle formed between the long axis of the object and the film. SID and OID affect size distortion, not shape distortion. The technical factors of milliamperage-seconds, kilovolts (peak), and FSS have no effect on distortion.

Carlton and McKenna-Adler, "Distortion," pp 421–429; Carroll, "Beam-Part-Film Alignment," 1998, pp 277–279.

82. **(B)** Bowel obstruction is considered a destructive pathology because it causes an increase in air or gas and a decrease in fluid, making the anatomic part easier to penetrate. Destructive diseases usually require a decrease in exposure of either 30 percent milliamperage-seconds or 5 percent kilovolts (peak). For bowel obstruction, a decrease in kilovolts (peak) of approximately 8 percent is recommended. Additive pathologies, on the other hand, increase fluid or tissue density in a body part. Examples include ascites, acromegaly, pulmonary edema, and Paget's disease.

Carlton and McKenna-Adler, "The Pathology Problem," pp 259–260; Carroll, "Pathology and Casts," 1998, pp 166–167.

83. **(A)** Steps to solve this problem are as follows:
    1. Solve for milliamperage-seconds. Rate them from 1 to 3, 3 being the greatest density (highest mAs). 2. Rate kilovolts from 1 to 4, giving the highest kilovolts a 4. 3. Rate the screen speed, the slowest being assigned a 1 and the fastest a 3. 4. Rate the grid ratio. The highest grid ratio would create the least film density, so give the 12:1 grid a 1, both 8:1 grids a 2, and the 6:1 grid a 3. 5. Rate the SIDs with the farthest distance a 1 and the closest distance a 3. The

lowest total would yield the least radiographic density as demonstrated below in the example:

	mAs	kV	Screen Speed	Grid Ratio	SID	Total
A.	40^1	70^2	200^1	$12{:}1^1$	$150\ cm^2$	$= 7$
B.	80^3	75^3	400^2	$6{:}1^3$	$200\ cm^1$	$= 12$
C.	60^2	80^4	800^3	$8{:}1^2$	$100\ cm^3$	$= 14$
D.	80^3	65^1	200^1	$8{:}1^2$	$200\ cm^1$	$= 8$

84. **(D)** All radiographs should be permanently identified (embedded into the radiographic emulsion) with at least the four following IDs: 1) the patient's name or medical record number; (2) the date; (3) the side marker, right or left; and (4) institution name. Other ID markings may be required by the institution, such as (1) the radiographer's initials, (2) the exact time of the examination, (3) age or birthday of the patient; and/or (4) the name of the attending physician. For certain examinations, it may also be necessary to identify cumulative times following a contrast medium injection or to identify the position of the patient (upright or decubitus).

Ballinger, "Preliminary Steps in Radiography," Vol I, p 16; Bontrager, "Imaging Principles," p 30; Carroll, "Evaluating Radiographs: Identification, Assessment and Labeling," 1993, p 15.

85. **(C)** The anode heel effect is a variation in intensity across the x-ray field caused by attenuation of x rays in the heel of the anode. As a result, there is less radiation intensity on the anode side of the beam than on the cathode side. Radiographers should bear this in mind when they position long body parts, such as the femur or thoracic vertebrae, at short SIDs. The size of the projected focal spot is also not constant across the radiograph. A smaller focal spot size exists on the anode side of the beam than on the cathode side. This variation leads to focal spot blur. The focal spot blur is small on the anode side and large on the cathode side. Images on the cathode side of the beam exhibit more blur and less spatial resolution.

Bushong, "Radiographic Quality," 1997, p 244; Carlton and McKenna-Adler, "Density," p 375; Carroll, "The Anode Bevel," 1998, pp 241–246; Cullinan, "Basic Operation of an X-Ray Tube," p 34.

86. **(B)** The fixed kilovolts (peak) chart is the most commonly used technique chart in contemporary diagnostic imaging departments. The optimum kilovolts (peak) is set for each anatomic body part to be examined. The adjustment for various degrees of thickness is made with the selection of milliamperage-seconds. One major benefit of using this method is that, on average, there is a reduction in patient dose. It also produces consistent radiographic quality and greater exposure latitude for a variety of patients.

Bushong, "Radiographic Technique," 1997, p 272; Carroll, "Simplifying and Standardizing Technique," 1998, pp 318–319; Wallace, "Radiographic Technique Charts," p 208.

87. **(C)** If the objective is to improve radiographic contrast, there are many methods the radiographer could try. The most notable are the use of higher-ratio grids; air-gap technique (increase in OID); increased collimation, which results in a smaller field size; and decreased kilovoltage. An increase in SID would most likely decrease contrast if it affected it at all. FSS has no visible effect on radiographic contrast.

Carlton and McKenna-Adler, "Contrast," p 398; Cullinan, "Recorded Detail," pp 122–123; Carroll, "Field Size Limitation," 1998, pp 139–140.

88. **(D)** Most modern imaging departments now incorporate the use of computer-assisted technology in the selection of technical factors. AECs use an electronic timer device. Although the name suggests that these devices are completely automatic, it is still the radiographer's responsibility to select the proper kilovolts (peak), sensitivity cell, and density setting for the particular examination, patient, and pathology. Patient positioning is critical with the use of this type of device to ensure that the anatomic structure of interest is properly placed over the sensing chamber. When the radiographer possesses good positioning skills, the vast majority of AEC exposures will produce radiographs of diagnostic quality. Positioning skills are not nearly as critical for obtaining a properly exposed radiograph when using the other types of technique charts.

Bushong, "Radiographic Technique," 1997, p 273; Carlton and McKenna-Adler, "Automatic Exposure Controls," p 508.

89. **(D)** On most x-ray units that incorporate AECs, there are also density controls that can adjust the density, usually in increments of 25 percent or 30 percent. These controls should be used in unusual situations only, such as when the ion-chamber cells cannot be adapted to the necessary positioning (e.g., for a PA projection of the chest when an image is produced that is slightly too dark for the lung fields and a decrease in density is desired even though the patient is correctly positioned) or when the machine's calibration is slightly off and temporary adjustments with the density controls are necessary. Density controls should not be used to compensate for patient part thickness or kilovolt (peak) changes because the machine automatically compensates for this. It

also is not recommended that the controls be used to compensate for very small or narrow body parts, such as the extremities and other peripheral anatomy and the newborn chest. Manual timing should be used for these procedures instead. If the AEC device is functioning properly, there should only be a rare need for the use of the density control.

Bushong, "Radiographic Technique," 1997, p 274; Carlton and McKenna-Adler, "Automatic Exposure Controls," p 507; Carroll, "Automatic Exposure Controls," 1998, pp 354–358.

90. **(A)** High-kilovolt technique charts, usually exceeding a setting of 100 kilovolt (peaks), are limited to examinations such as barium contrast studies, chest radiography, and pelvimetry.

Bushong, "Radiographic Technique," 1997, p 272.

91. **(C)** It is suggested that actual kilovolt (peak) values should fall within ±2 kVp of the selected kilovolt (peak) setting. If they are not in this range, the equipment should be recalibrated. Some sources say that the kilovolts (peak) may fluctuate as much as ±5 kVp before calibration is necessary. In any case, kilovolt (peak) accuracy should be tested at least once a year using a Wisconsin kilovolt (peak) test cassette or Adran-Crookes cassette. Most modern equipment is tested using a computerized dosimeter because it is more accurate and less time consuming. A star test pattern and a resolution bar pattern are both used to test the FSS. A resolution bar pattern may also be used to test the resolution of an imaging system in line-pairs per millimeter. A sensitometer is used for film processor quality control and exposes the quality control test film with an optical step wedge.

Carlton and McKenna-Adler, "Quality Control," p 446; Carroll, "Quality Control," 1998, p 394; Tortorici, "Kilovoltage and Quality Control," 1992, pp 90–91.

92. **(B)** It is very important when using intensifying screens that the sensitivity of the film be matched to the light emitted by the screen. This is termed *spectral matching*. If blue light–sensitive film gets placed into a cassette with a green light–emitting screen, the result is a loss of density because the film is less sensitive to the light emitted by this screen.

Bushong, "Intensifying Screens," 1997, p 197; Cullinan, "X-Ray Film," p 93; Wallace, "Intensifying Screens," pp 164–165.

93. **(C)** There are three main contributors to the production of scatter radiation: (1) use of higher kilovolts (peak), which causes more scatter radiation to be directed forward toward the film; (2) the thickness of the body part; and (3) the amount of tissue exposed or field size. Of these three causes of scatter radiation, field size limitation should be the radiographer's primary method of preventing scatter radiation. There are also two means to control scatter after it has been produced: (1) grids that absorb scatter and (2) the air-gap technique, which allows scatter to be directed away from the film.

Carroll, "Evaluating Radiographs: Fog & Noise," 1993, pp 275–277; Wallace, "Control of Scattered Radiation," p 116.

94. **(D)** There are two basic forms of distortion: size and shape distortion. Size distortion, or magnification, is caused by a short SID or a long OID. Shape distortion includes foreshortening and elongation and may be caused by misalignment among x-ray beam, anatomic part, and the image receptor.

Carlton and McKenna-Adler, "Distortion," p 417; Carroll, "Evaluating Radiographs: Shape Distortion," 1993, p 303; Wallace, "Shape Distortion," p 38.

95. **(A)** If two linear grids are inadvertently positioned with their lead strips running in the same direction, a "Moiré" artifact may appear. This type of artifact is comparable to zebra-like stripes on the image. A treelike artifact is caused from static due to low humidity in the darkroom. Mottling is a grainy appearance and is usually seen on high-speed screens with insufficient milliamperage-seconds. Because grids are used to absorb secondary radiation (which causes fog), and grid cutoff is essentially excessive absorption of the secondary and primary beam, a fogging artifact would not appear as a result of misalignment of the grid.

Carroll, "Evaluating Radiographs: Processing & Film Handling Artifacts," 1993, pp 47–63; Cullinan, "Control of Scatter Radiation," pp 78, 81–82; Thompson et al., "Improving Image Quality," p 329.

96. **(D)** The only factors that affect recorded detail in this problem are: (1) SID, (2) the OID, and (3) FSS. You can find the greatest recorded detail by using the formula for penumbra for each of the following given factors: OID/SOD × FSS = Penumbra

OID	SID	FSS	OID/SOD × FSS	Total
A. 20 cm	100 cm	2.0 mm	20/80 × 2	0.50 mm
B. 30 cm	180 cm	1.0 mm	30/150 × 1	0.20 mm
C. 15 cm	170 cm	2.0 mm	15/155 × 2	0.197 mm
D. 25 cm	200 cm	0.5 mm	25/175 × 0.5	0.07 mm

The technical factors that result in the least geometric unsharpness would produce the best recorded detail.

Bushong, "Radiographic Quality," 1997, p 244; Carlton and McKenna-Adler, "Recorded Detail," pp

406–407; Wallace, "Geometric Factors Affecting Recorded Detail," p 137.

97. **(C)** The primary purpose of filtration in all radiographic equipment is to reduce patient dose. The addition of filtration serves to remove the lower-energy x rays that are considered undiagnostic because they do not have sufficient energy to penetrate the patient. Therefore, this radiation offers no diagnostic value and simply exposes the patient to unnecessary radiation. In effect, using a filter will raise the average energy of the x-ray beam, giving it a higher quality and more penetrating ability. However, filtration does not increase intensity because the filter is removing radiation, not adding to it. Filtration has no effect on resolution and also does not absorb scatter radiation. Scatter is produced primarily in the patient, not the x-ray tube. Because filtration raises the average energy of the beam, more scatter radiation may penetrate the patient and reach the image receptor, causing a reduction in contrast.

Bushong, "X-Ray Emission," 1997, pp 144–145; Carlton and McKenna-Adler, "Filtration," pp 171–176.

98. **(D)** Scatter radiation is produced in the patient's body when primary photons from the x-ray tube interact with matter in the patient. Secondary radiation, which includes scatter, is any radiation resulting from interactions within the patient. Other problems created in the x-ray tube that are sometimes mistakenly referred to as "scatter" are: (1) off-focus radiation and (2) leakage radiation.

Carroll, "Interactions of X-Rays within the Patient," 1998, pp 55–56; Wallace, "Methods to Control Scatter," p 116.

99. **(C)** Commercial films use relative speed numbers to classify film-screen combinations. The technical factor that needs to be adjusted from one screen speed to another is milliamperage-seconds. The conversion formula is as follows:

$$\frac{mAs_1}{mAs_2} = \frac{RS_2}{RS_1}$$

$$mAs_2 = \frac{mAs_1 \times RS_1}{RS_2}$$

$$mAs_2 = \frac{50 \times 200}{400}$$

$$mAs_2 = 25 \text{ mAs}$$

Carlton and McKenna-Adler, "Film/Screen Combinations," p 345; Wallace, "Intensifying Screens," pp 165–167.

100. **(B)** If the kilovolts (peak) is changed by 15 percent, to maintain density, the milliamperage-seconds must be changed by a factor of 2. If the kilovolts (peak) is increased by 15 percent, the milliamperage-seconds should be divided by 2. If the kilovolts (peak) is decreased by 15 percent, the milliamperage-seconds should be multiplied by 2.

Carlton and McKenna-Adler, "Density," p 372; Carroll, "Kilovoltage-Peak," 1998, pp 107–110; Wallace, "mAs and kVp Relationship," p 93.

101. **(D)** Categorize each set of factors as follows: (1) assign the highest number to the factor contributing to the greatest radiographic density (highest mAs, largest kVp, fastest relative screen speed, and shortest SID); (2) add all of the numbers together; (3) the highest total equals the greatest radiographic density.

	mAs	kVp	Screen Speed	SID	Total
A.	20^1	80^2	100^2	200 cm^1	$= 6$
B.	30^2	75^1	200^3	100 cm^2	$= 8$
C.	100^4	80^2	50^1	200 cm^1	$= 8$
D.	60^3	85^3	200^3	100 cm^2	$= 11$

102. **(A)** Collimation reduces the amount of scatter radiation produced, resulting in a radiograph of shorter scale or higher contrast. It is important to remember that scatter radiation is produced in and from tissue. The more tissue that is exposed, the more scatter radiation that will be produced, and the lower the contrast.

Bushong, "Radiographic Technique," 1997, p 268; Carlton and McKenna-Adler, "Contrast," p 398; Carroll, "Field Size Limitation," 1998, p 138.

103. **(C)** If a film is transported from a hot developer solution to a cool fixer solution, the entire film shrinks, causing "wrinkling," or reticulation. Crescent marks are caused from rough handling of the film in the darkroom. Streaking on a processed radiograph may have several causes: chemical fog, dried chemical deposits, pressure fog, uneven drying, exposure to white light before complete fixing, or insufficient agitation while processing. A radiograph with a green tint is caused by insufficient fixing or washing.

Carlton and McKenna-Adler, "Agfa's Troubleshooting: Symptoms and Causes," p 698; McKinney, "Film Artifacts," p 188.

104. **(C)** The total milliamperage-seconds is found by multiplying the milliampere station times the timer setting:

$$mAs = mA \times Time; \quad \frac{mAs}{Time} = mA$$

$$\frac{40}{0.05} = 800 \text{ mA}$$

105. **(D)** Phenidone and hydroquinone are the two reducing agents in an automatic processor that

change the latent image into the manifest image. Potassium bromide is the restraining agent that keeps unexposed silver bromide crystals from developing and fogging the film. Sodium sulfite is the preservative in both the fixer and the developer solutions and functions to control aerial oxidation. The processing chemicals in the developer, known as "activators," serve to keep the solution at the correct pH levels of 10 to 11. The activator provides an alkaline solution that best serves the reducing agents. Activators also cause the film emulsion to swell, which allows chemicals to penetrate all of the exposed crystals on the film. The two main activators used in the developer solution are sodium carbonate and potassium carbonate.

McKinney, "Development," p 60; Wallace, "Radiographic Film and Development," p 144.

106. **(D)** The base-plus-fog level on the film is the density of the unexposed portion of the film after processing. The toe of the characteristic curve is the area of underexposure where the exposure to the film is too small to record any density on the film. To the human eye, this part of the film appears "clear." However, the toe never drops to zero on the curve because the film usually has a blue tint in the base that measures approximately 0.15 on the densitometer. In addition to the tint, the film may have been exposed to fog, which also has a measurable density. The toe area takes into account the base-plus-fog measurement.

Carlton and McKenna-Adler, "Sensitometry," p 319; Carroll, "Sensitometry and Darkroom Quality Control," 1998, p 532; Gray et al., "Photographic Quality Control," p 33; Wallace, "Radiographic Film & Development," p 148.

107. **(D)** When alternating from one screen speed to another or from one grid ratio to another, it is necessary to alter the technical factors. It is also necessary to increase the technical factors when going from a large field size to a small field size. For instance, when comparing radiography of the lumbar vertebrae with a lateral projection on an 11 × 14 in. film, it would be necessary to increase technique when radiographing the L5–S1 joint spaces on an 8 × 12 in. or cylinder "cone-down" view.

Carroll, "Field Size Limitation," 1998, pp 140–143, and "Intensifying Screens," pp 209–211; Carlton and McKenna-Adler, "Density," pp 367–381; Wallace, "Methods to Control Scatter," p 118, and "Technique Conversion and Comparison," pp 193–203.

108. **(D)** Automatic exposure control affects only the exposure time that controls the radiographic density. Kilovolts (peak) controls contrast. If kilo-

volts (peak) is adjusted on a machine with an AEC, the time will automatically adjust to maintain the density. Adjusting the kilovolts (peak) when using an AEC will change only the contrast on the radiograph, not the density. The kilovolts (peak) should not be varied when using AECs. Adjusting either the mA station or the backup time will not have an effect on either contrast or density in an AEC machine.

Carlton and McKenna-Adler, "Automatic Exposure Controls," p 507; Wallace, "Automatic Exposure Control," p 217.

109. **(B)** A wire-mesh test tool is used to measure film-screen contact caused by damaged cassette holders. A penetrometer is a step wedge and may be used to test the accuracy of the milliampere or kilovolt (peak) settings. Resolution of an image can be easily measured by a device known as a resolution grid. The grid measures in units of line-pairs per millimeter. When the width of the recorded line-pair measures above 0.2 mm, the level of unsharpness that exists in the image is unacceptable.

Thompson et al., "Geometrical Factors Affecting Image Quality," pp 299–300; Tortorici, "Film Holders and Intensifying Screens," 1992, p 269; Wallace, "Geometric Factors Affecting Recorded Detail," pp 131–132.

110. **(C)** Compensating filters are used to even out varying densities in the image of the anatomy of interest. They should be placed in a track under the collimator.

Carlton and McKenna-Adler, "Filtration," p 173; Cullinan, "Basic Operation of an X-Ray Tube," p 36; Wallace, "Methods to Control Scatter," p 121.

SECTION IV: RADIOGRAPHIC PROCEDURES AND RELATED ANATOMY

111. **(A)** The foot consists of 26 bones divided into three parts: (1) the phalanges, or bones of the toes; (2) the metatarsal bones, or bones of the instep; and (3) the tarsal bones, or bones of the ankle. The phalanges and metatarsal bones are numbered one to five beginning at the medial, or great toe side of the foot. There are seven tarsal bones in the ankle: calcaneus (os calcis), talus (astragalus), navicular (scaphoid), cuboid, and three cuneiforms. Beginning at the medial side of the foot, the cuneiforms are described as the medial, intermediate, and lateral. The cuboid lies on the lateral side of the foot between the calcaneus and the fourth and fifth metatarsal bones. The navicular lies on the medial side of the foot between the talus and the three cuneiforms.

Ballinger, Vol 1, p 181; Bontrager, p 175.

112. **(A)** The hand is in the correct anatomic position when the palmar surface faces up. When the hand is rotated so that the palmar surface faces down, the hand is in pronation. When the hand is rotated into the anatomic position, the hand is in supination. Abduction is movement of an arm or leg away from the body in a lateral direction. Adduction is movement toward the body, or midline.

Ballinger, Vol 1, pp 56–57; Bontrager, p 26.

113. **(B)** Both the Colles' and Smith's fractures are found in the distal radius and ulna. The Colles' fracture is characterized by posterior displacement of the radius, and the Smith's fracture by anterior displacement of the radius. The Pott's fracture is a fracture affecting the distal tibia and fibula of the lower leg. A Jefferson fracture is a comminuted fracture of the ring of the atlas, or first cervical vertebra, and is usually caused by sudden deceleration, as in a motor vehicle accident.

Eisenberg and Dennis, "Skeletal System," 1995, pp 102–109; Laudicina, "Osseous System & Joints," pp 180–181.

114. **(A)** For a PA projection of the skull, the OML should be adjusted perpendicular to the image receptor. This baseline is also known as the "radiographic baseline" because it is used so frequently in skull positioning. The IOML is also a common baseline and is sometimes called "Reid's baseline." If the frontal bone is of primary interest, the central ray should be directed perpendicular to the image receptor. For a PA axial projection (Caldwell method), the central ray is angled 15° caudad to exit through the nasion with the OML perpendicular to the film.

Ballinger, Vol 2, pp 233, 242; Bontrager, pp 345, 353.

115. **(D)** To best demonstrate the lungs as they appear fully expanded, the patient should be instructed to suspend respiration at the end of the second full inhalation. This technique should not cause the patient to strain unduly to take in a deep breath. It is easier for the patient to hold his or her breath on the second breath than the first. To best perform this method, it should be practiced with the patient prior to the exposure to make sure that the patient understands.

Ballinger, Vol 1, p 444; Bontrager, pp 66, 72.

116. **(B)** The Camp-Coventry method is a PA axial projection performed to demonstrate the intercondyloid fossa of the knee joint. It is performed with the patient prone and the lower leg elevated at an angle of 30°–40° to the table. The central ray is then directed perpendicular to the long axis of the lower leg and centered to the knee joint.

There are two other methods that may be used to evaluate the intercondylar fossa: the Holmblad method and the Beclere method.

Ballinger, Vol I, pp 250–255; Bontrager, p 210.

117. **(C)** For a dorsoplantar projection of the foot, to properly demonstrate the joint spaces, the central ray should be directed 10° toward the os calcis and should enter at the base of the third metatarsal bone.

Ballinger, Vol, 1, pp 198–199; Bontrager, p 193.

118. **(D)** When positioning a patient for an AP projection of the abdomen in the recumbent position, the cassette should be centered to the level of the iliac crests with the bottom margin of the cassette at the symphysis pubis. The central ray should enter at the level of the iliac crests and be centered to the cassette. For the upright position, the cassette should be centered 2 to 3 inches above the level of the crests of the ilia or high enough to include the diaphragm.

Ballinger, Vol 2, p 38; Bontrager, p 94.

119. **(C)** Breathing techniques are performed to blur the lung markings that may be obscuring the anatomy of interest. Lung markings are not normally a problem when imaging the cervicothoracic region. Breathing techniques are often recommended when radiographing the lower thoracic vertebrae in both the oblique and lateral positions. A breathing technique is also helpful in blurring the lung markings when radiographing the sternum in the oblique position.

Ballinger, Vol 1, pp 334, 355, 408; Bontrager, pp 263–266, 270, 314; Eisenberg et al., 1989, pp 154, 168–176.

120. **(C)** The superior and inferior articulating processes of the vertebral column join to form apophyseal joints. The superior process of the lower vertebra articulates with the inferior process of the upper vertebra. In the lumbar vertebrae, these joints can best be demonstrated on an oblique projection with the patient rotated at an angle of 45°. If the specific area of interest is the fifth lumbar facet, an additional projection may be necessary with a 30° rotation of the patient. When the oblique positions are performed in the RPO and LPO positions, the joints closer to the film are demonstrated. When the oblique positions are performed in the RAO and LAO positions, the joints farther from the film are demonstrated.

Ballinger, Vol 1, p 372; Bontrager, p 290; Eisenberg et al., 1989, p 188.

121. **(C)** The rugae are the folds of the stomach. The haustra are the folds of the large intestine. The

villi are located in the folds of the small intestine. The cilia are hairlike structures found in the lining of the bronchial tree of the lungs.

Scanlon and Sanders, "The Digestive System," pp 291–297, and "Tissues & Membranes," p 58.

122. **(B)** The human skeleton has two main divisions: the axial skeleton and the appendicular skeleton. The axial skeleton consists of the skull, vertebral column, and rib cage. The bones of the arms, legs, shoulder, and pelvic girdles make up the appendicular skeleton. There are a total of 206 bones in the adult skeleton.

Ballinger, Vol 1, p 43; Scanlon and Sanders, "The Skeletal System," p 88.

123. **(D)** The arm has one bone—the humerus. At its distal end is the articulating surface for the formation of the elbow joint with the bones of the forearm. On the lateral aspect is the capitulum, or capitellum, which articulates with the radial head. On the medial aspect is the trochlea, which articulates with the semilunar (trochlear) notch of the ulna.

Ballinger, Vol 1, p 62; Eisenberg et al., 1989, p 39.

124. **(B)** To allow for visualization of large amounts of free air, it is suggested that the patient be erect for a minimum of 5 minutes before the radiograph is produced. For small amounts of intraperitoneal gas, Ballinger recommends that the patient be kept in the left lateral position for 10 to 20 minutes before performing an acute abdominal series.

Ballinger, Vol 2, p 42; Bontrager, p 97; Eisenberg et al., 1989, p 212.

125. **(A)** The positioning term *decubitus* is defined as the act of or the position assumed in lying down. *Recumbent* is lying down in any position (i.e., dorsal recumbent, ventral recumbent, lateral recumbent). *Supine* is the position assumed in lying recumbent on the dorsal side. *Prone* is the position assumed when lying recumbent on the ventral side.

Ballinger, Vol 1, p 54; Bontrager, pp 17–19; Miller-Keane Encyclopedia and Dictionary of Medicine, Nursing and Allied Health, p 417.

126. **(D)** To demonstrate the apices of the lungs free of any superimposition, it may be necessary to perform an AP lordotic projection radiograph. For this projection, the patient is placed standing about 12 inches in front of the chest Bucky. The patient is then asked to lean backward against the cassette in extreme lordosis with the elbows and shoulders rolled forward. The height of the cassette should be placed about 3 to 4 inches above the patient's shoulders. The MSP should be placed perpendicular with the plane of the film. The apices of the lungs should be well demonstrated without superimposition of the clavicles.

Ballinger, Vol 1, p 468; Bontrager, p 78; Eisenberg et al., 1989, p 29.

127. **(B)** The routine oblique projection for the foot is the internal or medial oblique. This projection is done primarily to demonstrate the third through the fifth metatarsal joints free of superimposition. If the specific area of interest is the intertarsal joints between the first and second cuneiform bones or the space between the first and second metatarsal joints, an alternative projection is the lateral oblique, in which the foot is rotated 30° laterally (externally).

Ballinger, Vol 1, pp 200–201; Bontrager, p 194; Eisenberg et al., 1989, p 107.

128. **(B)** The colon, or large intestine, may be examined with the use of Gastrografin or a high-density barium sulfate suspension. The barium sulfate may also be mixed with air for a dual contrast enema examination. An enteroclysis study is a double-contrast study used to image the small bowel. The enteroclysis procedure is done by injecting a contrast medium into the duodenum under fluoroscopic control. The contrast medium and/or air is injected through either a Bilboa or a Sellink tube.

Ballinger, Vol 2, pp 119–122; Bontrager, pp 457, 459.

129. **(D)** The part of the pelvis that forms the cavity between the pelvic inlet and the pelvic outlet is termed the "true" pelvis, or lesser pelvis. The "false" pelvis, also called the greater pelvis, is the area superior to the pelvic brim. The filum terminale is the nerve tissue in the spinal canal that has branched from the end of the spinal cord. The fovea capitis is the depression in the center of the femoral head that serves as an attachment for a ligament.

Ballinger, Vol 1, p 275; Bontrager, p 225; Eisenberg et al., 1989, p 101.

130. **(C)** The shape of the average adult skull is termed "mesocephalic." Variations of the average-shaped skull are the "brachycephalic" and the "dolichocephalic." The important differentiation between these three skull shapes is the angle differences between the petrous pyramids and the MSP. In the mesocephalic skull, the petrous pyramids form an angle of 47° to the MSP. An angle greater than 47° (approximately 54°) to the MSP is found in the short, broad head of the brachycephalic skull shape. In the dolichocephalic skull, the head is long and narrow and forms an angle that is less than 47° to

the MSP, or approximately 40°. These skull shapes are important to note when positioning the skull for radiography.

Ballinger, Vol 2, p 234; Bontrager, p 343; Eisenberg et al., 1989, p 271.

131. **(B)** The bones of the cranium and face, with the exception of the mandible, are joined together by sutures or synarthrodial joints. Diarthrodial joints are freely movable joints, such as the shoulder, hip, and knee. Amphiarthrodial joints are partially movable joints as in the intervertebral joints of the vertebral column.

Ballinger, Vol 2, p 216; Bontrager, pp 10–13; Eisenberg et al., 1989, p 263; Tortora and Grabowski, "Articulations," p 217.

132. **(B)** If the patient's wrist is positioned in ulnar flexion, the navicular joint should be seen without distortion (no foreshortening) and with adjacent interspaces open on the radiograph.

Ballinger, Vol 1, p 89; Bontrager, p 129; Eisenberg et al., 1989, p 60.

133. **(B)** To properly demonstrate the ankle mortise, the ankle should be rotated from the vertical 15° to 20° medially. This rotation should place the malleoli parallel to the plane of the film, or equidistant to the film.

Ballinger, Vol 1, p 231; Bontrager, p 200.

134. **(D)** When performing a UGI series, a partial Trendelenburg (head down) position may be necessary for asthenic patients in order to fill the fundus. A full Trendelenburg position is useful in the evaluation of hiatal hernias.

Ballinger, Vol 2, p 110; Bontrager, p 444.

135. **(C)** The three most widely used projections for imaging the breast during mammography are the craniocaudal, mediolateral, and axillary. Most institutions, however, recommend the use of the mediolateral oblique projection instead of the true 90° mediolateral projection.

Ballinger, Vol 2, p 470; Bontrager, p 537; Eisenberg et al., 1989, pp 326–332.

136. **(B)** When radiographing the thoracic vertebrae, the lateral projection will best demonstrate the intervertebral foramina. The 70° oblique projection is used to demonstrate the apophyseal joints.

Ballinger, Vol 1, pp 358–360; Bontrager, p 276; Eisenberg et al., 1989, pp 182–183.

137. **(C)** An auricular surface on both lateral surfaces of the sacrum articulates with a similar surface on the ilium. The superior articulating process of the sacrum articulates with the inferior articulating process of L5. The base of the sacrum articulates

with the fifth lumbar vertebral body, forming the L5–S1 disk space.

Ballinger, Vol 1, p 323; Bontrager, p 281; Tortora and Grabowksi, "The Axial Skeleton," p 190.

138. **(C)** Microscopic examination of kidney tissue reveals the presence of approximately 1 million tiny structures called "nephrons." Nephrons are responsible for maintaining homeostasis by continually adjusting conditions that are necessary for survival. The nephron produces urine by three physiological activities: (1) filtration, (2) reabsorption, and (3) secretion. Filtration takes place in the renal corpuscle (made up of the glomerulus and Bowman's capsule), where water, electrolytes, sugar amino acids, and other compounds pass from the blood to the glomerulus into Bowman's capsule.

Ballinger, Vol 2, p 154; Gylys and Wedding, "Genitourinary System," pp 239–241; Mallett, "The Urinary System," pp 189–190; Tortora and Grabowski, "The Urinary System," p 874.

139 and 140. **(C)** and **(C)** In Figure 2–5, 1 represents the iliac crest, 2 the right sacroiliac joint, 3 the acetabulum, 4 the ischial tuberosity, 5 the pubic bone, 6 the sacrum, 7 the coccyx, and 8 the pubic symphysis.

Ballinger, Vol 1, pp 272–275; Bontrager, pp 222–225; Scanlon and Sanders, "The Skeletal System," p 122.

141. **(A)** Directing the central ray at an angle of 5° cephalad will prevent the joint space from being obscured by the magnified image of the medial femoral condyle.

Ballinger, Vol 1, p 243; Bontrager, p 208; Eisenberg et al., 1989, p 127.

142. **(A)** Some secretions into the mouth come from the minor salivary glands and the buccal glands. The three major pairs of salivary glands secrete most of the saliva. Their secretions pour into ducts that empty into the oral cavity. The parotid glands, which are located inferior and anterior to the ears, empty saliva through Stensen's duct. The submandibular glands, sometimes called the "submaxillary" glands, are found beneath the base of the tongue and empty their secretions through the Wharton's ducts. The ducts of the sublingual glands, located superior to the submandibular glands, are collectively called the Rivinus ducts.

Ballinger, Vol 2, p 3; Mallett, "The Digestive System," p 171; Tortora and Grabowski, "The Digestive System," p 772.

143. **(B)** It is important in positioning of the skull that the radiographer become familiar with all cranial

baselines. Drawing a line from various anterior landmarks to the midpoint of the EAM forms most baselines. The most superior of these lines is the glabellomeatal line. There is about a 7° to 8° difference between the glabellomeatal line and the OML (or radiographic baseline). There is also a 7° to 8° difference between the OML and the IOML. Knowing these differences is an important factor when making positioning adjustments.
Ballinger, Vol 2, p 233; Bontrager, p 345.

144. **(B)** The parietoacanthial projection (Waters method) is mainly performed to demonstrate the maxillary sinuses. It may also be useful in demonstrating the rotundum foramina, which are seen just inferior to the medial aspect of the orbital floor and superior to the roof of the maxillary sinuses.
Ballinger, Vol 2, p 382.

145. **(D)** The pedicles are short, thick projections that extend posteriorly from either side of the vertebral body. The laminae are broad, flat layers of bone that extend posteriorly from each pedicle to unite in the midline to form the spinous process. The transverse processes project laterally and slightly posteriorly from the junctions of the pedicles and laminae.
Ballinger, Vol 1, p 314; Eisenberg et al., 1989, p 164; Tortora and Grabowski, "The Axial Skeleton," p 186.

146. **(D)** When radiographing the entire cranium with a lateral projection, the central ray should enter at approximately 2 inches superior to the EAM. If a cone-down lateral projection of the sella turcica is desired, a centering point of approximately ¾ inch anterior and superior to the EAM is recommended.
Ballinger, Vol 2, pp 239, 263; Bontrager, pp 351, 355; Eisenberg et al., 1989, p 279.

147. **(A)** It is suggested that when positioning for a PA projection of the chest, a 14 × 17 in. cassette be placed in the crosswise position for hypersthenic patients. Hypersthenic patients make up 5 percent of the population and have a very broad and deep thorax, but are shallow in the vertical dimension.
Ballinger, Vol 1, p 452; Bontrager, pp 64, 72.

148. **(B)** When performing radiography of the abdomen with an AP projection, it is important to ensure that there is no rotation of the patient's body. The radiographer should determine that (1) the outer margins of the ribs are the same distance from the vertebral column, (2) the right and left iliac wings appear equal in size and shape, and (3) the obturator foramina appear equal in size and shape. For instance, the right

iliac wing will appear elongated if the patient is rotated toward the right side, and the right obturator foramen will appear foreshortened. If the patient is rotated toward the left side, the right iliac wing will appear foreshortened, and the right obturator foramen will appear elongated, or more fully open.
Ballinger, Vol 2, p 39; Bontrager, p 94; Carroll, "Evaluating Radiographs: Torso Positions," 1993, pp 110–112.

149. **(C)** When the patient is in the prone position, the central ray should be angled caudad to correct for inadequate chin extension on the Waters method. If a patient is being radiographed with the use of a head unit, the cassette may also be tilted toward the forehead to correct for this. If the central ray is angled cephalad or if the cassette is tilted away from the forehead, the petrous ridges will be projected higher than they should be. It must be noted, however, that any angulation of the central ray will obscure the air-fluid levels. If the demonstration of air-fluid levels is desired, the radiograph should be exposed with a horizontal beam and the patient erect if possible.
Carroll, "Evaluating Radiographs: Head Positions," 1993, pp 199–200; McQuillen-Martensen, p 413.

150. **(C)** An outline of a "scotty dog" should be clearly demonstrated on a correctly positioned 45° oblique of the lumbar vertebrae. The pedicle, represented by the "eye" of the scotty dog, should appear near the center of the vertebral body. The "nose" of the scotty dog (transverse process) should be pointed toward the side closer to the table on a posterior oblique (RPO or LPO) projection. In this projection, the nose of the scotty dog is facing the right side; thus this radiograph is an RPO projection.
Ballinger, Vol 1, pp 372–373; Bontrager, p 290.

151. **(B)** Chest radiographs are often obtained with the patient swallowing a bolus of high-density barium sulfate to outline the heart and aorta. The barium sulfate used in heart studies should be much thicker than that used to evaluate the stomach so that it will descend more slowly and adhere to the esophageal walls. According to Bontrager, the barium swallow for cardiac series is rarely performed today to evaluate heart size because it is being replaced by echocardiography (imaging with ultrasound). The echocardiogram is considered the ideal method to evaluate the size of the heart and vessels. Cardiac catheterization is not necessary for evaluating just the heart size because of the invasive nature of the procedure. Cardiac catheterization is usually reserved

for therapeutic measures such as angioplasty. The lordotic projection is specifically performed to demonstrate the apices of the lungs, not the heart size. Electrocardiograms evaluate the cardiac pulse rate and rhythm, not the heart size.

Ballinger, Vol 1, pp 455, 463; Bontrager, p 430.

152. **(D)** When radiographing the elbow in acute flexion with the central ray perpendicular to the forearm, the proximal ulna and the radius will be superimposed by the distal humerus. With the proper exposure factors, the radial head and neck should be clearly visible through the distal humerus. It is important to take two projections to visualize both the proximal ulna and the distal humerus: one with the central ray perpendicular to the forearm and one with the central ray perpendicular to the humerus.

Ballinger, Vol 1, p 109; Bontrager, p 140.

153. **(C)** The contrast medium used to image the gallbladder may be delivered to the liver by either the oral or the venous routes. When given orally, the contrast medium is absorbed by the small intestines and carried to the liver through the portal vein. When administered intravenously, it is most commonly injected into the antecubital vein, circulates throughout the bloodstream, then is absorbed by the liver via the hepatic artery and the portal vein. In either case, when the contrast medium has been delivered to the liver, the contrast medium is biochemically changed in the hepatic cells and then excreted by the liver with the bile to the gallbladder.

Ballinger, Vol 2, p 54; Bontrager, pp 484–485.

154. **(C)** Myelography is a good diagnostic tool for demonstrating lesions in the spinal canal that may impinge on the spinal cord. These lesions include herniated nucleus pulposus (HNP), cancerous or benign tumors, cysts, and possible bone fragments. The most common pathological finding of a myelogram is HNP (herniation of the inner portion of the vertebral disk).

Bontrager, p 620; Tortorici, "Myelography," 1995, p 76.

155. **(B)** When the leg is in the true anatomic position, the proximal femur is actually rotated posteriorly 15° to 20°. The femoral neck appears foreshortened and the lesser trochanter is visible. If the lower extremities are rotated 15° to 20° medially, the greater trochanter is seen in profile, and the femoral neck is parallel to the plane of the film. The lesser trochanter should not be visible at all.

Ballinger, Vol 1, pp 276–277; Bontrager, p 229–230; Eisenberg et al., 1989, pp 142–143.

156. **(B)** Hysterosalpingography is indicated in cases of infertility, habitual abortion, abnormal uterine bleeding, absence of menses, and suspected blockage of the uterine (fallopian) tubes. It may also be useful in demonstrating intrauterine and pelvic masses, fistulae, and congenital abnormalities. As a therapeutic tool, an HSG may restore the patency of the ducts in cases of blockage in the fallopian tubes. An HSG would be contraindicated if the patient has a history of PID or active uterine bleeding.

Tortorici, "Hysterosalpingography," 1995, p 55.

157. **(C)** The thyroid cartilage is located at the level of the fifth cervical vertebra. The jugular notch is located at the level of the second and third thoracic vertebral interspace. The sternal angle is located at the level of the fourth and fifth thoracic vertebral interspace. The xyphoid process is located at the level of the 10th thoracic vertebra.

Ballinger, Vol 1, p 40; Bontrager, p 52; Eisenberg et al., 1989, pp 17–18.

158. **(B)** The lithotomy position gets its name from the medical term "lith," which means stone, and the term "tome," which means to cut. It is the position assumed for surgical removal of a kidney stone. In the Trendelenburg position, the patient is supine and the head is lower than the feet. Fowler's position is the opposite of the Trendelenburg position and has the patient supine with the feet lower than the head. Sims' position is the position assumed by the patient during insertion of an enema tip.

Bontrager, p 17.

159. **(D)** The carpal bridge procedure is recommended for the demonstration of (1) fractures of the scaphoid, (2) lunate dislocations, (3) calcifications and foreign bodies in the dorsum of the wrist, and (4) chip fractures of the dorsal aspect of the carpal bones.

Ballinger, Vol 1, pp 96–97; Bontrager, p 133.

160. **(A)** To best demonstrate the joint space of the sacroiliac joint, the patient must be positioned 25° to 30° degrees oblique. If the patient is supine, the side that is elevated is demonstrated. If the patient is prone, the side closer to the film is demonstrated. Therefore, the left sacroiliac joint is best demonstrated by the 25° to 30° RPO and the 25° to 30° LAO projections. An obliquity of 45° would be too steep and would obscure the joint space.

Ballinger, Vol 1, pp 380–383; Bontrager, pp 243–244; Eisenberg et al., 1989, pp 196–197.

161. **(D)** There are basically two broad categories of surface markings that may be found on the outer

surfaces of bones. They are (1) *depressions,* which receive bony prominences and allow for passages of vessels and nerves, and (2) *projections,* which serve as points of articulation or as attachments for tendons and ligaments. Condyles are rounded processes at the end of bones that serve as points of articulation. Tuberosities, tubercles, or trochanters are roughened areas on bone which serve as points of attachment for muscles, ligaments, and tendons. A meatus and a foramen are both openings in bones that allow the passage of nerves or blood vessels.

Mosby's Medical, Nursing and Allied Health Dictionary, p 377; Tortora and Grabowski, "The Skeletal System: The Axial Skeleton," pp 166–167.

162. **(B)** The mastoid portion forms the inferior and posterior part of the temporal bone. The mastoid air cells are contained within the mastoid process of the temporal bone.

Ballinger, Vol 2, pp 226–227; Bontrager, p 391; Eisenberg et al., 1989, p 266.

163. **(B)** The wall of the large intestine is divided into four layers: (1) the serous coat, (2) the muscular coat, (3) the submucous layer, and (4) the mucous coat. The muscular coat consists of an inner layer of circular fibers and an outer layer of longitudinal fibers arranged in three bands over the greater part of the large intestine. These bands, called *teniae coli,* are shorter than the outer layers. The result is that between the teniae coli the wall of the large intestine is pouched or sacculated. The recesses of the sacculations are called *haustra. Escherichia coli,* sometimes called *E. coli* for short, is a bacterium found in the large intestine. The *gyri* are folds of the brain.

Ballinger, Vol 2, p 87; Bontrager, p 449.

164. **(C)** Chronic alcoholism may lead to a deterioration of the liver, which eventually leads to cirrhosis. In fact, for as many as 90 percent of patients with this condition, a history of alcohol abuse is present.

Eisenberg and Dennis, "Gastrointestinal System," 1995, p 160; Laudicina, "Hepatobiliary System,"p 92.

165. **(D)** Most adult patients require a second radiograph centered 2 or 3 inches higher on the RPO if the left colic (splenic) flexure is to be included. For the AP axial projection, or "butterfly" position, the central ray should enter 2 inches inferior and 2 inches medial to the right anterosuperior iliac spine.

Bontrager, p 475; Carroll, "Evaluating Radiographs: Torso Positions," 1993, p 120.

166 and 167. **(B)** and **(D)** In Figure 2–7, 1 represents the gallbladder, 2 the cystic duct, 3 the common bile duct, 4 the duodenal loop, 5 the hepatopancreatic ampulla (ampulla of Vater), 6 the liver, 7 the common hepatic duct, 8 the pylorus, 9 the pyloric sphincter, 10 the pancreas, and 11 the pancreatic duct.

Ballinger, Vol 2, p 33; Bontrager, p 418; Eisenberg et al., 1989, p 209; Scanlon and Sanders, "The Digestive System, " 1999, p 364; Tortorici, "Endoscopic Retrograde Cholangiopancreatography," 1995, p 46.

168. **(C)** The instep is best demonstrated with a weight-bearing lateral projection that demonstrates the longitudinal arch of the foot. The mortise joint is best demonstrated in the 15° to 20° medial oblique projection of the ankle. The os calcis or calcaneus is best demonstrated with a 40° cephalad angle with the plantodorsal projection. The subtalar joint is best demonstrated by a PA axial oblique projection with the ankle in the exaggerated lateral position and with the central ray angled 5° anterior and 23° caudal.

Ballinger, Vol 1, pp 208, 215, 220; Bontrager, p 200.

169. **(C)** An AP oblique projection of the urinary tract should demonstrate the kidneys, ureters, and bladder filled with iodinated contrast medium. The elevated kidney should be placed parallel to the film, and the kidney closer to the film should be placed perpendicular. To accomplish this, the patient must turn from the supine position so that the midcoronal plane forms an angle of 30° with the plane of the film.

Ballinger, Vol 1, p 172; Bontrager, p 523.

170. **(B)** The axillary portion of the ribs is best demonstrated with the patient in the oblique position. In the anterior oblique (RAO and LAO) position, the elevated side is better demonstrated. In the posterior oblique position (RPO and LPO), the side closer to the film is better demonstrated.

Ballinger, Vol 1, pp 428–431.

SECTION V: PATIENT CARE

171. **(A)** It is essential that the radiographer closely monitor a patient who has just been injected with an iodinated contrast medium because usually in the first 5 minutes the patient will suffer a reaction. The reaction may range from mild (metallic taste, warm sensation) to moderate to severe (anaphylactic shock, death). All patients, however, should be monitored for at least 1 hour after the injection because delayed reactions can occur.

Kowalczyk, "Medication Administration," p 191; Tortorici, "Contrast Media," 1995, p 25.

172. **(B)** In cases of medical negligence or failure to acquire informed consent, the burden of proof is placed on the patient and requires the use of expert testimony. In the case of negligence, the patient must prove four points: (1) that the radiographer has a *duty to provide care,* (2) that the radiographer *breached that duty,* (3) that the patient was *injured,* and (4) that the radiographer's breach of duty caused the injury (*proximate cause*).

Tortorici, "Medical Legal Implications," 1995, p 12; Obergfell, "Medical Negligence and Malpractice," pp 61–62.

173. **(B)** When radiographers are involved in sterile procedures, either in the radiology department or in the surgical suite, it is essential that the instruments remain sterile. To prevent contamination, appropriate steps must be taken. Some sterile instruments may be wrapped, whereas others will be sealed. Items that are wrapped are opened differently from those that are sealed. To open a wrapped sterile package, the package should be placed so that the top flap opens away from the individual opening the package.

Ehrlich and McCloskey, "Infection Control," pp 167–171; Kowalczyk, "Infection Control & Aseptic Technique," p 94; Torres, "Surgical Asepsis," pp 109–111, 174; Tortorici, "Sterile Technique," 1995, p 167.

174. **(A)** When preparing an injection site for the Seldinger technique, a local anesthetic is usually administered to prevent vasospasm and to localize the anesthetic effect to an immediate area. Lidocaine is the usual choice for a local anesthetic but may also be used in combination with epinephrine. Epinephrine helps to reduce bleeding and causes vasoconstriction.

Ballinger, Vol 2, p 520, and Vol 3, p 96; Kowalczyk, "Medication Administration," p 178; Tortorici, "Catheterization Methods and Patient Management," 1995, pp 182–183.

175. **(C)** Infections may be transmitted by four different means: (1) direct or indirect *contact,* (2) *airborne,* (3) *vehicle,* and (4) *vector.* Contaminated inanimate objects that contain pathogens would be an example of indirect contact. These objects are called *fomites* and may be objects such as a bedpan, needle, or catheter. Infection by airborne transmission occurs when dust particles or droplets containing the pathogen are inhaled. Transmission by a vehicle is also by inanimate items, but these items differ from fomites in that they produce pathogens because of improper storage or handling. Examples are water, blood, drugs, and spoiled food. A vector is a disease-carrying insect or animal that transmits germs to humans.

An example of a disease that may be transmitted via a vector would be malaria.

Ehrlich and McCloskey, "Infection Control," pp 146–147; Kowalczyk, "Infection Control and Aseptic Technique," pp 81–82.

176. **(D)** There is some debate among medical professionals as to how the patient should be prepared during the 24-hour period preceding an OCG. Most agree that the patient should be NPO at least 12 hours preceding the procedure. It is also highly recommended that the patient avoid laxatives during this period so that the contrast medium in the form of oral tablets will be properly absorbed by the small intestine. Smoking and chewing gum are also to be avoided during this 12-hour period.

Ballinger, Vol 2, p 60; Bontrager, p 488.

177. **(C)** Suction is needed for clearing the airway of any mucus or phlegm that may be obstructing the airway in a patient with tracheostomy tube. Resuscitation is an artificial means of reviving either the respiration through rescue breathing or the cardiac heart rhythm through chest compressions. Intubation is the insertion of a tube into any hollow organ, as into the larynx or trachea through the glottis, for entrance of air or to dilate a stricture. Patients who are given general anesthesia are often intubated to provide artificial respiration. In bronchography (radiography of the bronchial tree), a patient may also need to be intubated.

Ehrlich and McCloskey, "Bedside Radiography: Special Conditions & Environments," p 303; Kowalczyk, "Patient Care in Critical Situations," pp 204–207; Taber's Cyclopedic Medical Dictionary, p 1017.

178. **(C)** Negligence, the parent of malpractice, is a failure to fulfill the expected standard of care. Although the *standard of care* may vary somewhat from institution to institution, providing a safe environment for the patient is within the *standards of care* for all health-care professionals, including radiographers. In the cases of slipping and falling, this type of negligence is categorized as *contributory negligence.* The radiographer is held responsible for the patient's injuries because the radiographer should have anticipated the fall or should have tried to help prevent it in some way. Therefore, a breach of this duty would be considered negligence.

Gurley and Callaway, "Medicolegal Considerations," p 178; Obergfell, "Medical Negligence & Malpractice," pp 56–58; Wilson, "Medical Legal Issues for the Practice of Medical Imaging," pp 152–154.

179. **(B)** One of the most important responsibilities of the radiographer in ensuring quality of patient

care and reducing unnecessary radiation exposure is to verify the identity of the patient before the examination begins. This should be the first step of a radiographic examination. Once the patient has been identified, it is then necessary to verify the examination requested by checking the orders in the patient's chart or by carefully reading the prescription written by the referring physician. Placing a cassette in the Bucky tray or obtaining an accurate history on the patient would be pointless if it is performed on the wrong patient or the wrong examination has been ordered.

Gurley and Callaway, "Patient Care and Management," p 166.

180. **(B)** Protective, or reverse, isolation is used to protect immunosuppressed patients. Types of conditions that may affect the immune system include leukemia, burns, and acquired immunodeficiency syndrome. Patients with hepatitis B should not require any special isolation procedures because every patient in the hospital is treated as potentially infectious through universal precautions. Universal precautions should protect the radiographer from any blood-borne pathogens, such as the hepatitis B virus.

Adler and Carlton, "Infection Control," p 210; Ehrlich and McCloskey, "Infection Control," pp 163, 165; Kowalczyk, "Infection Control and Aseptic Technique," pp 87–88.

181. **(A)** The abbreviation *PRN* stands for "as needed." The abbreviations *bid* and *qid* stand for "twice daily" and "four times a day," respectively. The medical term *NPO* stands for "nothing by mouth." All are abbreviations for Latin terms.

Gylys and Wedding, pp 381–389; Mosby's Medical, Nursing and Allied Health, pp 1728–1732.

182. **(B)** Hypoglycemia is a condition of low blood sugar that is usually caused by a diabetic patient being NPO for several hours. It may occur in other patients as well. It is not caused as a result of a contrast medium injection. Anaphylaxis is a severe, life-threatening condition that is a direct result of an allergic reaction that may be induced by an injection of an iodinated contrast medium. Urticaria, otherwise known as "hives," is a moderate allergic reaction to a contrast medium and must be carefully monitored because it may be a warning of the onset of more severe symptoms. Urticaria is usually treated with diphenhydramine (Benadryl). Hypovolemic shock is a type of shock that results from a loss of a large amount of blood. This does not usually result from the administration of an iodinated contrast medium.

Kowalczyk, "Patient Care in Critical Situations," pp 211–213; Tortorici, "Contrast Media," 1995, p 26.

183. **(D)** There are four major categories of microorganisms that lead to infectious disease: (1) bacterial, (2) viral, (3) fungal, and (4) parasitic (protozoa). Ehrlich and McCloskey also mention a fifth category called prions, which are a poorly understood mechanism of infection and may be linked to causing Alzheimer's disease in humans.

Adler and Carlton, "Infection Control," p 196; Ehrlich and McCloskey, "Infection Control," p 138; Kowalczyk, "Infection Control and Aseptic Technique," p 78; Torres, "Infection Control and Institutional Safety," pp 41–45.

184. **(D)** Osteogenesis imperfecta is an inherited congenital disorder sometimes called the brittle bone disease. Patients with this condition suffer multiple fractures and are often misdiagnosed as being child abuse victims. Care should be taken when handling these patients because of the osteoporotic condition of their bone tissue. Osteomyelitis is an infection of the bone and bone marrow that may arise secondary to a fracture. Osteomyelitis most often begins as an abscess in bone called Brodie's abscess. Osteochondritis dissecans has several forms, one of which is Osgood-Schlatter disease in which the tibial tubercle separates from the tibial shaft. Erythrocythemia is an increase in the number of red blood cells in the circulating blood.

Eisenberg and Dennis, "Skeletal System," 1995, p 69–95; Laudicina, "Osseous System & Joints," pp 134, 145–146, 159; Taber's Cyclopedic Dictionary, p 671.

185. **(C)** Barium sulfate is not water-soluble, so the body cannot naturally absorb it. It should never be injected into the bloodstream, the subarachnoid space, or in any location where it may leak into the peritoneal cavity. Thus, if bowel perforation is suspected, barium contrast would be contraindicated. Barium has a tendency to clump up and harden in the bowel, causing constipation and, in severe cases, obstruction. It is therefore very important to properly care for the bowel after any barium study of the gastrointestinal tract. Usually, the recommendations are to drink plenty of liquids and to take a cathartic that will help to cleanse the bowel. In some institutions, administration of cathartics is the responsibility of the radiographer. If this is the case, the time and dosage administered must be charted for all inpatients to provide proper documentation.

Ehrlich and McCloskey, "Preparation and Examination of the Gastrointestinal Tract," pp 244–245; Kowalczyk, "Medication Administration," p 190; Torres, "Pharmacology for Radiographers," p 262.

186. **(B)** When an adult is found unresponsive, the most likely cause is cardiac arrest. This requires immediate medical assistance. The radiographer should request assistance immediately on establishing unresponsiveness; if the radiographer is alone, he or she should call a "code" before attempting to open the airway. Once the emergency medical system has been activated, the radiographer may then proceed to open the airway, check for breathing, attempt to ventilate, check for pulse, and so forth, in the proper sequence of ABCs (airway, breathing, circulation) as set forth by the American Heart Association. In children, the most likely cause of unresponsiveness is respiratory arrest. It is therefore more important to attempt to open the airway and immediately start cardiopulmonary resuscitation, if necessary, prior to calling a code blue on a pediatric patient.

Adler and Carlton, "Medical Emergencies," pp 263–264; American Heart Association, pp 28–29, 40; Torres, "Medical Emergencies in Radiographic Imaging," pp 160–166.

187. **(A)** Iodinated contrast agents are by far the most commonly used radiographic contrast agents. They are ideal because they have a high atomic number, making them very radiopaque, a property similar to bony tissue. Iodinated contrast agents may be water soluble or oil based so they may be administered orally, intravenously, intrathecally, or intravaginally. They may also be ionic or nonionic. Nonionic iodinated contrast has become more popular because of its reduced osmolality and thus reduced toxicity to the body. The only drawback to the nonionic versus the ionic contrast is the tremendous difference in cost. Although iodinated contrast medium has relatively low toxicity even in its ionic form, this is not the principal reason for its use as a contrast agent.

Adler and Carlton, "Contrast Media," p 309; Ehrlich and McCloskey, "Contrast Media and Special Imaging Techniques," pp 264–265; Kowalczyk, "Medication Administration," pp 190–192.

188. **(B)** An informed consent form may be required for certain invasive procedures performed in the radiology department. Examples of these may be arteriography, HSG, and myelography. The physician is the only health-care professional recognized by the law who may obtain consent from a patient. The form either should come with the patient if he or she is an outpatient or should be included in the patient's chart. However, it is the radiographer's responsibility to ensure that the form is filled out properly and that the patient is truly informed about the procedure prior to beginning the procedure. If the radiographer, on questioning the patient, discovers that the patient was not properly informed, the radiographer should take the time to fully explain the procedure in lay terms. The form should include the patient's name, the procedure name, a brief description of the procedure using lay terms, the person who will be performing the procedure, the benefits and risks of the procedure, and at least three signatures. Signatures required are those of the patient or patient's legal guardian, the person performing the consultation (the physician), and a witness who will not be participating in the procedure. Such an individual may include a ward clerk, a hospital chaplain, or other nonrelated health-care worker.

Obergfell, "Standard of Care, Patient Rights, and Informed Consent," pp 86–89; Tortorici, "Medical Legal Implications," 1995, p 10.

189. **(D)** Arthrography is a radiographic examination of diarthrodial joints; it is not a good diagnostic tool for bone pathology. Both computed tomography scan and magnetic resonance imaging may be good diagnostic tools for bone metastases in a localized region of the body. However, a radionuclide bone scan is able to image the entire skeleton on one view and is therefore the best diagnostic imaging tool for metastatic bone disease.

Eisenberg and Dennis, "Skeletal System," 1995, p 82; Mace and Kowalczyk, "The Skeletal System," p 83; Laudicina, "Neoplasia," p 275.

190. **(B)** Elisabeth Kübler-Ross first established the fact that people who have suffered a loss adapt to it gradually through a grieving process. She described the process as the individual experiencing five different stages: (1) denial, (2) anger, (3) bargaining, (4) depression, and (5) acceptance. It is important for the radiographer to assess the grieving patient prior to beginning care to determine which phase the patient may be experiencing.

Ehrlich and McCloskey, "Professional Communications," pp 76–77; Kowalczyk, "Communication," p 37; Torres, "The Patient in Radiographic Imaging," pp 32–33.

191. **(D)** If the radiographer has injected contrast media through an IV drip and notices signs of swelling in the surrounding tissue, it is his or her responsibility to remove the needle and to immediately provide either a warm or cold compress. One reference cites using a moist cloth heated with hot water (as hot as the skin can tolerate).

Adler and Carlton, "Pharmacology," p 292; Ehrlich and McCloskey, "Medications and Their Administration," p 209; Kowalczyk, "Medication Administration," p 188; Torres, "Drug Administration," p 293.

192. **(B)** It is the function of the colon to absorb water from waste products before they are expelled from the body. This absorption may greatly increase during a barium enema procedure because of the introduction of barium or gastroview and/or cleansing enemas prior to the procedure. All of this excess fluid may be absorbed into the bloodstream, causing a condition known as hypervolemia. Hypervolemia is a very serious condition and may lead to pulmonary edema, renal failure, and death. Hypervolemia may be avoided by adding 2 tsp of table salt to each liter of enema solution. It is important to follow the manufacturer's recommendations for enema preparation.

Adler and Carlton, "Contrast Media," pp 304, 308; Ehrlich and McCloskey, "Preparation and Examination of the Gastrointestinal Tract," p 253.

193. **(C)** Because barium sulfate is an inert compound, it does not react chemically with the body. Allergies from the barium itself are most likely not the problem. Reports of allergic reactions during barium enema examinations may either be attributed to the preservatives in the barium preparation or to the latex enema tip. Allergies to latex or rubber products are on the rise. Some of these reported reactions to latex enema tips and latex gloves have been fatal. As a result, some new nonlatex products are being manufactured, but they are very expensive. It has been suggested that radiographers take a thorough history of each patient and then reserve these nonlatex products for only the high-risk patients. Those patients who are considered high risk for allergies to rubber or latex also have allergies to fruit, especially avocados and bananas. To best protect the patient, the radiographer should consider those patients with any history of allergies high risk.

Adler and Carlton, "Contrast Media," p 308; Ehrlich and McCloskey, "Medications and Their Administration," p 194; Torres, "Care of Patients during Imaging Examinations of the Gastrointestinal System," p 207.

194. **(C)** An indwelling catheter is designed to be left in place for prolonged periods. The urinary drainage bag should be kept below the level of the patient's bladder to reduce the risk of urinary tract infections. Placing the bag below the level of the radiographic table, at the foot end of the table, or attached to the stretcher or wheelchair may not always place it properly below the patient's bladder. The radiographer should always be aware of this during transport.

Adler and Carlton, "Aseptic Techniques," pp 233–234; Ehrlich and McCloskey, "Patient Care during Urologic Procedures," p 328; Kowalczyk, "Tubes, Catheters, and Vascular Access Lines," p 153.

195. **(B)** The system of universal (standard) precautions assumes that all patients are potentially infectious. Universal precautions means using gloves on every patient, especially when coming in direct contact with patient's body fluids (wounds, blood, pus, sputum, etc.). Hand washing should routinely be performed between procedures and between patients. The CDC sets the guidelines, and many organizations enforce these. Those enforcing the universal precautions system include the Joint Commission on Accreditation for Health Care Organizations (JCAHO) and the Occupational Safety and Health Administration (OSHA).

Adler and Carlton, "Infection Control," pp 209–210; Ehrlich and McCloskey, "Infection Control," pp 152–153; Kowalczyk, "Infection Control and Aseptic Technique," pp 86–87.

196. **(B)** After being injected with an iodinated contrast media, the patient may have various reactions ranging from mild to moderate to severe. Examples of mild reactions would be a warm sensation and a metallic taste in the mouth. Examples of moderate reactions would be skin erythema, urticaria (hives), rhinitis, or facial edema. Severe reactions would include convulsions, cyanosis, anaphylactic shock, cardiac arrest, renal failure, and respiratory arrest.

Adler and Carlton, "Contrast Media," p 313; Kowalczyk, "Medication Administration," p 191; Tortorici, "Contrast Media," 1995, p 25.

197. **(C)** The greatest risk when lifting heavy objects is injury to the lower back. It is therefore of utmost importance to use proper body mechanics during the transport of patients. Lift using the legs and do not bend at the waist. Also remember that the best way to move a heavy object is to push it.

Adler and Carlton, "Transfer Techniques," p 143; Ehrlich and McCloskey, "Safety, Transfer and Positioning," pp 91–92; Kowalczyk, "Patient Assessment and Assistance," p 122.

198. **(D)** The rate of compressions for a one-rescuer adult victim should be 15 compressions to every 2 ventilations. This should be completed for four complete cycles of 15:2 before reassessing the patient for the return of a pulse and spontaneous breathing.

Adler and Carlton, "Medical Emergencies," p 265; American Heart Association, pp 30–31; Kowalczyk, "Patient Care in Critical Situations," p 206; Torres, "Medical Emergencies in Radiographic Imaging," p 162.

199. **(A)** The oral route is the easiest, safest, and most desirable route for drug administration for the patient.

Kowalczyk, "Medication Administration," p 170; Ehrlich and McCloskey, "Medications and Their Administration," p 192; Torres, "Pharmacology for Radiographers," p 245.

200. **(A)** Orthostatic, or postural, hypotension is a sudden drop in blood pressure when a person changes from a supine or sitting position to the upright position. This drop in blood pressure may lead to a feeling of dizziness or faintness. It is important for the radiographer to closely monitor a patient who has been recumbent for a long time and is then asked to stand, especially if the patient is on any medication.

Adler and Carlton, "Transfer Techniques," pp 142, 148; Ehrlich and McCloskey, "Safety, Transfer and Positioning," p 96; Torres, "Care of Patients with Special Problems," p 183.

BIBLIOGRAPHY

Adler, AM, and Carlton, RR: Introduction to Radiography and Patient Care. WB Saunders, Philadelphia, 1993.

American Heart Association: Basic Life Support for Healthcare Providers. AHA, Dallas, TX, 1997.

Ballinger, PW: Merrill's Atlas of Radiographic Positions and Radiologic Procedures, ed 8, 3 vols. Mosby–Year Book, St Louis, 1995.

Bontrager, KL: Textbook of Radiographic Positioning and Related Anatomy, ed 4. Mosby–Year Book, St Louis, 1997.

Bushong S: Radiologic Science for Technologists: Physics, Biology and Protection, ed 6. Mosby–Year Book, 1997.

Carlton, R, and McKenna-Adler, A: Principles of Radiographic Imaging: An Art and a Science, ed 2. Delmar, Albany, NY, 1996.

Carroll, QB: Evaluating Radiographs. Charles C Thomas, Springfield, IL, 1993.

Carroll, QB: Fuchs's Radiographic Exposure, Processing and Quality Control, ed 6. Charles C Thomas, Springfield, IL, 1998.

Centers for Disease Control and Prevention: Infection Control Standards and Guidelines for Healthcare Workers. Author, Atlanta, GA, 1997.

Cullinan, AM: Producing Quality Radiographs, ed 2. Lippincott, Philadelphia, 1994.

Curry, TS, et al: Christensen's Physics of Diagnostic Radiology, ed 4. Lea & Febiger, Philadelphia, 1990.

Dennis, CA, and Eisenberg, RL: Applied Radiographic Calculations. WB Saunders, Philadelphia, 1993.

Dowd, SB, and Tilson, ER: Practical Radiation Protection and Applied Radiobiology, ed 2. WB Saunders, Philadelphia, 1999.

Ehrlich, RA, and McCloskey, ED: Patient Care in Radiography, ed 5. Mosby, St Louis, 1999.

Eisenberg, RL, and Dennis, CA: Comprehensive Radiographic Pathology, ed 2. Mosby, St Louis, 1995.

Eisenberg, RL, et al: Radiographic Positioning. Little, Brown & Co, Boston, 1989.

Gray, JE, et al: Quality Control in Diagnostic Imaging. University Park Press, Baltimore, 1983.

Gurley, LT, and Callaway, WJ: Introduction to Radiologic Technology, ed 4. Mosby, St Louis, 1996.

Gylys, BA, and Wedding, ME: Medical Terminology: A Systems Approach, ed 4. FA Davis, Philadelphia, 1999.

Hendee, WR: Medical Radiation Physics: Roentgenology, Nuclear Medicine and Ultrasound, ed 2. Year Book Medical Publishers, Chicago, 1979.

Hiss, SS: Understanding Radiography, ed 3. Charles C Thomas, Springfield, IL, 1993.

Ireland, SJ: Integrated Mathematics of Radiographic Exposure. St. Louis, Mosby, 1994.

Kowalczyk, N: Integrated Patient Care for the Imaging Professional. Mosby, St Louis, 1996.

Laudicina, P: Applied Pathology for Radiographers. WB Saunders, Philadelphia, 1989.

Mace, JD, and Kowalczyk, N: Radiographic Pathology, ed 2. Mosby–Year Book, St Louis, 1994.

Mallett, M: Anatomy and Physiology for Students of Medical Radiation Technology. Burnell, Mankato, MN, 1981.

Malott, JC, and Fodor, J: The Art and Science of Medical Radiography, ed 7. Mosby, St Louis, 1993.

McKinney, WEJ: Radiographic Processing and Quality Control. Lippincott, Philadelphia, 1988.

McQuillen-Martensen, K: Radiographic Critique. WB Saunders, Philadelphia, 1996.

Memmler, RL, and Wood, DL: The Human Body in Health and Disease, ed 5. JB Lippincott, Philadelphia, 1983.

Miller, BF: Miller-Keane Encyclopedia and Dictionary of Medicine, Nursing, and Allied Health, ed 6. WB Saunders, Philadelphia, 1997.

Mosby's Medical, Nursing and Allied Health Dictionary, ed 3. Mosby, St Louis, 1993.

National Council on Radiation Protection and Measurements (NCRP): Limitation of Exposure to Ionizing Radiation, Report No. 116. Author, Bethesda, MD, 1993.

NCRP: Medical X-Ray Electron Beam and Gamma-Ray Protection for Energies up to 50 MeV (Equipment Design, Performance and Use), Report No. 102. Author, Bethesda, MD, 1989.

NCRP: Quality Assurance for Diagnostic Imaging, Report No. 99. Author, Bethesda, MD, 1988.

NCRP: Radiation Protection for Medical and Allied Health Personnel, Report No.105. Author, Bethesda, MD, 1989.

Obergfell, AM: Law and Ethics in Diagnostic Imaging and Therapeutic Radiology. WB Saunders, Philadelphia, 1995.

Papp, J: Quality Management in the Radiologic Sciences. Mosby, St Louis, 1998.

Scanlon, VC, and Sanders, T: Essentials of Anatomy and Physiology, ed 3. FA Davis, Philadelphia, 1999.

Selman, J: The Fundamentals of X-Ray and Radium Physics, ed 8. Charles C Thomas, Springfield, IL, 1994.

Sheldon, H: Boyd's Introduction to the Study of Disease, ed 10. Lea & Febiger, Philadelphia, 1988.

Snopek, AM: Fundamentals of Special Radiographic Procedures, ed 3. WB Saunders, Philadelphia, 1992.

Springhouse Medication Administration and I.V. Therapy Manual: Process and Procedures. Springhouse Corporation, Springhouse, PA, 1988.

Statkiewicz-Sherer, MA, et al: Radiation Protection in Medical Radiography, ed 3. Mosby, St Louis, 1998.

Sweeney, RJ: Radiographic Artifacts: Their Cause and Control. Lippincott, Philadelphia, 1983.

Taber's Cyclopedic Medical Dictionary, ed 18. FA Davis, Philadelphia, 1997.

Thompson MA, et al: Principles of Imaging Science and Protection. WB Saunders, Philadelphia, 1994.

Torres, LS: Basic Medical Techniques and Patient Care in Imaging Technology, ed 5. Lippincott, Philadelphia, 1997.

Tortora, GJ, and Grabowski, SR: Principles of Anatomy and Physiology, ed 7. HarperCollins, New York, 1993.

Tortorici, MR: Concepts in Medical Radiographic Imaging: Circuitry, Exposure and Quality Control. WB Saunders, Philadelphia, 1992.

Tortorici, MR, and Apfel, PJ: Advanced Radiographic and Angiographic Procedures. FA Davis, Philadelphia, 1995.

Travis, EL: Primer of Medical Radiobiology, ed 2. Year Book, Chicago, 1989.

Wallace, JE: Radiographic Exposure: Principles and Practice. FA Davis, Philadelphia, 1995.

Wilson, BG: Ethics and Basic Law for Medical Imaging Professionals. FA Davis, Philadelphia, 1997.

Wolbarst, AB: Physics of Radiology. Appleton & Lange, Norwalk, CT, 1993.

SIMULATION TEST #2

NAME_____
       Last   First   Middle

ADDRESS _____
            Street

_____
       City   State   Zip

. . . .

MAKE
ERASURES
COMPLETE

PLEASE USE NO. 2 PENCIL ONLY.

↓ BEGIN HERE

Radiation Protection and Radiobiology

01 Ⓐ Ⓑ Ⓒ Ⓓ	21 Ⓐ Ⓑ Ⓒ Ⓓ	41 Ⓐ Ⓑ Ⓒ Ⓓ	61 Ⓐ Ⓑ Ⓒ Ⓓ
02 Ⓐ Ⓑ Ⓒ Ⓓ	22 Ⓐ Ⓑ Ⓒ Ⓓ	42 Ⓐ Ⓑ Ⓒ Ⓓ	62 Ⓐ Ⓑ Ⓒ Ⓓ
03 Ⓐ Ⓑ Ⓒ Ⓓ	23 Ⓐ Ⓑ Ⓒ Ⓓ	43 Ⓐ Ⓑ Ⓒ Ⓓ	63 Ⓐ Ⓑ Ⓒ Ⓓ
04 Ⓐ Ⓑ Ⓒ Ⓓ	24 Ⓐ Ⓑ Ⓒ Ⓓ	44 Ⓐ Ⓑ Ⓒ Ⓓ	64 Ⓐ Ⓑ Ⓒ Ⓓ
05 Ⓐ Ⓑ Ⓒ Ⓓ	25 Ⓐ Ⓑ Ⓒ Ⓓ	45 Ⓐ Ⓑ Ⓒ Ⓓ	65 Ⓐ Ⓑ Ⓒ Ⓓ
06 Ⓐ Ⓑ Ⓒ Ⓓ	26 Ⓐ Ⓑ Ⓒ Ⓓ	46 Ⓐ Ⓑ Ⓒ Ⓓ	66 Ⓐ Ⓑ Ⓒ Ⓓ
07 Ⓐ Ⓑ Ⓒ Ⓓ	27 Ⓐ Ⓑ Ⓒ Ⓓ	47 Ⓐ Ⓑ Ⓒ Ⓓ	67 Ⓐ Ⓑ Ⓒ Ⓓ
08 Ⓐ Ⓑ Ⓒ Ⓓ	28 Ⓐ Ⓑ Ⓒ Ⓓ	48 Ⓐ Ⓑ Ⓒ Ⓓ	68 Ⓐ Ⓑ Ⓒ Ⓓ
09 Ⓐ Ⓑ Ⓒ Ⓓ	29 Ⓐ Ⓑ Ⓒ Ⓓ	49 Ⓐ Ⓑ Ⓒ Ⓓ	69 Ⓐ Ⓑ Ⓒ Ⓓ
10 Ⓐ Ⓑ Ⓒ Ⓓ	30 Ⓐ Ⓑ Ⓒ Ⓓ	50 Ⓐ Ⓑ Ⓒ Ⓓ	70 Ⓐ Ⓑ Ⓒ Ⓓ
11 Ⓐ Ⓑ Ⓒ Ⓓ	31 Ⓐ Ⓑ Ⓒ Ⓓ	51 Ⓐ Ⓑ Ⓒ Ⓓ	71 Ⓐ Ⓑ Ⓒ Ⓓ
12 Ⓐ Ⓑ Ⓒ Ⓓ	32 Ⓐ Ⓑ Ⓒ Ⓓ	52 Ⓐ Ⓑ Ⓒ Ⓓ	72 Ⓐ Ⓑ Ⓒ Ⓓ
13 Ⓐ Ⓑ Ⓒ Ⓓ	33 Ⓐ Ⓑ Ⓒ Ⓓ	53 Ⓐ Ⓑ Ⓒ Ⓓ	73 Ⓐ Ⓑ Ⓒ Ⓓ
14 Ⓐ Ⓑ Ⓒ Ⓓ	34 Ⓐ Ⓑ Ⓒ Ⓓ	54 Ⓐ Ⓑ Ⓒ Ⓓ	74 Ⓐ Ⓑ Ⓒ Ⓓ
15 Ⓐ Ⓑ Ⓒ Ⓓ	35 Ⓐ Ⓑ Ⓒ Ⓓ	55 Ⓐ Ⓑ Ⓒ Ⓓ	75 Ⓐ Ⓑ Ⓒ Ⓓ
16 Ⓐ Ⓑ Ⓒ Ⓓ	36 Ⓐ Ⓑ Ⓒ Ⓓ	56 Ⓐ Ⓑ Ⓒ Ⓓ	76 Ⓐ Ⓑ Ⓒ Ⓓ
17 Ⓐ Ⓑ Ⓒ Ⓓ	37 Ⓐ Ⓑ Ⓒ Ⓓ	57 Ⓐ Ⓑ Ⓒ Ⓓ	77 Ⓐ Ⓑ Ⓒ Ⓓ
18 Ⓐ Ⓑ Ⓒ Ⓓ	38 Ⓐ Ⓑ Ⓒ Ⓓ	58 Ⓐ Ⓑ Ⓒ Ⓓ	78 Ⓐ Ⓑ Ⓒ Ⓓ
19 Ⓐ Ⓑ Ⓒ Ⓓ	39 Ⓐ Ⓑ Ⓒ Ⓓ	59 Ⓐ Ⓑ Ⓒ Ⓓ	79 Ⓐ Ⓑ Ⓒ Ⓓ
20 Ⓐ Ⓑ Ⓒ Ⓓ	40 Ⓐ Ⓑ Ⓒ Ⓓ	60 Ⓐ Ⓑ Ⓒ Ⓓ	80 Ⓐ Ⓑ Ⓒ Ⓓ

Equipment Operation and Maintenance

Image Production and Evaluation

081 Ⓐ Ⓑ Ⓒ Ⓓ

Radiographic Procedures and Related Anatomy

111 Ⓐ Ⓑ Ⓒ Ⓓ

141 Ⓐ Ⓑ Ⓒ Ⓓ

Patient Care

171 Ⓐ Ⓑ Ⓒ Ⓓ

082 Ⓐ Ⓑ Ⓒ Ⓓ   112 Ⓐ Ⓑ Ⓒ Ⓓ   142 Ⓐ Ⓑ Ⓒ Ⓓ   172 Ⓐ Ⓑ Ⓒ Ⓓ

083 Ⓐ Ⓑ Ⓒ Ⓓ   113 Ⓐ Ⓑ Ⓒ Ⓓ   143 Ⓐ Ⓑ Ⓒ Ⓓ   173 Ⓐ Ⓑ Ⓒ Ⓓ

084 Ⓐ Ⓑ Ⓒ Ⓓ   114 Ⓐ Ⓑ Ⓒ Ⓓ   144 Ⓐ Ⓑ Ⓒ Ⓓ   174 Ⓐ Ⓑ Ⓒ Ⓓ

085 Ⓐ Ⓑ Ⓒ Ⓓ   115 Ⓐ Ⓑ Ⓒ Ⓓ   145 Ⓐ Ⓑ Ⓒ Ⓓ   175 Ⓐ Ⓑ Ⓒ Ⓓ

086 Ⓐ Ⓑ Ⓒ Ⓓ   116 Ⓐ Ⓑ Ⓒ Ⓓ   146 Ⓐ Ⓑ Ⓒ Ⓓ   176 Ⓐ Ⓑ Ⓒ Ⓓ

087 Ⓐ Ⓑ Ⓒ Ⓓ   117 Ⓐ Ⓑ Ⓒ Ⓓ   147 Ⓐ Ⓑ Ⓒ Ⓓ   177 Ⓐ Ⓑ Ⓒ Ⓓ

088 Ⓐ Ⓑ Ⓒ Ⓓ   118 Ⓐ Ⓑ Ⓒ Ⓓ   148 Ⓐ Ⓑ Ⓒ Ⓓ   178 Ⓐ Ⓑ Ⓒ Ⓓ

089 Ⓐ Ⓑ Ⓒ Ⓓ   119 Ⓐ Ⓑ Ⓒ Ⓓ   149 Ⓐ Ⓑ Ⓒ Ⓓ   179 Ⓐ Ⓑ Ⓒ Ⓓ

090 Ⓐ Ⓑ Ⓒ Ⓓ   120 Ⓐ Ⓑ Ⓒ Ⓓ   150 Ⓐ Ⓑ Ⓒ Ⓓ   180 Ⓐ Ⓑ Ⓒ Ⓓ

091 Ⓐ Ⓑ Ⓒ Ⓓ   121 Ⓐ Ⓑ Ⓒ Ⓓ   151 Ⓐ Ⓑ Ⓒ Ⓓ   181 Ⓐ Ⓑ Ⓒ Ⓓ

092 Ⓐ Ⓑ Ⓒ Ⓓ   122 Ⓐ Ⓑ Ⓒ Ⓓ   152 Ⓐ Ⓑ Ⓒ Ⓓ   182 Ⓐ Ⓑ Ⓒ Ⓓ

093 Ⓐ Ⓑ Ⓒ Ⓓ   123 Ⓐ Ⓑ Ⓒ Ⓓ   153 Ⓐ Ⓑ Ⓒ Ⓓ   183 Ⓐ Ⓑ Ⓒ Ⓓ

094 Ⓐ Ⓑ Ⓒ Ⓓ   124 Ⓐ Ⓑ Ⓒ Ⓓ   154 Ⓐ Ⓑ Ⓒ Ⓓ   184 Ⓐ Ⓑ Ⓒ Ⓓ

095 Ⓐ Ⓑ Ⓒ Ⓓ   125 Ⓐ Ⓑ Ⓒ Ⓓ   155 Ⓐ Ⓑ Ⓒ Ⓓ   185 Ⓐ Ⓑ Ⓒ Ⓓ

096 Ⓐ Ⓑ Ⓒ Ⓓ   126 Ⓐ Ⓑ Ⓒ Ⓓ   156 Ⓐ Ⓑ Ⓒ Ⓓ   186 Ⓐ Ⓑ Ⓒ Ⓓ

097 Ⓐ Ⓑ Ⓒ Ⓓ   127 Ⓐ Ⓑ Ⓒ Ⓓ   157 Ⓐ Ⓑ Ⓒ Ⓓ   187 Ⓐ Ⓑ Ⓒ Ⓓ

098 Ⓐ Ⓑ Ⓒ Ⓓ   128 Ⓐ Ⓑ Ⓒ Ⓓ   158 Ⓐ Ⓑ Ⓒ Ⓓ   188 Ⓐ Ⓑ Ⓒ Ⓓ

099 Ⓐ Ⓑ Ⓒ Ⓓ   129 Ⓐ Ⓑ Ⓒ Ⓓ   159 Ⓐ Ⓑ Ⓒ Ⓓ   189 Ⓐ Ⓑ Ⓒ Ⓓ

100 Ⓐ Ⓑ Ⓒ Ⓓ   130 Ⓐ Ⓑ Ⓒ Ⓓ   160 Ⓐ Ⓑ Ⓒ Ⓓ   190 Ⓐ Ⓑ Ⓒ Ⓓ

101 Ⓐ Ⓑ Ⓒ Ⓓ   131 Ⓐ Ⓑ Ⓒ Ⓓ   161 Ⓐ Ⓑ Ⓒ Ⓓ   191 Ⓐ Ⓑ Ⓒ Ⓓ

102 Ⓐ Ⓑ Ⓒ Ⓓ   132 Ⓐ Ⓑ Ⓒ Ⓓ   162 Ⓐ Ⓑ Ⓒ Ⓓ   192 Ⓐ Ⓑ Ⓒ Ⓓ

103 Ⓐ Ⓑ Ⓒ Ⓓ   133 Ⓐ Ⓑ Ⓒ Ⓓ   163 Ⓐ Ⓑ Ⓒ Ⓓ   193 Ⓐ Ⓑ Ⓒ Ⓓ

104 Ⓐ Ⓑ Ⓒ Ⓓ   134 Ⓐ Ⓑ Ⓒ Ⓓ   164 Ⓐ Ⓑ Ⓒ Ⓓ   194 Ⓐ Ⓑ Ⓒ Ⓓ

105 Ⓐ Ⓑ Ⓒ Ⓓ   135 Ⓐ Ⓑ Ⓒ Ⓓ   165 Ⓐ Ⓑ Ⓒ Ⓓ   195 Ⓐ Ⓑ Ⓒ Ⓓ

106 Ⓐ Ⓑ Ⓒ Ⓓ   136 Ⓐ Ⓑ Ⓒ Ⓓ   166 Ⓐ Ⓑ Ⓒ Ⓓ   196 Ⓐ Ⓑ Ⓒ Ⓓ

107 Ⓐ Ⓑ Ⓒ Ⓓ   137 Ⓐ Ⓑ Ⓒ Ⓓ   167 Ⓐ Ⓑ Ⓒ Ⓓ   197 Ⓐ Ⓑ Ⓒ Ⓓ

108 Ⓐ Ⓑ Ⓒ Ⓓ   138 Ⓐ Ⓑ Ⓒ Ⓓ   168 Ⓐ Ⓑ Ⓒ Ⓓ   198 Ⓐ Ⓑ Ⓒ Ⓓ

109 Ⓐ Ⓑ Ⓒ Ⓓ   139 Ⓐ Ⓑ Ⓒ Ⓓ   169 Ⓐ Ⓑ Ⓒ Ⓓ   199 Ⓐ Ⓑ Ⓒ Ⓓ

110 Ⓐ Ⓑ Ⓒ Ⓓ   140 Ⓐ Ⓑ Ⓒ Ⓓ   170 Ⓐ Ⓑ Ⓒ Ⓓ   200 Ⓐ Ⓑ Ⓒ Ⓓ

SIMULATION EXAMINATION 3

Questions

Directions: (Questions 1 to 200) For each of the following items, select the best answer among the four possible choices (A, B, C, or D). For ease of scoring, it is suggested that you use the bubble sheet provided in the back of this examination. Make sure to answer all questions. You should allow yourself a maximum of three hours to take this examination.

Refer to the scale in the back of the book to determine a passing score in each section. It is not necessary that you pass each section, but you must receive a total "scaled" score of 75 to pass the examination.

SECTION I: RADIATION PROTECTION AND RADIOBIOLOGY

1. If the patient is required to hold the cassette during an exposure, any portion of the body other than the area of clinical interest that may be struck by the primary beam must be covered by at least:
   A. 0.25-mm lead (Pb) equivalent
   B. 0.5-mm Pb equivalent
   C. 2.5-mm Pb equivalent
   D. 5.0-mm Pb equivalent

2. Which of the following types of radiation-induced cancers appears to exhibit a threshold?
   A. Leukemia
   B. Skin cancer
   C. Breast cancer
   D. Thyroid cancer

3. Early biological effects of radiation that may be observable are:
   A. Produced by high radiation doses
   B. Experienced regularly by radiographers
   C. Caused by chronic low doses
   D. Seen in a patient following a nuclear medicine "bone scan"

4. What concept do the initials RBE represent?
   A. The amount of radiation necessary to double the amount of genetic mutations in a population
   B. The amount of energy deposited by radiation in a micron of tissue
   C. The comparison of various types of radiation and their resulting biologic effects
   D. The maximum amount of radiation that a radiographer may be exposed to annually

5. What is the result if the radiographer repeats a radiograph using a decrease in kilovolts (peak) (kVp)?
   A. An increase in radiographic density
   B. An increase in patient's skin dose
   C. An increase in the radiographer's dose
   D. An increase in recorded detail

6. What is the maximum radiation dose in a single month that the fetus of a pregnant radiographer is allowed to receive?
   A. 0.5 mSv (0.05 rem)
   B. 5 mSv (0.5 rem)
   C. 50 mSv (5 rem)
   D. 150 mSv (15 rem)

113

7. When radiation interacts with matter through the process of photoelectric interaction, the incident photon is:
   A. Scattered with reduced energy
   B. Scattered with no change in energy
   C. Completely absorbed by an inner-shell electron
   D. Completely absorbed by the atomic nucleus

8. A radiation detection device that measures the amount of current flow resulting from an interaction between ionizing radiation and an appropriate gas is known as a(an)
   A. Scintillation detector
   B. Ionization chamber
   C. Thermoluminescent dosimeter (TLD)
   D. Cloud chamber

9. Which of the following effects may increase from chronic doses of radiation exposure?
   1. Leukemia
   2. Nonspecific shortening of the life span
   3. Cataractogenesis
   A. 1 and 2 only
   B. 1 and 3 only
   C. 2 and 3 only
   D. 1, 2, and 3

10. Which of the following protective measures may radiographers use to protect the patient from unnecessary radiation exposure?
    1. High-kilovolt (peak) exposure factors
    2. Reducing the field size
    3. Slow-speed screens
    A. 1 and 2 only
    B. 1 and 3 only
    C. 2 and 3 only
    D. 1, 2, and 3

11. What is the recommended minimum lead equivalent for protective gloves worn by the radiographer during a fluoroscopic procedure?
    A. 0.25-mm Pb equivalent
    B. 0.50-mm Pb equivalent
    C. 2.5-mm Pb equivalent
    D. 5.0-mm Pb equivalent

12. When kilovolts (peak) is increased with a compensating reduction in milliamperage-seconds, a decrease in _____ results.
    A. Scatter radiation reaching the film
    B. Radiographic density
    C. Quantum mottle
    D. Patient dose

13. The reduction in radiation intensity as x rays pass through matter is referred to as:
    A. Transmutation
    B. Isotropic propagation
    C. Attenuation
    D. Quantum mottle

14. Examples of somatic effects of radiation include:
    1. Skin erythema
    2. Thyroid cancer
    3. Leukopenia
    A. 1 and 2 only
    B. 1 and 3 only
    C. 2 and 3 only
    D. 1, 2, and 3

15. According to the National Council on Radiation Protection and Measurement (NCRP), to what level should the primary barrier reduce the radiation intensity in a controlled area that is limited to occupational personnel?
    A. 10 mR/wk
    B. 50 mR/wk
    C. 100 mR/wk
    D. 500 mR/wk

16. What should the minimum source-skin distance (SSD) be on a fixed fluoroscopic unit?
    A. 30 cm (12 in.)
    B. 38 cm (15 in.)
    C. 45 cm (18 in.)
    D. 60 cm (24 in.)

17. Which of the following is the best method of protection from ionizing radiation for the radiographer?
    A. Increased lead shielding
    B. Increased distance
    C. Increased time
    D. Increased filtration

18. What are the possible results when a fetus is exposed to radiation in utero?
    1. Spontaneous abortion
    2. Neonatal death
    3. Congenital anomalies
    A. 1 and 2 only
    B. 1 and 3 only
    C. 2 and 3 only
    D. 1, 2, and 3

19. Which of the following types of equipment would be most effective at reducing the genetic significant dose to the population?
    A. Linear tomographic machines
    B. Fluoroscopic machines
    C. Positive beam limitation (PBL)
    D. Computed tomography (CT) machines

20. Radiation that leaves the x-ray tube housing by any other means than through the window or tube port is referred to as:
    A. Leakage radiation
    B. Primary radiation
    C. Scatter radiation
    D. Remnant radiation

21. Which of the following x-ray interactions occurs most often with x-ray photons of energies in excess of 100 kiloelectron volts (keV)?
    A. Photoelectric effect
    B. Compton scattering
    C. Pair production
    D. Photodisintegration

22. Which of the following radiation detectors is sometimes referred to as a "cutie pie"?
    A. Victoreen condenser R-meter
    B. Geiger-Müller detector
    C. Ionization chamber–type survey meter
    D. Proportional counter

23. If the intensity of a radiation source is 100 mR/h at a distance of 1 m, what is the intensity at a distance of 3 m from the source?
    A. 11 mR/h
    B. 30 mR/h
    C. 300 mR/h
    D. 900 mR/h

24. Which of the following statements is true regarding the biologic effects of ionizing radiation?
    A. Damage to an exposed individual may not be passed on to the progeny.
    B. No effects are seen below dose-equivalent limits.
    C. Mutated cells only occur following high-radiation dose levels.
    D. The body has the ability to repair most damage.

25. Figure 3–1 graphically depicts the mean survival time for the acute radiation syndrome. Which area on the graph would estimate the dose received by a victim suffering from the gastrointestinal (GI) syndrome?
    A. Area A
    B. Area B
    C. Area C
    D. Area D

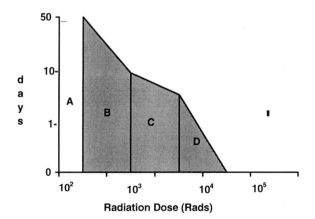

FIGURE 3–1. Graph of mean survival time for acute radiation syndrome (ARS).

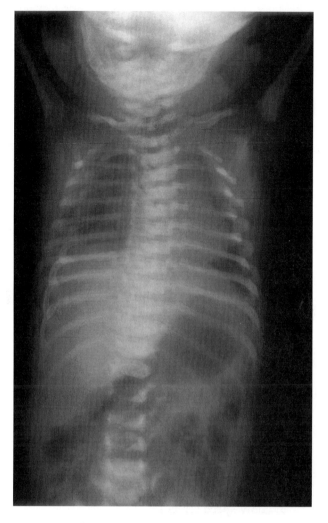

FIGURE 3–2. Neonatal chest radiograph.

26. The effective dose-equivalent limit for the general population is limited to:
    A. 0.2 mSv/yr (0.02 rem/yr)
    B. 4 mSv/yr (0.4 rem/yr)
    C. 5 mSv/yr (0.5 rem/yr)
    D. 50 mSv/yr (5 rem/yr)

27. Which of the following radiation protection principles has been violated as evidenced by the radiograph of a neonatal chest in Figure 3–2?
    A. Failure to provide adequate shielding
    B. Failure to collimate
    C. Failure to use a detail speed screen
    D. Failure to use adequate kilovolts (peak)

28. How far below the collimator should the patient's skin surface be placed to protect the patient from possible exposure to electrons produced by photon interaction with the collimator?
    A. 8 cm (3.14 in.)
    B. 12 cm (4.7 in.)
    C. 15 cm (5.9 in.)
    D. 20 cm (7.9 in.)

29. A cumulative timing device on the fluoroscopic tube should emit an audible sound to alert radiological practitioners of fluoroscopic exposure ON time. This device should sound after the fluoroscope has been activated for:
    A. 2 minutes
    B. 5 minutes
    C. 8 minutes
    D. 10 minutes

30. Several factors are used when determining the appropriate lead thickness in walls. The use factor is based on:
    A. How often the x-ray beam is in use
    B. How many people will occupy the area in a given time
    C. What total amount of milliamperage-seconds is used during a week's time
    D. What percentage of time the primary x-ray beam will be striking a barrier

SECTION II: EQUIPMENT OPERATION AND MAINTENANCE

31. What is the formula that is used to calculate heat units in a high-frequency generator?
    A. mA × Time × kVp   *single phase*
    B. mA × Time × kVp × 1.35   *6 pulse*
    C. mA × Time × kVp × 1.41   *12 pulse*
    D. mA × time × kVp × 1.45   *high*

32. General-purpose x-ray tubes typically have an inherent filtration of:
    A. 0.10-mm aluminum (Al) equivalent
    B. 0.15-mm Al equivalent
    C. 1.0-mm Al equivalent
    D. 2.5-mm Al equivalent

33. The filter in the developer section of an automatic processor is used for:
    A. Silver reclamation
    B. Removing the film gelatin
    C. Removing the buildup of algae
    D. Eliminating cross-contamination of chemicals

34. A fine, tightly coiled thread of tungsten that is mounted in the cathode of the x-ray tube is called the
    A. Focusing cup
    B. Filament
    C. Autotransformer
    D. Phototimer

For questions 35 and 36, refer to Figure 3–3:

35. In Figure 3–3, the part of the image intensifier labeled number 4 is the
    A. Input phosphor
    B. Output phosphor
    C. Electrostatic lenses
    D. Photocathode

36. In Figure 3–3, the part of the image intensifier labeled number 1 is the
    A. Electrostatic lenses
    B. Input phosphor
    C. Output phosphor
    D. Photocathode

37. Any material that allows the free flow of electrons is called a(an)
    A. Resistor
    B. Transducer
    C. Insulator
    D. Conductor

38. In an automatic processor, which of the following is used to prevent cross-contamination of chemicals?
    A. Crossover assembly rack
    B. Splash guards
    C. Squeegee rollers
    D. Replenishment microswitch

39. What is the purpose of the vidicon or plumbicon in an image intensifier?
    A. When activated, can expose several frames per second
    B. Converts the light image to an electronic signal that is sent to the cathode-ray tube (CRT)
    C. Is coupled with the input phosphor for direct viewing of the image
    D. Focuses the electronic signal from the input side to the output side

40. The milliamperage meter in a x-ray circuit is located between the _____ and the _____.
    A. Step-up transformer; x-ray tube
    B. Step-down transformer; x-ray tube
    C. Rheostat; rectification system
    D. Autotransformer; timer

41. Approximately 99 percent of the kinetic energy of the high-speed electron stream is converted to _____ when it strikes the target on the anode.
    A. X-radiation
    B. Gamma radiation
    C. Thermal radiation
    D. Light waves

For questions 42 and 43, refer to Figure 3–4:

42. If a particular examination generates 350,000 heat units (HU) in the anode of the x-ray tube, determine how long it will take the anode to cool completely.
    A. 3 minutes
    B. 5 minutes
    C. 6 minutes
    D. 8 minutes

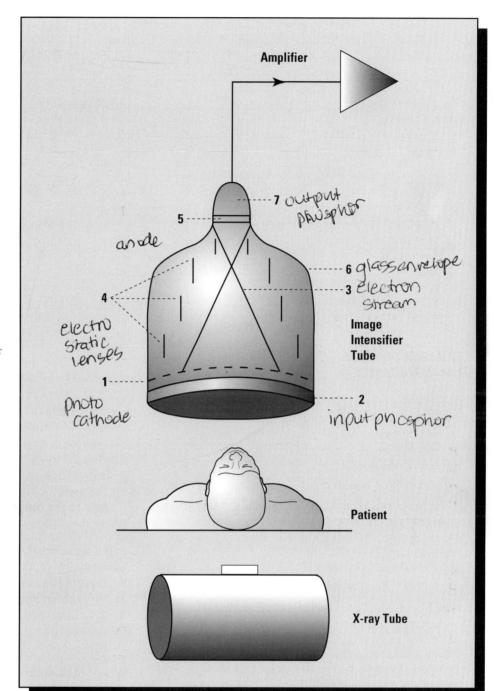

FIGURE 3–3. Image intensifier tube.

The following handwritten labels appear on the figure:

Amplifier

7 output phosphor

5

anode

6 glass envelope

3 electron stream

4

electro static lenses

Image Intensifier Tube

1

photo cathode

2

input phosphor

Patient

X-ray Tube

43. If the anode has reached its maximum heat capacity of 500,000 HU, how long will the radiographer have to wait before attempting an exposure using technical factors of 83 kVp, 800 mA, and 1.5 seconds?
   A. 1.5 minutes
   B. 2 minutes
   C. 3 minutes
   D. 5 minutes

44. The kilovolt (peak) setting needed to produce an x-ray beam with a minimum wavelength of 0.10 Å is:
   A. 60 kVp
   B. 80 kVp
   C. 100 kVp
   D. 125 kVp

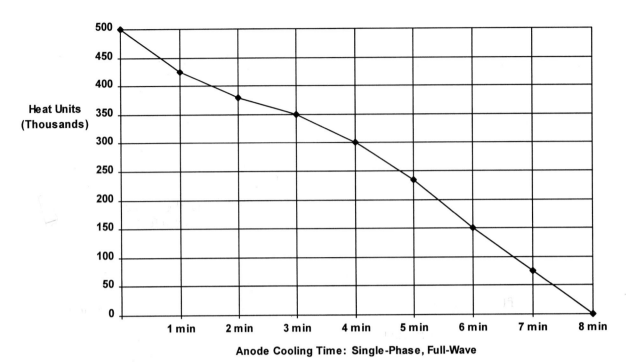

FIGURE 3–4. Anode-cooling curve.

45. An apparatus located in a circuit that acts as an insulator of electricity in one direction but conducts electricity in the opposite direction is called a:
    A. Capacitor
    B. Rectifier
    C. Transformer
    D. Rheostat

46. Which of the following meters registers only during the actual x-ray exposure?
    A. Milliammeter
    B. Prereading kilovolt meter
    C. Kilovolt meter
    D. Prereading milliammeter

47. What corrective action should be taken if a wire-mesh test performed by the quality control technologist displays an area of localized blurring on the image?
    A. Retake a radiograph using a test phantom to pinpoint the problem.
    B. The cassette should be repaired or discarded.
    C. Replace the viewbox illuminator bulbs, and reset the photometer.
    D. Post a note on the cassette to inform all radiographers to adjust technique accordingly.

48. All electromagnetic radiation travels at a velocity of:
    A. 3×10^8 m/s
    B. 3×10^{10} m/s
    C. 18,000 m/s
    D. 186,000 m/s

49. In the x-ray tube, the speed at which electrons are accelerated from the cathode to the anode side is determined by:
    A. Heat of the filament
    B. Voltage applied to the tube
    C. Heat of the anode
    D. Angle of the tube target

50. A special imaging technique in which various selected planes of the body can be demonstrated on a radiograph is known as:
    A. Stereoradiography
    B. Cinefluorography
    C. Tomography
    D. Sonography

51. Which of the following may be classified as basic types of x-ray generators?
    1. Half-phase
    2. Single-phase
    3. High-frequency

    A. 1 and 2 only
    B. 1 and 3 only
    C. 2 and 3 only
    D. 1, 2, and 3

52. The filament transformer in the x-ray tube is an example of a(an)
    A. Autotransformer
    B. Step-up transformer
    C. Step-down transformer
    D. Capacitor discharge

53. In an automatic processor, only the silver halide crystals that contain _____ are reduced to black metallic silver by the developing solution.
    A. Ionic bonds
    B. The latent image
    C. Negative surface electrification
    D. Oxidized silver bromide

54. Which of the following interactions of x rays with matter is more likely to occur with an inner-shell electron?
    A. Compton scattering
    B. Classical scattering
    C. Pair production
    D. Photoelectric effect

55. What is the primary function of the quality control test known as the star test pattern?
    A. To check the film-screen contact
    B. To test the accuracy of the phototimer
    C. To measure the size of the focal spot
    D. To check linearity or reproducibility

56. Which of the following would be a possible fluoroscopic milliampere setting?
    A. 3 mA
    B. 30 mA
    C. 300 mA
    D. 3000 mA

57. For which of the following is a manual spinning top used to check the accuracy of the timer?
    1. Single-phase
    2. 3-phase
    3. High-frequency

    A. 1 only
    B. 2 only

C. 3 only
D. 1, 2, and 3

58. What type of radiation is produced when a high-speed electron is decelerated as it approaches the nucleus of a target atom?
    A. Compton scattering
    B. *Bremsstrahlung*
    C. Characteristic
    D. Remnant

59. The chemical properties of an element may be determined by the number of electrons in its outer shell. This is referred to as the atom's
    A. Atomic number
    B. Valence number
    C. Atomic weight
    D. Electrical charge

60. According to Figure 3–5, which of the following sets of technical factors would be considered "safe"?
    A. 75 mA, 2 seconds, 70 kVp
    B. 100 mA, 2 seconds, 60 kVp
    C. 100 mA, 1 second, 60 kVp
    D. 125 mA, 0.5 second, 50 kVp

SECTION III: IMAGE PRODUCTION AND EVALUATION

61. In which of the following radiographic procedures would a small focal spot be of greatest benefit?
    A. Skull radiography
    B. Chest radiography
    C. Nephrotomography
    D. Magnification radiography

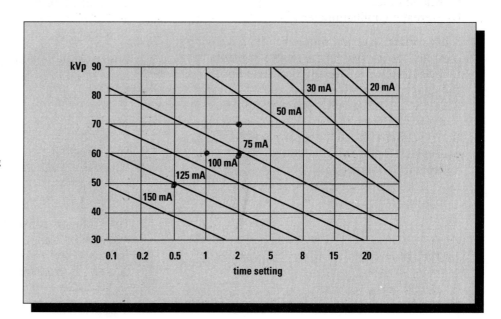

FIGURE 3–5. X-ray tube rating chart.

62. What technical factors would be required for a 400-speed imaging system if an optimum technique required technical factors of 400 mA, 0.25 second, and 65 kVp while using a 200-speed imaging system?
    A. 400 mA, 0.50 second, 65 kVp
    B. 200 mA, 0.50 second, 65 kVp
    C. 400 mA, 0.50 second, 75 kVp
    D. 200 mA, 0.25 second, 65 kVp

63. While performing a lateral projection of the lumbar vertebrae on an asthenic patient, the radiographer activates both side cells on an automatic exposure control (AEC) device. The resultant radiograph would most likely appear to have:
    A. Excessive radiographic density
    B. Insufficient radiographic density
    C. Motion due to excessive exposure time
    D. Grid lines because side cells fail to activate the reciprocating Bucky

64. A dual-emulsion film exiting from an automatic processor with a wet or tacky surface may be caused by:
    1. Depletion of hardener in the fixer
    2. Depletion of hardener in the developer
    3. Dryer temperature too low

    A. 1 and 2 only
    B. 1 and 3 only
    C. 2 and 3 only
    D. 1, 2, and 3

65. Which of the following would require an increase in technical factors for the radiograph?
    A. Emphysema
    B. Osteolytic lesion
    C. Hemothorax
    D. Osteoporosis

66. Which of the following properties should a phosphor exhibit in order for the phosphor to be effective in an intensifying screen?
    1. High x-ray absorption
    2. High conversion efficiency
    3. Phosphorescence

    A. 1 and 2 only
    B. 1 and 3 only
    C. 2 and 3 only
    D. 1, 2, and 3

67. Which of the following will increase resolution or recorded detail?
    A. A large space charge
    B. A strongly positive anode
    C. A large phosphor crystal
    D. A small focal spot

68. Which of the following sets of technical factors would result in the image with the shortest scale of contrast?

mA	Exposure Time	kVp	FSS
A. 100	0.5	65	1.0
B. 200	0.3	75	1.0
C. 300	0.1	80	0.5
D. 100	0.2	85	0.5

69. If a satisfactory radiograph were taken using technical factors of 75 kVp, 400 mA, and 0.25 second at a 72-inch source-image receptor-distance (SID), what new technical factors would be necessary if the SID was changed to 40 inches?
    A. 75 kVp, 400 mA, 0.075 second
    B. 75 kVp, 400 mA, 0.75 second
    C. 85 kVp, 400 mA, 0.25 second
    D. 65 kVp, 400 mA, 0.25 second

70. Which of the following technical factors primarily regulates the quantity of x-ray photons delivered to the patient in a given exposure?
    A. Kilovolts at peak value
    B. Milliamperage-seconds
    C. SID
    D. Focal spot size (FSS)

71. If an object is placed at a distance of 10 inches from the image receptor with a SID of 40 inches, what is the size of the object if the image size measures 15 inches?
    A. 3.75 inches
    B. 5 inches
    C. 11.25 inches
    D. 20 inches

72. Which two sets of milliamperes and time represent an example of the reciprocity law?
    1. 200 mA, 0.05 second
    2. 400 mA, 0.03 second
    3. 500 mA, 0.02 second
    4. 600 mA, 0.05 second

    A. 1 and 3
    B. 2 and 4
    C. 1 and 4
    D. 2 and 3

73. When compensating wedge filters are used, the thickest end of the filter should always be placed:
    A. Toward the thicker anatomy
    B. Toward the patient's feet
    C. Toward the patient's head
    D. Toward the thinner anatomy

74. A positive contrast medium readily absorbs radiation because of its:
    A. Thickness
    B. Viscosity
    C. Atomic number
    D. Density

75. Which of the following technical factors will produce the greatest radiographic density?

	mA	Exposure Time	kVp	Screen Speed
A.	400	0.01 s	94	100
B.	500	0.008 s	94	200
C.	200	0.04 s	90	50
D.	100	0.02 s	80	200

6. If a focused grid is used outside of its intended SID range, the result will most likely be:
   A. Top of the film underexposed
   B. Both sides of the film underexposed
   C. One side of the film underexposed
   D. The center of the film underexposed

77. What type of phosphor material was in Roentgen's laboratory when he discovered x rays?
   A. Cesium iodide
   B. Calcium tungstate
   C. Barium platinocyanide
   D. Lithium fluoride

78. What is the ultimate outcome if a radiographer needs to repeat a radiograph with an increase in radiographic contrast?
   A. Creation of greater difference between the black and white optical densities of adjacent structures
   B. An increase in the range of gray tones that may be visible in the image
   C. Production of a radiograph with long scale and greater latitude
   D. An increase in the kilovolt (peak) setting

79. The number of grid strips or grid lines per unit value is known as:
   A. Grid ratio
   B. Line-pairs per millimeter
   C. Interspatial ratio
   D. Grid frequency

80. Which of the following sets of technical factors will result in the best recorded detail?

	mAs	kVp	SID	OID	FSS	Screen Speed
A.	25	70	100 cm	10 cm	0.6 mm	200
B.	12	80	180 cm	10 cm	0.6 mm	100
C.	15	70	180 cm	20 cm	0.6 mm	200
D.	20	80	100 cm	20 cm	1.2 mm	100

81. The instrument used to measure varying degrees of film exposure and that is essential to a quality assurance program is called a
   A. Sensitometer
   B. Densitometer
   C. Penetrometer
   D. Oscilloscope

82. Manufacturers of x-ray film have found that when silver iodide and _____ are added to the silver bromide crystals in the film emulsion, the crystals become more sensitive to the x-ray photon energy range.
   A. Silver nitrate
   B. Potassium bromide
   C. Mustard oil
   D. Gelatin colloid suspension

83. What is the purpose of radiographic contrast in an image?
   A. To reduce the possible parallax effect from dual-emulsion films
   B. To aid in the visibility of detail of the image
   C. To diminish the effects of impurities in the film emulsion
   D. To overcome the inherent base plus fog in the film

84. Blurring of the radiographic image caused by movement of either the patient or the x-ray tube during exposure is called:
   A. Geometric unsharpness
   B. Shape distortion
   C. Motion unsharpness
   D. Radiographic parallax

85. Which of the following will serve to reduce radiographic noise in an image?
   1. Use of a lower-kilovolt (peak) setting
   2. Use of a lower-milliampere setting
   3. Use of slower-speed imaging receptors

   A. 1 and 2 only
   B. 1 and 3 only
   C. 2 and 3 only
   D. 1, 2, and 3

86. What is the exposure time if the milliampere setting is at 400 and the milliampere meter on the operating console measures 60?
   A. 0.10 second
   B. 0.15 second
   C. 0.45 second
   D. 0.67 second

87. Which of the following contrast media, when added to the body, decreases the tissue density of the body part?
   A. Carbon dioxide
   B. Gastroview
   C. Barium sulfate
   D. Pantopaque

88. What is the main purpose of using the line focus principle in an x-ray tube?
   A. To decrease the heat capacity
   B. To decrease the maximum milliamperes
   C. To decrease the anode heel effect
   D. To decrease the effective FSS

89. Which set of technical factors would produce a radiograph with the least optical density?

mA	Exposure Time
A. 200 mA	1/10 s
B. 400 mA	1/40 s
C. 300 mA	1/20 s
D. 100 mA	1/3 s

90. What is the area of the image if the area of an object is 10 inches when using a magnification factor (MF) of ×2?
    A. 2 inches
    B. 10 inches
    C. 20 inches
    D. 40 inches

91. Which of the following radiographic qualities will be improved with the use of a compression band when radiographing a cooperative patient for an abdomen?
    A. Recorded detail
    B. Density
    C. Contrast
    D. Shape distortion

92. Of the following quality assurance tests, which will determine the accuracy of the kilovolt (peak) settings?
    A. Wire-mesh test
    B. Wisconsin test cassette
    C. Pinhole camera
    D. Star test pattern

93. When is it advisable for the radiographer to use a grid?
    1. When kilovolts (peak) exceeds 70
    2. When radiographing body parts thicker than 12 cm
    3. When the anatomy contains mostly soft tissue (low atomic number)

    A. 1 and 2 only
    B. 1 and 3 only
    C. 2 and 3 only
    D. 1, 2, and 3

94. Which of the following sets of technical factors would result in the greatest magnification?
    A. 40-inch SID, 5-inch object-image receptor-distance (OID)
    B. 60-inch SID, 10-inch OID
    C. 72-inch SID; 25-inch OID
    D. 80-inch SID; 30-inch OID

95. Which of the following sensitometric measurements should evaluate the consistency of film contrast in a quality control program?
    A. Medium density
    B. Density difference
    C. Base-plus-fog
    D. Maximum density

96. Which of the following statements is correct if it is necessary to increase contrast in a radiograph?
    A. Increase the range of optical densities between adjacent structures.
    B. Increase the amount of gray shades that are visible in the image.
    C. Produce a radiograph with a longer scale of contrast.
    D. Increase the average energy of the x-ray beam (kilovolts [peak]).

97. Which of the following statements are true regarding radiographic pathology?
    1. Certain pathology may actually increase tissue mass and density.
    2. Metastasis makes the tissue density more radiopaque.
    3. Atrophy makes the tissue more radiolucent.

    A. 1 and 2 only
    B. 1 and 3 only
    C. 2 and 3 only
    D. 1, 2, and 3

98. What relationship does the milliamperage have to the x-ray intensity?
    A. Inversely proportional
    B. Directly proportional
    C. Exponentially proportional
    D. Inverse-square

99. What is the purpose of a small focal spot?
    A. Increases the heat capacity of the x-ray tube
    B. Increases the efficiency of x-ray production
    C. Increases the amount of milliamperage available
    D. Increases the resolution on the radiograph

100. Making adjustments in the kilovolts (peak) is the best way to control:
    A. Radiation quantity
    B. Magnification
    C. Scale of contrast
    D. Braking radiation

101. What is the best way to measure the quality of an x-ray beam?
    A. Spinning top test
    B. Step wedge
    C. Half-value layer (HVL)
    D. Star test pattern

102. What may be the result when the processor development time is excessive?
    A. Speed decreases
    B. Fog increases
    C. Contrast increases
    D. Latitude decreases

103. The use of a longer SID will result in:
    A. An increase in patient dose
    B. The need for reduced kilovolts (peak)
    C. Greater magnification
    D. Less geometric blur

104. The light photons emitted from intensifying screens form a radiographic image in the film by interacting with the
    A. Atoms in the iodine and gelatin of the film emulsion
    B. Atoms in silver halide crystals
    C. Black metallic silver
    D. Blue-tinted dye in the base

105. At lower diagnostic energies (less than 70 keV), the majority of x-ray interactions will:
    A. Be Compton scattering events
    B. Penetrate the patient and expose the film
    C. Be photoelectric events
    D. Require reduced milliamperage-seconds

106. As the milliamperage-seconds are increased:
    A. X-ray quantity will increase proportionately
    B. X-ray quality will increase proportionately
    C. X-ray quantity will be greatly reduced
    D. The optical density will decrease inversely

107. A 16 × 8 cm aperture diaphragm is located 10 cm below the x-ray source at a 40-cm SID. What is the size of the exposed field?
    A. 4 cm × 2 cm
    B. 8 cm × 4 cm
    C. 32 cm × 16 cm
    D. 64 cm × 32 cm

108. Which one of the following collimator field sizes would provide the greatest radiation protection to the patient?
    A. 15-cm diameter circular field
    B. 12 × 12 cm square field
    C. 14 × 10 cm rectangular field
    D. 12 × 13 cm rectangular field

109. Which of the following film-screen-system image qualities is comparable to the brightness (window level) of a computed radiographic image?
    A. Density
    B. Contrast
    C. Recorded detail
    D. Distortion

110. One type of film used to record an image from a computer screen is:
    A. Periapical film
    B. Occlusal film
    C. Roll film
    D. Laser film

SECTION IV: RADIOGRAPHIC PROCEDURES AND RELATED ANATOMY

111. A standard posteroanterior (PA) chest radiograph is usually obtained with a horizontal x-ray beam at a SID of:
    A. 3 ft
    B. 6 ft
    C. 7 ft
    D. 9 ft

112. Which of the following radiographic projections best demonstrates medial or lateral displacement of fractures of the nasal bones?
    A. Lateral
    B. Oblique
    C. Inferosuperior axial
    D. Parietoacanthial

113. How should the central ray be angled for an anteroposterior (AP) projection of the sacrum?
    A. Perpendicular to the plane of the film
    B. Parallel to the sacroiliac joints
    C. 15° cephalad
    D. 10° caudad

114. How much should the radiographer rotate the patient from the vertical position to demonstrate the apophyseal joints of the thoracic vertebrae?
    A. 20°
    B. 30°
    C. 45°
    D. 70°

115. Where is the proper central ray centering point for an AP projection of the hand?
    A. Second metacarpophalangeal joint
    B. Base of the third metacarpal
    C. Base of the fourth metacarpal
    D. Third metacarpophalangeal joint

116. How much angulation of the central ray would be required for a tangential projection of the os calcis?
    A. 20°
    B. 30°
    C. 40°
    D. 45°

117. What type of specialized examination is represented by the radiograph in Figure 3–6?
    A. Hysterosalpingogram
    B. Cystogram
    C. Voiding cystourethrogram
    D. Retrograde pyelogram

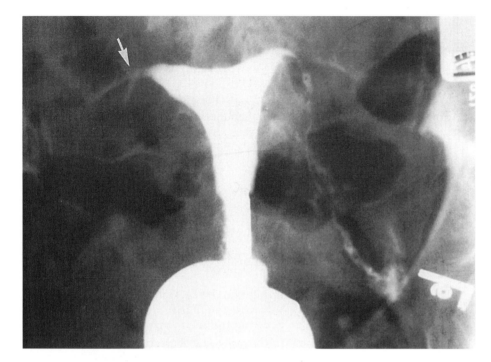

FIGURE 3–6. (From Tortorici, MR, and Apfel, PJ: Advanced Radiographic and Angiographic Procedures: With an Introduction to Specialized Imaging. FA Davis, Philadelphia, 1995, p 58, with permission.)

118. The best radiographic demonstration of a pneumothorax would be achieved by a
   A. Lateral projection of the chest in the erect position
   B. Lateral projection of the chest in the ventral decubitus position
   C. PA projection of the chest with expiration
   D. PA projection of the chest with inspiration

119. Which of the following is a necessary criterion for demonstrating the intercondyloid fossa?
   A. The knee should be flexed 90°.
   B. The central ray should be directed perpendicular to the knee joint.
   C. The patient's lower leg should be rotated medially 45°.
   D. The central ray should be directed perpendicular to the lower leg.

120. How does the stomach lie in the asthenic patient?
   A. Low and vertical
   B. Low and horizontal
   C. High and vertical
   D. High and horizontal

121. From which chamber of the heart does the aorta arise?
   A. Right atrium
   B. Left atrium
   C. Right ventricle
   D. Left ventricle

122. To demonstrate the swallowing function during a radiological procedure, how should the patient be positioned at the start of a fluoroscopic examination of the esophagus?

   A. Oblique or lateral erect position
   B. Left lateral decubitus position
   C. Recumbent left anterior oblique (LAO) position
   D. Recumbent right anterior oblique (RAO) position

123. The sense of equilibrium, or balance, is controlled by an organ(s) in the inner ear called the
   A. Cochlea
   B. Semicircular canals
   C. Malleus, incus, and stapes
   D. Canaliculi

124. What is the longest blood vessel in the human body?
   A. Aorta
   B. Femoral artery
   C. Great saphenous vein
   D. Inferior vena cava

125. What is the average degree of separation between the orbitomeatal line (OML) and the glabellomeatal line in an adult?
   A. 1°
   B. 5°
   C. 6°
   D. 8°

126. Posterior displacement of the fibula in a lower leg fracture would best be demonstrated with the
   A. AP projection
   B. Lateral projection
   C. Medial oblique projection
   D. Lateral oblique projection

127. The best method to localize lymphatic vessels for pedal lymphangiography is to use:
 A. A blue-staining dye
 B. Ethiodized oil
 C. A scalpel and a scope
 D. A water-soluble iodinated medium

128. In the anterior oblique position of the cervical vertebrae, the central ray should be directed:
 A. Perpendicular to C4
 B. 15° cephalad to C4
 C. 15° caudad to C4
 D. 25° cephalad to C4

129. Which of the following structures are best demonstrated on the lateral projection of the thoracic vertebrae?
 A. Intervertebral foramina
 B. Apophyseal articulations
 C. Transverse processes
 D. Laminae

130. What is the name of the flexure that lies between the transverse colon and the ascending colon?
 A. Splenic
 B. Ileocecal
 C. Hepatic
 D. Sigmoid

131. How many degrees should the central ray be angled for a PA projection of the clavicle?
 A. 0° perpendicular to midshaft
 B. 15° cephalad to midshaft
 C. 15° caudal to midshaft
 D. 25° cephalad to midshaft

132. Which structure of the nephron is responsible for blood filtration?
 A. Glomerulus
 B. Major calyx
 C. Afferent arteriole
 D. Renal tubule

133. Which projection or position places the gallbladder closest to the image receptor?
 A. Supine
 B. Prone
 C. Erect LAO
 D. Recumbent left posterior oblique (LPO)

134. Which projection performed during sialography will demonstrate an unobstructed view of the sublingual area?
 A. Axial
 B. Lateral
 C. Tangential
 D. Verticosubmental

135. At what level of the patient should the central ray be directed for an AP projection of the pharynx and larynx?
 A. C3–4
 B. Thyroid cartilage
 C. Mandibular rami
 D. Laryngeal prominence

136. Which anatomic landmark indicates that the humerus is correctly positioned for the lateral projection?
 A. The greater tubercle is seen in profile.
 B. The epicondyles are superimposed.
 C. The humeral head is seen in profile.
 D. The lesser tubercle is superimposed over the humeral head.

137. Which anatomic term refers to a body part on the opposite side of the body?
 A. Lateral
 B. Abduction
 C. Ipsilateral
 D. Contralateral

138. Where should the central ray be directed for the lateral projection of the foot?
 A. To the center of the longitudinal arch
 B. To the midpoint of the calcaneus
 C. To the base of the third metatarsal
 D. To the head of the fifth metatarsal

139. Where should the patella be demonstrated on the medial AP oblique projection of the knee?
 A. Over the medial condyle of the femur
 B. Over the lateral condyle of the femur
 C. Superimposed over the tibiofibular articulation
 D. Centered between the tibial condyles

140. Which anatomic structure is best demonstrated by an AP axial projection of the mandible with the central ray directed 35° caudal to the OML?
 A. Mandibular symphysis
 B. Body of the mandible
 C. Mandibular condyles
 D. Angles of the mandible

141. Which method for controlling motion should not be used when radiographing foreign bodies in the patient?
 A. Use of a minimum exposure time
 B. Use of compression bands
 C. Use of suspended respiration
 D. Placement of the affected part in contact with the image receptor

142. When imaging trauma patients, which method should the radiographer use?
 A. Always remove splints prior to making an exposure.
 B. Always move the patient onto the radiographic table prior to making an exposure.
 C. Ensure proper alignment of baselines by flexing the patient's neck.
 D. Communicate consistently with all cooperative patients.

143. What is the most common radiographic finding of arthrography?
    A. Bursitis
    B. Synovial cysts
    C. Torn ligament(s)
    D. Torn meniscus(i)

144. For which projection of the chest should the mid-sagittal plane (MSP) be adjusted parallel to the image receptor?
    A. AP erect
    B. Lateral erect
    C. Lateral decubitus
    D. AP axial lordotic

145. Where should the top border of the cassette be placed for the AP projection to demonstrate the ribs above the diaphragm?
    A. At the cervical prominens
    B. At the level of the sternal notch
    C. 1½ inches above the shoulders
    D. 1½ inches above the sternal notch

146. Which set of vertebrae contains the articulating facets, or demifacets?
    A. Cervical
    B. Thoracic
    C. Lumbar
    D. Sacrum and coccyx

147. Which bony structures join to form the obturator foramen?
    A. Ilium and pubic bone
    B. Ilium and ischium
    C. Pubic bone and ischium
    D. Ischium, ilium, and pubic bone

148. Where should the radiographer center the central ray for an AP projection of the pelvis?
    A. At the level of the iliac crest
    B. 3 inches superior to the symphysis pubis
    C. 2 inches inferior to the greater trochanter
    D. At the soft-tissue depression above the greater trochanter

149. What are the articulations located between the bones of the hand and the bones of the fingers?
    A. Carpometacarpal joints
    B. Interphalangeal joints
    C. Metacarpophalangeal joints
    D. Metacarpocarpal joints

150. Which position or projection would best demonstrate the occipital bone?
    A. PA axial (Caldwell method) projection
    B. AP semiaxial (Grashey-Towne) projection
    C. Lateral projection
    D. Submentovertical projection

151. A Baker's cyst is associated with:
    A. Carpal tunnel syndrome
    B. Collateral ligaments of the ankle
    C. Popliteal area of the bursa
    D. Quadriceps femora

152. Conventional radiographs of the lumbar area during myelography include:
    A. AP and lateral projections
    B. AP, RPO, LPO, and lateral projections
    C. Lateral projection and right and left lateral decubitus positions
    D. Translateral projection only after spot film fluoroscopy

153. What is the lower outer margin of the lung at the junction of the ribs and diaphragm called?
    A. Apex
    B. Mediastinum
    C. Parietal junction
    D. Costophrenic angle

154. What is the most anterior portion of the tibia called?
    A. Tibial plateau
    B. Tibial spine
    C. Tibial condyle
    D. Tibial tuberosity

155. If all patients were positioned with their head under the anode end of the x-ray tube, which one of the following projections would benefit most from the anode heel effect?
    A. AP projection of the thoracic vertebrae
    B. AP projection of the femur
    C. Lateral projection of the thoracic vertebrae
    D. AP projection of the lumbar vertebrae

156. Which projection of the cervical vertebrae requires the central ray to be angled 15° to 20° cephalad?
    A. AP axial
    B. Anterior oblique
    C. AP (open-mouth)
    D. AP (Judd method)

157. Where is the fovea capitis located?
    A. Occipital bone
    B. Proximal femur
    C. Distal tibia
    D. Innominate bone

158. What is the preferred term when referring to the AP projection of the foot?
    A. PA
    B. Tangential
    C. Dorsoplantar
    D. Plantodorsal

159. The lateral border of the scapula may also be referred to as the
    A. Inferior border
    B. Superior border
    C. Vertebral border
    D. Axillary border

160. Referring to Figure 3–7, critique the radiograph of this lateral projection of the wrist:
    A. The hand is overly pronated, causing rotation.
    B. The hand is too far supinated, causing rotation.
    C. The shoulder, elbow, and wrist joints are not all in the same plane
    D. There is nothing wrong with the positioning—the patient has a fractured ulna.

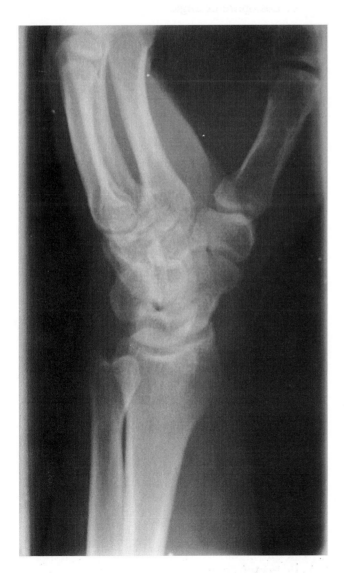

FIGURE 3–7. (Courtesy of UAMS Department of Radiologic Technology.)

161. In which body position should the patient be placed to demonstrate the right shoulder for a PA projection of the scapular "Y"?
    A. Right anterior oblique (RAO)
    B. RPO
    C. LAO
    D. LPO

162. Which organ has mucosal folds in it that are referred to as haustra?
    A. Stomach
    B. Small intestine
    C. Liver
    D. Colon

163. What anatomic structure is of primary interest when the head is in the lateral position and the central ray enters at the zygoma?
    A. Facial bones
    B. Paranasal sinuses
    C. Sella turcica
    D. Mandible

164. Referring to the macroscopic view of the renal system in Figure 3–8, the structure labeled number 5 is the
    A. Renal cortex
    B. Renal medulla
    C. Renal column
    D. Renal pelvis

165. In the same figure, the structure labeled number 1 is the
    A. Renal artery
    B. Renal vein
    C. Renal pelvis
    D. Renal cortex

166. Spina bifida is best demonstrated on an AP projection of the lumbar vertebrae and can be characterized as:
    A. Pedicles not fusing to the vertebral body
    B. Posterior laminae not fusing
    C. Pedicles and laminae not fusing
    D. Laminae and transverse processes not fusing

167. What is the medical term for swallowing?
    A. Peristalsis
    B. Digestion
    C. Deglutition
    D. Mastication

168. In conventional tomography, the objective plane should be at the same level as the
    A. Tabletop
    B. OID
    C. Amplitude
    D. Fulcrum

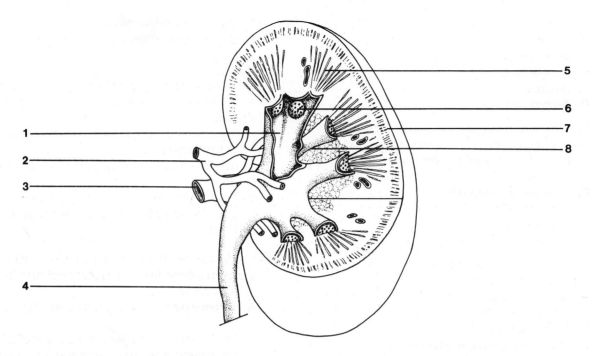

FIGURE 3–8. Macroscopic view of the kidney. (From Scanlon, VC, and Sanders, T: Student Workbook for Essentials of Anatomy and Physiology, ed 3. FA Davis, Philadelphia, 1999, p 305, with permission.)

169. What is the proper medical term for the first cervical vertebra?
    A. Odontoid
    B. Dens
    C. Axis
    D. Atlas

170. For the shoulder to be in external rotation, how should the humeral epicondyle plane be positioned in reference to the film?
    A. Parallel
    B. Perpendicular
    C. 45° medial rotation
    D. 45° lateral rotation

SECTION V: PATIENT CARE

171. When monitoring a patient's vital signs, what condition is indicated by a diastolic pressure above 90 mm Hg?
    A. Anaphylaxis
    B. Hypoglycemia
    C. Bradycardia
    D. Hypertension

172. Isolation that is used for patients who have a depressed immune system is known as:
    A. Enteric isolation
    B. Protective isolation
    C. Respiratory isolation
    D. Contact isolation

173. If a patient is recumbent on the radiographic table and says that he or she feels "faint," what action should the radiographer take?
    A. Sit the patient upright slowly.
    B. Contact the referring physician.
    C. Place the patient in the Fowler's position.
    D. Place the patient in the Trendelenburg position.

174. The most common complication of arthrography is:
    A. Reaction to the contrast medium
    B. Injury to the joint capsule
    C. Infection
    D. Injury to the menisci

175. What type of disease process is indicated by a positive Venereal Disease Research Laboratory (VDRL) analysis of a cerebrospinal fluid (CSF) sample taken from a spinal puncture?
    A. Arachnoiditis
    B. Brain tumor
    C. Syphilis
    D. Meningitis

176. Which of the following may cause a loss of patency in an IV line?
    A. Poor circulation
    B. Malnutrition
    C. Improper height of IV solution
    D. Improper needle selection

177. The term used to describe the reduction of the spread of microorganisms is:
A. Lethargy
B. Contracture
C. Isolation
D. Asepsis

178. How should the linen be handled in cases of suspected salmonella contamination?
A. It should be placed in a red contamination bag.
B. It should be placed in the dirty linen as usual.
C. It should be stored in a separate dirty linen compartment for 24 hours.
D. It should be placed in a bag and sent to the incinerator immediately.

179. A percutaneous endoscopic gastrostomy (PEG) tube may be used for:
A. Gas decompression
B. Intentional irrigation
C. Nutrition support
D. Suctioning gastric secretions

180. Swelling caused by excessive fluid in tissues is called:
A. Hyperemesis
B. Edema
C. Cyanosis
D. Cirrhosis

181. The only safe soap recommended for a cleansing enema is:
A. Liquid detergent
B. Oatmeal soap
C. Lye soap
D. Castile soap

182. The radiographer who is performing a contrast study on a patient with a stoma should recognize that the patient has suffered a major bodily change and may be experiencing the
A. Grieving process
B. Degenerative process
C. Self-evaluation process
D. Self-actualization process

183. Signs and symptoms indicating that a patient might need suctioning are:
1. Audible rattling and gurgling sounds
2. Gagging
3. Difficulty breathing

A. 1 and 2 only
B. 1 and 3 only
C. 2 and 3 only
D. 1, 2, and 3

184. The first signs and symptoms of an anaphylactic reaction are usually:
A. Choking, dyspnea, and cyanosis
B. Hypertension, pallor, and facial paralysis
C. Itching, sneezing, and apprehension
D. Hypotension; dilated pupils; and weak, rapid pulse

185. If the agitated patient refuses to continue with a radiographic examination, the radiographer should:
A. Reassure the patient and attempt to talk him or her through it
B. Call for security and force the patient to cooperate
C. Ask the patient to be more cooperative
D. Stop the procedure and inform the person in charge

186. Special caution should be taken when caring for a patient whose brain or spinal cord may be injured because:
A. Extreme pain can be caused by moving the patient
B. The infection rate is high in this type of injury
C. The patient is agitated easily and may become combative
D. The patient has lost mobility and any manipulation may cause further damage

For the following scenario, answer questions 187 to 189:

A 42-year-old male patient has an open reduction of the lower leg performed in the operating room. Three days later, he is brought to the radiology department for a follow-up radiograph. As the radiographer brings the patient into the room, the patient suddenly begins to complain of mild chest pain and he appears short of breath. The radiographer takes the patient's vital signs and notes that his blood pressure is 120/80 mm Hg and his pulse rate is 120 beats per minute. The radiographer immediately summons help.

187. The patient's symptoms indicate that he may be suffering from:
A. A stroke
B. A convulsion
C. A pulmonary embolus
D. Hypovolemic shock

188. The patient's blood pressure indicates that he is:
A. In shock
B. Hypertensive
C. Hypoglycemic
D. Stable; the pressure is normal

189. The patient's pulse rate indicates that he has:
A. An athletic lifestyle
B. Bradycardia
C. Tachycardia
D. An infarct

190. What is the minimum required height for hanging the enema bag in relation to the table during a lower gastrointestinal examination?
    A. 30 inches
    B. 40 inches
    C. 50 inches
    D. It depends on size of patient

191. What is the average respiratory rate for an adult at rest?
    A. 8 to 10 breaths per minute
    B. 12 to 20 breaths per minute
    C. 25 to 30 breaths per minute
    D. 80 to 90 breaths per minute

192. The most common cause of trauma among elderly patients is:
    A. Back injuries
    B. Falls
    C. Burns
    D. Domestic violence

193. The usual rate of flow for oxygen administration through a nasal cannula is:
    A. 1 to 5 L/s
    B. 1 to 5 L/min
    C. 6 to 10 L/s
    D. 6 to 10 L/min

194. Log rolling is a method of moving patients with a suspected:
    A. Head injury
    B. Vertebral column injury
    C. Extremity fracture
    D. Bowel obstruction

195. A device that may be used to measure the oxygen content of blood is the
    A. Pulse oximeter
    B. Stethoscope
    C. Sphygmomanometer
    D. Oxygen flow-rate meter

196. Instruments needed to assess vital signs include:
    1. Thermometer
    2. Tongue depressor
    3. A watch with a second hand

    A. 1 and 2 only
    B. 1 and 3 only
    C. 2 and 3 only
    D. 1, 2, and 3

197. A common device used for high-pressure steam sterilization is called the
    A. Thermal ventilator
    B. Vector chamber
    C. Autoclave
    D. Inhalator

198. Examples of a disease that may be transferred by vector include:
    1. Malaria
    2. Lyme disease
    3. Human immunodeficiency virus (HIV)

    A. 1 and 2 only
    B. 1 and 3 only
    C. 2 and 3 only
    D. 1, 2, and 3

199. According to the Centers for Disease Control and Prevention (CDC), what type of isolation precautions should be used for HIV-positive patients?
    A. Strict
    B. Respiratory
    C. Enteric
    D. Standard (universal)

200. Which of the following is required for a patient who is in insulin shock but is still conscious?
    A. Food or liquid with sugar
    B. Food or liquid with salt
    C. An insulin injection
    D. A blood transfusion

Answers and Explanations

Each rationale is followed by references to texts listed in the bibliography at the end of this chapter.

SECTION I: RADIATION PROTECTION AND RADIOBIOLOGY

1. **(B)** In certain radiographic examinations, it may be necessary for the patient to hold the cassette during the exposure. Examples include when attempting to obtain a "sunrise" view of the patella or an axiolateral "shoot-through" projection of the hip. In these cases, if the primary beam will strike any part of the patient's body other than the area of interest, the use of a shielding device of at least 0.5-mm Pb equivalent is required.
    Dowd and Tilson, "Health Physics," p 188; NCRP Report No. 102, p 8.

2. **(B)** Skin cancer induced by radiation seems to follow a threshold dose-response relationship. It usually begins with the development of radiodermatitis. The threshold is approximately 500 rad.
    Bushong, "Late Effects of Radiation," 1997, p 486; Dowd and Tilson, "Late Effects of Radiation," p 148.

3. **(A)** Acute or early radiation effects are typically seen in cases of very high radiation doses or in tissues that are especially sensitive to radiation, such

as white blood cells. A total body dose as low as 25 rad can cause a drop in the white blood cell count. A dose of 25 rad is five times more than the annual dose limit for occupational workers and is much higher than a patient may receive from a typical nuclear medicine bone scan. An "early effect" is a biologic effect that appears within days or weeks as a result of a substantial dose.

Bushong, "Early Effects of Radiation," 1997, p 464; Carlton and McKenna-Adler, "Radiation Protection Concepts and Equipment," p 145; Dowd and Tilson, "Early Effects of Radiation," pp 128–130; Statkiewicz-Sherer et al., "Radiation Biology," p 116.

4. **(C)** Response A refers to the *doubling dose,* or the amount of radiation that would double the genetic effects in the population. Response B is the definition of linear energy transfer (LET). Response D is the definition for the dose-equivalent limit as set forth by the NCRP. RBE stands for "relative biologic effectiveness" and is a formula that is used to compare the differences in biologic effects among various types of radiation. In the formula, a 250-keV x-ray source is the constant by which all other types of radiation may be compared:

$$\frac{\text{Dose of 250-keV x-ray source to produce a biologic effect}}{\text{Dose of test radiation to produce the same effect}}$$

Bushong, "Molecular and Cellular Radiobiology," 1997, p 459; Dowd and Tilson, "Principles of Radiobiology," pp 106–109; Statkiewicz-Sherer et al., "Radiation Biology," p 96; Travis, "Basic Biologic Interactions of Radiation," p 31.

5. **(B)** Decreasing the kilovolts (peak) from one radiograph to another will result in a less intense beam and will also have the negative effect of reduced penetration. Reduced penetration means that less radiation will reach the image receptor (reduced optical density) and more radiation will be absorbed by the patient's skin. Because reduced kilovolts (peak) means reduced energy or penetrating power, the radiographer's dose will also be decreased. Alterations in the kilovolts (peak) will have a negligible effect on the recorded detail of the image.

Bushong, "X-Ray Emission," 1997, p 141, and "Radiation Protection Procedures," p 526; Dowd and Tilson, "Protecting the Patient in Radiography," pp 219–221; Statkiewicz-Sherer et al., "Protection of the Patient during Diagnostic Radiological Procedures," pp 162–163.

6. **(A)** According to the latest NCRP report, the embryo and fetus should not receive more than 0.5 mSv/mo (0.05 rem/mo). The total dose equivalent to the fetus for the entire gestation period should not exceed 5 mSv (0.5 rem).

Bushong, "Health Physics," 1997, p 503; Dowd and Tilson, "Health Physics," p 183; NCRP Report No. 116, p 56.

7. **(C)** The photoelectric effect is characterized by total absorption of the incident photon by an orbital electron, not the nucleus of the atom. The photoelectric effect accounts for radiographic contrast due to the differences in the tissue density. The tissues with higher atomic numbers will tend to undergo more photoelectric effects than either the Compton or coherent effects.

Bushong, "X-Ray Interaction with Matter," 1997, pp 151–154; Carlton and McKenna-Adler, "X-Ray Interactions," p 192; Dowd and Tilson, "Interactions of Radiation with Matter," pp 67–70.

8. **(B)** Both scintillation detectors and TLDs operate on the principle of the luminescence of a phosphorescent crystal. A cloud chamber operates on the principle of a physical change and is useless for the measurement of radiation or dosimetry. The ionization chamber operates on the principle of electric current because x rays and other types of ionizing radiation can free electrons from their shells, thereby causing a charge "in air" or in a gas chamber. A pocket dosimeter is a type of ion chamber and may be used for personnel monitoring when an immediate reading is necessary.

Bushong, "Designing for Radiation Protection," 1997, pp 516–520; Dowd and Tilson, "Ionizing Radiation," pp 48–49; Statkiewicz-Sherer et al., "Radiation Monitoring," pp 226–228.

9. **(B)** Some of the epidemiological studies on long-term exposure to low doses of radiation have shown that these doses may increase the incidence of leukemia, cataract formation (which is a cumulative effect), and also nonspecific shortening of the life span. Early studies showed that radiation workers' lives might have been cut short because of their radiation exposure. The latest data on atomic bomb survivors, radium-dial watch painters, and x-ray patients show that such an effect on shortened life span does not exist.

Bushong, "Late Effects of Radiation," pp 478–480; Dowd and Tilson, "Late Effects of Radiation," pp 144–156.

10. **(A)** The use of the technical factors high kilovolts (peak) and low milliamperage-seconds is better for the patient in terms of reducing the skin dose. This technique must be weighed against the effect on image quality for a particular examination. Most radiology departments use an optimum kilovolts (peak) for each specific anatomic part. Reducing the film size has a great effect on reducing the patient's dose; it also increases the quality of the im-

age by allowing less scatter radiation to be produced within the patient. The use of slower-speed screens will also increase image quality by improving the recorded detail, but the patient dose will increase because a larger dose will be needed to maintain the same optical density.

Carlton and McKenna-Adler, "Minimizing Patient Dose," pp 210–221; Dowd and Tilson, "Protecting the Patient in Radiography," pp 219–221; Statkiewicz-Sherer et al., "Protection of the Patient during Diagnostic Radiological Procedures," pp 161–163.

11. **(A)** The NCRP recommends that gloves worn by the radiographer or radiologist should be lined with a lead equivalent of at least 0.25 mm.

Gurley and Callaway, "Radiation Safety and Protective Measures," p 242; NCRP Report No. 102, p 18(q); Statkiewicz-Sherer et al., "Protecting Occupationally Exposed Personnel during Diagnostic Radiological Procedures," p 200.

12. **(D)** Scatter radiation *increases* with an increase in kilovolts (peak) because a greater percentage of Compton events are occurring. Quantum mottle may *increase* with a decrease in milliamperage-seconds because there may be an insufficient number of x rays produced to interact with the film emulsion. When the kilovolts (peak) is increased and the milliamperage-seconds is decreased using the 15 percent rule, the optical density should not be affected. A technique of higher kilovolts (peak) and lower milliamperage-seconds will lower the patient dose because the patient will absorb fewer x rays due to the photoelectric effect.

Carlton and McKenna-Adler, "Minimizing Patient Dose," pp 210–212; Dowd and Tilson, "Protecting the Patient in Radiography," pp 219–221; Statkiewicz-Sherer et al., "Protection of the Patient during Diagnostic Radiological Procedures," pp 161–163.

13. **(C)** *Attenuation* can be defined as the reduction of x-ray photons as they travel through matter. This loss can be in the form of either absorption through the photoelectric effect or scatter through the Compton effect. *Transmutation* is the natural decay process of radioactive materials as they change from unstable elements into stable end-products. For instance, the stable end-product of uranium is lead. *Isotropic propagation* (transmitted in all directions) is how x rays are produced at the target. *Quantum mottle* is a grainy appearance of the radiograph when insufficient milliamperage-seconds are used with a high-speed film-screen combination.

Bushong, "X-Ray Interaction with Matter," 1997, p 159; Carlton and McKenna-Adler, "X-Ray Interactions," p 191; Dowd and Tilson, "Interactions of Radiation with Matter," p 64; Statkiewicz-Sherer et al.,

"Basic Interactions of X-Radiation with Matter," pp 21–29.

14. **(D)** Biologic effects of radiation can basically be divided into two main categories: (1) somatic effects, which are seen in the exposed individual, and (2) genetic effects, which are seen in the progeny of the exposed individual whose gametes (sperm or ova) may have been damaged. Data on genetic effects on human populations are nonconclusive, although genetic effects induced from radiation have been observed in animal populations. There are much more data available on somatic effects suffered by exposed individuals. Some documented examples include (1) various types of cancer, especially leukemia and thyroid cancer, (2) cataractogenesis, (3) acute radiation syndrome, (4) skin erythema, (5) alopecia, (6) nausea and vomiting, (7) reduction in the white blood cell count (leukopenia), and (8) effects to the developing embryo and fetus.

Carlton and McKenna-Adler, "Radiation Protection Concepts and Equipment," p 145; Statkiewicz-Sherer et al., "Radiation Biology," pp 115–131; Travis, "Late Effects of Radiation," p 176.

15. **(C)** A controlled work area, such as the control booth, is an area that should be limited to radiation workers only (radiologists and radiographers). The level of radiation should be limited in this area to the dose-equivalent limit that the occupational worker is allowed annually. This dose limit is 5 rem/y, or 5000 mrem/y; 5000 mrem divided by a 50-week work year equals 100 mrem/wk. Uncontrolled areas are those to which the public has access, such as a back hall of a radiographic room. These areas should be limited to ¹⁄₁₀ the occupational dose, or 10 mrem/wk.

Bushong, "Designing for Radiation Protection," p 514; NCRP Report No. 116; Statkiewicz-Sherer et al., "Protecting Occupationally Exposed Personnel during Diagnostic Radiological Procedures," p 194.

16. **(B)** The design of fluoroscopic units limits the SSD because the skin doses can be quite high during a fluoroscopic examination. The limitations for a fixed unit are more restrictive than for a mobile unit such as a C-arm. A fixed unit should be designed to maintain a minimum SSD of 38 cm (15 in.). Mobile units must be designed to maintain a minimum SSD of 30 cm (12 in.).

Bushong, "Designing for Radiation Protection," p 511; NCRP Report No. 105; Statkiewicz-Sherer et al., "Protection of the Patient during Diagnostic Radiological Procedures," p 167.

17. **(B)** Increasing filtration may benefit the patient as it removes the lower-energy photons that would otherwise be deposited in the patient's tis-

sue. Filtration does not reduce the radiographer's dose. Increasing the exposure time will increase both the patient's and the radiographer's dose. Although increasing lead shielding will decrease dose to a certain degree, the best method of reducing the radiographer's exposure is to increase distance from the source, thereby taking advantage of the inverse-square law.

Dowd and Tilson, "Protecting the Radiographer," p 199; Statkiewicz-Sherer et al., "Protecting Occupationally Exposed Personnel," p 228; Thompson et al., "Radiation Protection," p 476.

18. **(D)** When an embryo or fetus is exposed to radiation in utero, three possible effects may be seen: (1) spontaneous abortion or neonatal death, (2) congenital defects, and (3) long-term late effects, such as childhood malignancy, sterility, or leukemia. The time of gestation when the radiation occurred is the most important factor in determining which effect may be induced. Spontaneous abortion or miscarriage is more likely to occur as a result of radiation exposure to the fetus during the preimplantation stage, which occurs between 0 to 10 days postconception. Neonatal death or congenital defects are more likely to be seen when irradiation occurs during the major organogenesis period, spanning between 2 and 8 weeks postconception. Long-term late effects, such as childhood malignancy and sterility, are a more likely to occur if the exposure was received during the fetal stage of development, when the developing baby is more resistant to radiation.

Bushong, "Late Effects of Radiation," pp 489–491; Dowd and Tilson, "Late Effects of Radiation," pp 158–162; Travis, "Total Body Radiation Response," pp 149–154.

19. **(C)** The genetic significant dose is the dose that takes into account the amount of radiation received by the gonads of individuals who may be undergoing radiation procedures (diagnostic or therapeutic). The dose actually received by these irradiated individuals is averaged for the entire population to estimate the potential genetic risks for future generations within that population. As radiographers, we should be acutely aware of this genetic risk and should do everything within our power to limit the radiation dose to the patient's gonads. We can accomplish this by using faster-speed film-screen combinations, higher-kilovolt (peak) and lower–milliamperage-second techniques, and shielding for the gonads whenever possible; avoiding repeats; and using tight collimation. Tomography, fluoroscopy, and CT machines are very high-dose diagnostic procedures and should be used only when absolutely necessary.

PBL is a device that is standard equipment with most modern radiographic units. It ensures that the collimation of the beam will be limited to the size of the image receptor. Most machines with PBL have an override mechanism attached to the unit. The important principle is that the beam size should be no larger than the image-receptor size. The smaller the field size, the less risk there is to the patient and to future generations.

Bushong, "Designing for Radiation Protection," 1997, p 510; Dowd and Tilson, "Protecting the Patient in Radiography," p 231; Statkiewicz-Sherer et al., "Protection of the Patient during Diagnostic Radiological Procedures," p 154.

20. **(A)** Primary radiation is the radiation that leaves the x-ray tube through the port window of the tube housing. Scatter radiation is radiation that has come in contact with matter such as human tissue. Remnant radiation is the portion of the exit beam that leaves the patient to expose the image receptor. Leakage radiation is any radiation that leaves the tube housing other than through the port window. Leakage radiation is not part of the useful beam and leads to unnecessary exposure to both the radiographer and the patient.

Bushong, "The X-Ray Tube," p 108; Carlton and McKenna-Adler, "The X-Ray Tube," p 124; Dowd and Tilson, "The Production of X-Radiation," p 25.

21. **(B)** The two most dominant interactions of diagnostic x-ray photons are the photoelectric effect and the Compton effect. The photoelectric effect is more likely to occur in tissues with high atomic numbers and with incident photons of lower energies. The Compton effect is more likely to occur in tissues with low atomic numbers and with higher-energy incident x rays. There will be reduced subject contrast in tissues that contain more water, such as fat and muscle as in the abdomen. Lower-kilovolt (peak) technical factors will produce images with shorter-scale (higher) contrast. An incident photon with an energy level as high as 100 keV would most likely interact through the Compton effect.

Bushong, "X-Ray Interaction with Matter," pp 151–154; Carlton and McKenna-Adler, "X-Ray Interactions," p 194; Dowd and Tilson, "Interactions of Radiation with Matter," p 72.

22. **(C)** The "cutie pie" is actually an acronym that stands for Q = t × π, or Quantity of radiation = Time of exposure × 3.14. *Pi* is designated because the quantity is measured inside a cylinder. There are several types of gas-filled detectors with charged electrodes that are sensitive to reading ionizing events. Only the ionization chamber is

sensitive to the specific energy range of diagnostic x-radiation and measures in units of milliroentgen per hour. Other types of gas-filled detectors include Geiger-Müller counters and proportional counters. Only the ionization chamber is specifically designed to measure the output of diagnostic x-ray tubes and fluoroscopes.

Bushong, "Designing for Radiation Protection," p 516; Carlton and McKenna-Adler, "Radiation Protection Concepts and Equipment," p 149; Hendee, "Ionization Chambers," p 187; Selman, "Protection in Radiology: Health Physics," p 539.

23. **(A)** To find the answer to this question, the inverse-square law should be used:

$$\frac{I_1}{I_2} = \frac{D_2{}^2}{D_1{}^2} ; \frac{100 \text{ mR}}{x} = \frac{3^2}{1^2} ; \frac{100 \text{ mR}}{9} = x;$$

$$x = 11.1 \text{ mR}$$

Carlton and McKenna-Adler, "The Prime Factors," p 185.

24. **(D)** Radiation damage may be passed on to an individual's progeny if the individual received exposure to the gonads (sperm or ova). This damage is referred to as a genetic effect. Radiation damage can occur below the dose-equivalent limits as set forth by the NCRP. Stochastic effects, or nonthreshold effects (cancer and genetic effects), may occur at even the smallest doses. Mutations in cells, especially white blood cells, have been observed after very small exposures, including occupational doses. Even though damage does occur, the cells and tissue of the body do have the capability of repairing the damage. This is sometimes referred to as "sublethal" damage because the cells are able to recover fully from the damage induced by the radiation.

Bushong, "Molecular and Cellular Radiobiology," pp 457–458; Statkiewicz-Sherer et al., "Radiation Biology," pp 119–120; Travis, "Cell and Tissue Responses to Radiation," p 104.

25. **(C)** Figure 3–1 depicts the mean survival time of a person experiencing the acute radiation syndrome in relation to the radiation dose received. Area A is a nonlethal total body dose, which does not exceed 200 rad. Between 200 and 1000 rad, the victim's mean survival time would range from approximately 60 days to 4 days and corresponds to the hematopoietic syndrome (Area B). Area C depicts lethality within 4 days following a dose of between 1000 and 5000 rad and would correspond to the GI syndrome. Area D is lethality to the central nervous system when the dose exceeds 5000 rad. Death from the central nervous system syndrome would occur in less than 3 days.

Bushong, "Early Effects of Radiation," p 467; Dowd and Tilson, "Early Effects of Radiation," pp 128–130; Travis, "Total Body Radiation Response," p 139; Statkiewicz-Sherer et al., "Radiation Biology," pp 116–119.

26. **(C)** According to NCRP Report No. 116, the public should be limited to $\frac{1}{10}$ the occupational dose. The occupational dose-equivalent limit is 50 mSv/yr (5 rem/yr). The public therefore must be limited to less than 5 mSv/yr (0.5 rem/yr.).

Bushong, "Health Physics," p 503; Dowd and Tilson, "Health Physics," p 183; NCRP Report No. 116.

27. **(B)** The radiograph of a neonatal chest in Figure 3–2 is an example of poor collimation. Too much tissue is exposed that is not part of the anatomy of interest. Although it is hoped that the infant was properly protected with a gonadal shield, it is impossible to tell from this radiograph if proper shielding was used. It is also impossible to tell what speed screen was used without having any knowledge of the equipment or technical factors used. The kilovolts (peak) appears to be adequate because all of the anatomy is demonstrated. If proper collimation had been used, the radiograph would have reduced density and increased contrast and would therefore be of better quality.

Carlton and McKenna-Adler, "Beam Restriction," p 243; Dowd and Tilson, "Protecting the Patient in Radiography," pp 231–232; Statkiewicz-Sherer et al., "Protection of the Patient during Diagnostic Radiological Procedures,": pp 150–155.

28. **(C)** The NCRP recommends that the patient's skin surface should not be placed any closer than 15 cm from the collimating device. This distance ensures that electrons produced by photon interaction with the collimator do not strike the patient's skin surface and cause unnecessary damage.

NCRP Report No. 102; Statkiewicz-Sherer et al., "Protection of the Patient during Diagnostic Radiological Procedures," p 152.

29. **(B)** The cumulative timer on a fluoroscopic unit functions to remind the physician of the amount of time that a patient has been exposed to the fluoroscopic x-ray beam. It is the radiographer's responsibility to ensure that the timer is reset prior to the beginning of every procedure so that the physician can more accurately estimate the fluoroscopic ON time for each patient. The timer should activate an audible alarm every 5 minutes as a reminder.

Bushong, "Designing for Radiation Protection," p 512; NCRP Report No. 102; Statkiewicz-Sherer et al., "Protection of the Patient during Diagnostic Radiological Procedures," p 168.

30. **(C)** How often the x-ray beam is in use is referred to as the workload factor and is measured in milliamperage-minutes per week. How many people will occupy the area (occupancy factor) is dependent on whether it is considered a controlled or uncontrolled area. The use factor is the proportional amount of time that the primary beam is directed at a particular barrier.

Bushong, "Designing for Radiation Protection," pp 514–515; Statkiewicz-Sherer et al., "Protecting Occupationally Exposed Personnel during Diagnostic Radiological Procedures," p 202.

SECTION II: EQUIPMENT OPERATION AND MAINTENANCE

31. **(D)** The heat units that are produced in a x-ray machine vary slightly from one type of generator to another. To correctly calculate heat units, it is important to know what the constant value is for each generator. The basic formula for heat units is as follows: HU = kVp × mA × Time × Generator-type constant. The generator-type constant for single-phase, full-wave equipment is 1. The generator-type constant for a 3-phase, 6-pulse machine is 1.35. The generator-type constant for a 3-phase, 12-pulse generator is 1.41, and the generator-type constant for a high-frequency generator is 1.45.

Carlton and McKenna-Adler, "The X-Ray Tube," pp 126–127.

32. **(C)** Most x-ray tubes have an inherent filtration between 0.5-mm and 1-mm Al equivalent. This inherent filtration consists primarily of the window of the glass envelope.

Carlton and McKenna-Adler, "Filtration," p 172; Curry et al., "Filters," p 87; Thompson et al., "Factors Affecting the X-Ray Spectrum," p 228.

33. **(B)** The purpose of a filter in an automatic processor is to remove debris that could clog the system. In the developer, a filter is often used so that gelatin will not coat the transport rollers. Removal of algae by a filter is not recommended because the algae can easily penetrate most mesh sizes. Cross-contamination of chemicals is prevented by the use of splash guards, which keep the fixer from splashing back into the developer tank.

Bushong, "Processing the Latent Image," p 185; Carlton and McKenna-Adler, "Radiographic Processing," p 299; McKinney, "Circulation/Filtration System," p 105.

34. **(B)** The tightly coiled wire that is found in the x-ray tube is the filament. The filament acts as a re-

sistor for the purpose of boiling off electrons through thermionic emission. The focusing cup surrounding the filament is usually made of molybdenum, not tungsten. The autotransformer is a tightly coiled loop of wire that is located in the operating console and is responsible for the selection of kilovolts (peak). The automatic exposure control (AEC) device is usually located in the x-ray table, not the x-ray tube.

Bushong, "The X-Ray Tube," p 110; Carlton and McKenna-Adler, "The X-Ray Tube," p 112; Curry et al., "Production of X-Rays," p 11; Selman, "X-Ray Tubes and Rectifiers," p 205.

35 and 36. **(C)** and **(D)** In Figure 3–3, the number 1 is the photocathode, 2 the input phosphor, 3 the electron stream, 4 the electrostatic lenses that focus the electrons across the tube, 5 the anode that attracts the electrons, 6 the glass envelope, and 7 the output phosphor.

Bushong, "Fluoroscopy," p 324; Carlton and McKenna-Adler, "Fluoroscopy," p 537; Thompson et al., "Fluoroscopy: Viewing with Motion," p 364.

37. **(D)** Any material that allows the free flow of electrons is called a *conductor*. Examples of conductors include copper, aluminum, tungsten, and water. *Insulators* are materials that do not allow the free flow of electrons. Examples include rubber, glass, and wood. A *transducer* allows the conduction of sound waves, as in ultrasound. A *resistor* resists the flow of electrons and is a useful device in circuits such as light bulbs, toasters, or filaments inside the x-ray tube.

Bushong, "Electricity," p 61; Carlton and McKenna-Adler, "Electricity," p 48; Selman, "Electrostatics," p 57.

38. **(B)** Cross-contamination from the fixer tank into the developer may occur from splashing the chemicals during transport of the film. To prevent cross-contamination, all automatic processors should be equipped with special splash guards. Splashing or evaporation of developer into the fixer tank is not a major concern because the developer is regularly transported into the fixer tank by each sheet of film. On the other hand, fixer contamination in the developer is very significant because it requires complete extraction of the contaminated chemicals, washing, and replenishing of the entire development solution (which is messy, time consuming, and costly). It is therefore recommended that the splash guards always be in place during operation of the processor. It is also recommended that because solutions may evaporate when the processor is not in use, the lid be opened slightly to prevent cross-contamination.

Carlton and McKenna-Adler, "Radiographic Processing," p 299; Carroll, "Automatic Processors," 1998, p 504.

39. **(B)** The vidicon and plumbicon are two different types of television camera tubes that are used with modern image intensifiers. These tubes are coupled with the output phosphor and convert the light image into an electronic signal that is then sent to the CRT for dynamic imaging during fluoroscopy. Frame cameras may also be coupled with the output phosphor to produce static images during fluoroscopy. Television camera tubes are not used for this purpose. No device is capable of viewing an image directly from the input phosphor. The electrostatic lenses are the devices that focus the electron stream from the photocathode on the input side to the output phosphor.

Bushong, "Fluoroscopy," p 327; Carlton and McKenna-Adler, "Fluoroscopy," p 543.

40. **(A)** The milliamperage meter records only the current flowing during the exposure. Therefore, it must be placed on the secondary side of the step-up transformer where the amperage is stepped down for production of the x-ray beam. The milliamperage meter is located between the step-up transformer and the x-ray tube. The step-down transformer and the rheostat are both parts of the filament circuit, not the x-ray tube circuit.

Bushong, "The X-Ray Machine," p 105; Selman, "X-Ray Circuits," pp 250–251; Thompson et al., "X-Ray Machine Operation: The X-Ray Circuit," p 188; Tortorici, "Production of X-Rays," 1992, p 70.

41. **(C)** When projectile electrons from the cathode strike the anode, three things may occur: (1) *excitation* of the target electrons, which causes heat or thermal radiation to be emitted; (2) creation of *Bremsstrahlung* radiation, or the deceleration of the projectile electrons as they pass by the atomic nuclei of the target atoms; and (3) creation of *characteristic* radiation that results when a target atom has been ionized by the projectile electron. Of these three, excitation, which results in thermal radiation or heat, accounts for more than 99 percent of the energy conversion at the target in the diagnostic range. Less than 1 percent of the electron kinetic energy is converted to either Bremsstrahlung or characteristic radiation in the useful beam.

Bushong, "X-Ray Production," pp 128–130; Carlton and McKenna-Adler, "X-Ray Production," p 133; Curry et al., "Production of X-Rays," p 30; Selman, "X-Rays (Roentgen Rays)," p 160.

42. **(B)** The 350,000-HU level intersects the anode-cooling curve at approximately 3 minutes. From

that point on, the curve requires an additional 5 minutes (8 − 3 = 5) to complete cooling. It takes 5 minutes for complete cooling of the anode.

Bushong, "The X-Ray Tube," p 123; Carlton and McKenna-Adler, "The X-Ray Tube," pp 126–127; Wolbarst, "X-Ray Tubes," pp 91–92; Selman, "X-Ray Tubes & Rectifiers," p 222.

43. **(A)** Every time an exposure is made, hundreds or thousands of heat units are produced at the anode. Each x-ray unit should have its own radiographic rating chart as well as its own anode-cooling chart, and each chart should be readily available to the radiographer near the control panel. The anode will usually cool very rapidly in the first 2 minutes after the exposure if no other exposures have been made. To read this graph, first find the saturation point, which for this chart is 500,000 HU and is located at the top of the vertical axis. Then, calculate the heat units for this single-phase machine with the technical factors given (83 kVp × 800 mA × 1.5 s = 99,600 HU). Next, subtract 99,600 from the saturation point (500,000 − 99,600 = 400,400). The anode would have to cool to approximately 400,000 HU before it could accommodate an exposure of 99,600 HU. Find 400,000 HU on the same axis and follow it across horizontally until it intersects with the cooling curve. The intersection for 400,000 HU is at approximately 1.5 minutes.

Bushong, "The X-Ray Tube," p 123; Carlton and McKenna-Adler, "The X-Ray Tube," pp 126–127; Selman, "X-Ray Tubes and Rectifiers," p 222; Wolbarst, "X-Ray Tubes," pp 91–92.

44. **(D)** The size of a photon's wavelength is inversely proportional to its energy. Some electromagnetic waves may be measured in meters, such as radio waves and microwaves. X- and gamma radiation have very high energy levels and very short wavelengths. A more convenient unit for measuring the size of an x-ray photon's wavelength is the angstrom (Å), which corresponds to 10^{-10} m. For the diagnostic energy range of between 25 and 125 keV, the corresponding wavelengths range from 0.1 to 0.5 Å. To calculate the exact size of the wavelength when the energy of an x-ray photon is known, use the following formula:

$$E = \frac{12.4}{\lambda} ; E = \frac{12.4}{0.1} ; E = 124 \text{ keV}$$

The 12.4 is found by multiplying Planck's constant (*h*) times the speed of light constant (*c*). For this question, 125 keV is the only energy level capable of producing x rays with a minimum wavelength of 0.1 Å.

Bushong, "Electromagnetic Radiation," p 54; Curry

et al., "Radiation," p 7; Thompson et al., "Radiation: Its Atomic and Nuclear Origins," p 64; Wolbarst, "Atoms & Photons," p 52.

45. **(B)** For the production of x rays to occur, it is necessary to have the ability to produce electrons traveling at a high rate of speed. The only way to accomplish this is to step up the energy of the incoming line voltage to several thousand volts or kilovolts. This is done with a transformer that operates only on AC. Unfortunately, x-ray tubes cannot function on AC and therefore must have a device located between the step-up transformer and the x-ray tube that is capable of changing AC to pulsating DC. This is accomplished by several rectifiers. Rectifiers are usually semiconductors, such as solid-state diodes. Semiconductors allow the current to flow in one direction but not in the opposite direction. When current passes through a rectified it is changed from AC to pulsating DC.

Bushong, "Electromagnetism," p 84; Carlton and McKenna-Adler, "Electromagnetism," pp 77–84. Curry et al., "X-Ray Generators," p 43; Selman, "Rectification," p 139.

46. **(A)** The milliamperage meter records only the current flowing during the exposure because it is measuring the tube current. The "prereading voltmeter" and the "kilovolt meter" are synonymous terms. The kilovolt meter is located on the primary side of the step-up transformer on most units and reads the kilovolts (peak) prior to the exposure and is sometimes referred to as the prereading voltmeter. Although there is a filament ammeter, which reads the current supplied to the cathode, it does not measure in units of milliamperes and is not referred to as a prereading milliammeter.

Bushong, "The X-Ray Machine," p 105; Selman, "X-Ray Circuits," pp 250–251; Thompson et al., "X-Ray Machine Operation: The X-Ray Circuit," p 188; Tortorici, "Production of X-Rays," 1992, p 70.

47. **(B)** Poor screen-film contact is usually caused by a warped or bent cassette. It may also be caused by a foreign object in the cassette. Large cassettes are more likely to suffer poor screen-film contact. The wire-mesh test is the most precise method of detecting poor film-screen contact because it is easier to assess the sharpness of the wire in the test tool than the sharpness of human tissue or a phantom. Poor film-screen contact may be a simple problem to fix. Replacing the felt or foam pad lining the cassette or removing the foreign object from the cassette may be all that is needed. If the cassette is warped beyond repair, it should be discarded.

Carroll, "Quality Control," 1998, p 404; Cullinan, "X-Ray Equipment Maintenance," p 261; Gray et al.,

"Basic Tests," pp 55–58; Tortorici, "Film Holders and Intensifying Screens," 1992.

48. **(A)** All electromagnetic radiation travels at a constant velocity called the "speed of light." This constant is equivalent to 186,400 miles/s in the English system of measure or 3×10^8 m/s in the International Systems of Units (SI units) or 3×10^{10} cm/s in the CGS system. The speed of light constant in a mathematical equation is usually designated by the symbol *c*, as in: $E = mc^2$.

Bushong, "Electromagnetic Radiation," p 44; Curry et al., "Radiation," p 5; Wolbarst, "Electric and Magnetic Fields and Electromagnetic Waves," p 36.

49. **(B)** The speed at which electrons are accelerated to the target is determined by the potential difference (kilovolts [peak]) between the negative charge placed on the cathode and the positive charge placed on the anode. These charges are determined by the kilovoltage applied to the tube. The heat of the filament, controlled by the milliamperage selector, determines how many electrons are boiled off, not how fast they are accelerated. The heat created in the anode and the target angle have nothing to do with how fast the electrons are accelerated from the cathode side.

Bushong, "X-Ray Emission," pp 127–128; Selman, "X-Rays (Roentgen Rays)", p 155; Thompson et al., "Factors Affecting the X-Ray Spectrum," p 226.

50. **(C)** Although sonography allows the technologist the ability to image in various planes of the body, it does not record these images onto a radiograph. A radiograph records radiation, specifically x rays. Stereoradiography allows the radiologist or physician to image an area of the body in a three-dimensional plane by virtue of the alignment of two radiographs taken in close proximity to each other. These images are then placed in a special stereoscopic lens to view the anatomy in three dimensions, not in selected planes. Cinefluorography records dynamic images (at 30 frames per second or more) from the fluoroscope onto roll film, similar to a movie reel. Tomography is the only imaging modality that records selected planes of the body onto a radiograph.

Bushong, "Tomography," p 282; Carlton and McKenna-Adler, "Tomography," p 554; Curry et al., "Body Section Radiography," p 242.

51. **(C)** There are several types of generators and current forms that produce x rays. Among the most common are (1) single-phase, half-wave rectified, (2) single-phase, full-wave rectified, (3) 3-phase, 6-pulse, (4) 3-phase, 12-pulse, (5) high-frequency, (6) falling-load generators, and (7) capacitor discharge generators. There is no such classification of generator as half-phase.

Bushong, "The X-Ray Unit," pp 100–104; Carlton and McKenna-Adler, "X-Ray Equipment," pp 99–105; Curry et al., "X-Ray Generators," pp 42–53; Tortorici, "Rectification."

52. **(C)** The filament of the x-ray tube requires a large current to provide an adequate source of electrons. A step-down transformer is used to decrease the voltage and to increase the current, or amperes. Most filament transformers supply the filament with a current of about 3 to 6 A. This is compared with the step-up transformer, which is used to increase the voltage and decrease the current supplied to the x-ray tube during the exposure. The tube current operates between 25 and 1200 mA.

Bushong, "The X-Ray Unit," p 97; Carlton and McKenna-Adler, "X-Ray Equipment," p 98; Curry et al., "X-Ray Generators," p 40.

53. **(B)** The photosensitive crystals in the film emulsion consist of positive silver ions (Ag^+) bonded with negative halide ions of either bromine (Br^-) or iodine (I^-). The halide atoms are usually more concentrated on the surface of the crystal, imparting the surface with a negative electrification prior to exposure. When either x-ray photons or light photons strike the crystal lattice, electrons are released through the process of ionization. The ionic bonds of the silver (Ag^+) and halide atoms are broken and the surface electrification is neutralized in the area of the exposure. As a result, free electrons migrate to the "sensitivity speck." A crystal that does not contain a sensitivity speck is incapable of being developed. The sensitivity speck that contains silver ions with no negative surface electrification is said to contain the "latent image" and is ready for development. During development positive silver ions can be converted to atomic silver ($Ag^+ + e^- \rightarrow Ag$). The developing agents of hydroquinone and phenidone contain excess electrons and will be attracted to the positive silver ions near the sensitivity speck in those areas of the crystal where the surface electrification has been neutralized.

Bushong, "Radiographic Film," pp 167–169; Carlton and McKenna-Adler, "Radiographic Film," pp 284–286; Carroll, "Image Receptor Systems," 1998, pp 223–225; Curry et al., "Physical Characteristics of X-Ray Film and Film Processing," pp 139–141.

54. **(D)** Interactions of x rays with matter are based on two important factors: (1) the energy of the incident photon and (2) the atomic number of the tissue being irradiated. Only two interactions are important in the diagnostic range of 30 to 150 kVp: the photoelectric and Compton effects. The Compton effect is more likely to occur when a higher-energy x-ray photon interacts with the outer-shell electron in lower atomic number tissues such as fat or water. The photoelectric effect usually occurs when lower-energy incident photons interact with the inner-shell (K-shell) electron in higher atomic number substances such as bone, barium, or iodine. Classical scattering occurs at very low energy levels, below 20 keV, and may interact with the entire atom, when it is known as "Rayleigh scattering," or with just a single electron, when it is called "Thomson scattering." Pair production can only occur at very high energy levels (above 1.02 megaelectron-volts) and involves interaction with the nuclear force field, not the electron cloud.

Bushong, "X-Ray Interaction with Matter," pp 150–155; Carlton and McKenna-Adler, "X-Ray Interactions," pp 192–198; Curry et al., "Basic Interactions between X-Rays and Matter," pp 61–68.

55. **(C)** The star test pattern is one of the many test tools that may be used to check the FSS. It is usually the quality control test tool of choice because it can accurately test the small FSSs and is much easier to use than other devices, such as the pinhole camera. A wire-mesh test is a device used to check film-screen contact. Testing the accuracy of the AEC device usually requires the use of a phantom, film, and densitometer. Calibration of x-ray equipment for linearity or reproducibility is usually performed with an ionization chamber such as a cutie pie.

Bushong, "Quality Assurance and Quality Control," p 410; Carlton and McKenna-Adler, "Quality Control," p 444; Carroll, "Quality Control," 1998, pp 400–401; Thompson et al., "Quality Control," pp 407–408.

56. **(A)** Fluoroscopic tubes operate with tube currents that may range from 0.5 to 5 mA. These settings are used for dynamic imaging when the tube is expected to operate for longer periods of time at greatly reduced milliamperes. For static spot filming, the milliampere stations are usually close to that of routine radiographic tubes: between 200 and 300 mA.

Carlton and McKenna-Adler, "Fluoroscopy," p 536; Carroll, "Fluoroscopic Imaging," 1998, p 428; Dowd, "The Production of X-radiation," p 25; Thompson et al., "Fluoroscopy: Viewing Motion with X-ray," p 363.

57. **(A)** For single-phase machines, a device called a manual spinning top may be used in conjunction with radiographic film to test the accuracy of the timer setting. In single-phase equipment, the voltage drops to zero for every impulse in the cycle. There are 120 impulses per second for full-wave and 60 impulses per second for half-wave

rectified machines. A tiny hole in the spinning top is used to record each impulse in the cycle for single-phase equipment. When performing the test, if the dots overlap, the top is spinning too fast. If the dots are too close together, the top is not spinning fast enough. The manual spinning top should not be used to measure the accuracy of 3-phase or high-frequency timers because in this type of equipment, the voltage is nearly constant and never drops to zero. Instead of a series of dots, the radiograph will demonstrate an arc or semicircle. A synchronous spinning top with an electronic motor should be used with 3-phase equipment. The spinning top must be set to spin at exactly 1 revolution per second. If the arc measures 180°, or half a circle, the time is half a second. If the arc measures 90°, the time is ¼ second. An ion chamber may also be used to check the accuracy of the timer in all types of x-ray equipment.

Carroll, "Quality Control," 1998, p 388; Carlton and McKenna-Adler, "Quality Control," p 446; Thompson et al., "Quality Control," pp 406–407.

58. **(B)** Two types of radiation are produced at the target when high-speed electrons interact with the tungsten atoms: (1) Bremsstrahlung and (2) characteristic radiation. *Bremsstrahlung*, also called "braking radiation," occurs when the projectile electrons from the filament are slowed down as they pass by the tungsten nucleus and change direction. The angle of deflection determines the energy of the x-ray photon that is produced. *Characteristic radiation* occurs when the projectile electron collides with a K-shell electron, causing ionization of the tungsten atom in the target. When outer-shell electrons attempt to fill the "hole" in the K shell, characteristic radiation is given off. The radiation is "characteristic" of the atom that was ionized by the type of energy emitted. The tungsten atom typically gives off characteristic radiation at very specific energy levels of 69.5 keV. *Compton scattering* does not involve a projectile electron and a target atom, but rather occurs when an x-ray photon interacts with matter, such as human tissue. *Remnant radiation* usually refers to radiation that exits the patient's body to expose the image receptor.

Bushong, "X-Ray Production," p 130; Carlton and McKenna-Adler, "X-Ray Production," pp 133–134; Carroll, "X-Rays and Radiographic Variables," 1998, pp 9–12; Hendee, "Interactions of Electrons," p 45.

59. **(B)** The atomic number of an atom is determined by the number of protons in its nucleus, represented by the letter "Z." For instance, the Z number of tungsten is 74 because there are 74 protons

in each atom of the element tungsten. The atomic mass number, represented by the letter "A," is determined by the number of protons and neutrons in the nucleus of an atom. The stable isotope for tungsten has an A number of 184 because it has 74 protons and 110 neutrons, or 184 nucleons. An element with atoms of various mass numbers is called an isotope. Some of these isotopes may be unstable and are called radioactive isotopes because they give off various forms of energy such as alpha, beta, or gamma. If an atom of an element has a net electrical charge it is said to be an ion because either it is missing an electron and has a net positive charge or it has an extra electron and has a net negative charge. The valence number of an atom is determined by the number of electrons in the outer shell of the atom. It is the valence number that determines the chemical properties of the element. On the periodic table, elements are grouped vertically according to their valence numbers. For example, radium-dial watch painters ingested radium that was deposited in their cortical bone tissue because radium has the same valence number as calcium and therefore possesses similar chemical properties.

Bushong, "The Atom," pp 31–33; Hendee, "The Atom," p 3; Selman, "The Structure of Matter," pp 50–51.

60. **(D)** Tube rating charts, also called radiographic rating charts, are designed by equipment manufacturers so radiographers can set safe combinations of exposure factors. Many radiographers will never need to use these charts because there are built-in safety features in most modern equipment that will not allow an unsafe exposure to be taken. Most tube rating charts are drawn so that the kilovolt (peak) setting is on the vertical axis and the timer setting is on the horizontal axis. The milliampere station is the diagonal line that crosses the entire graph. Some tube rating charts have the milliampere setting on the vertical axis and the kilovolt (peak) setting on the diagonal axis. In either case, the principle is the same: Any intersection of the vertical and horizontal axes that falls on or below the diagonal line is considered a "safe" combination of technical factors. If the intersection occurs above the diagonal line, it is an "unsafe" combination of technical factors. The first three combinations (A, B, and C) fall above the diagonal line and are therefore unsafe. Only the fourth combination (D) intersects on the diagonal line and is a safe combination of technical factors to use for this particular machine.

Bushong, "The X-Ray Tube," pp 121–122; Carlton

and McKenna-Adler, "The X-Ray Tube," p 126; Curry et al., "Production of X-Rays," p 22; Hendee, "Ratings for X-Ray Tubes," p 70; Thompson et al., "X-Ray Tube Components and Design," p156.

SECTION III: IMAGE PRODUCTION AND EVALUATION

61. **(D)** Recorded detail on a radiographic image is primarily affected by three factors: (1) SID, (2) OID, and (3) FSS. A small focal spot is usually desirable whenever detail, or image sharpness, may be compromised by the other two factors. Magnification radiography requires that the anatomic part be a certain distance from the image receptor. An increased OID will result in a loss of recorded detail. For this reason, most radiographic rooms such as mammography or angiography suites are used specifically for magnification purposes and come equipped with microfocal spot sizes usually less than 0.3 mm.

Bushong, "Alternative Film Procedures," pp 289–291; Carlton and McKenna-Adler, "Technical Aspects of Mammography," p 585; Carroll, "Distance Ratios," 1998, p 275; Thompson et al., "Geometrical Factors Affecting Image Quality," pp 290–291.

62. **(D)** Whenever the speed of the imaging system is altered from one radiograph to another, it is necessary to change the milliamperage-seconds. To calculate the change, use the following formula:

$$\frac{mAs_1}{mAs_2} = \frac{Relative\ speed_2\ (RS_2)}{Relative\ speed_1\ (RS_1)}$$

mAs_1 = Original mAs

mAs_2 = New mAs

RS_2 = New screen speed

RS_1 = Original screen speed

$$\frac{100}{x} = \frac{400}{200}; x = \frac{(200)(100)}{400}; x = 50\ mAs$$

Carlton and McKenna-Adler, "Density," p 380; Dennis and Eisenberg, "Radiographic Calculations," p 94; Wallace, "Intensifying Screens," pp 165–166.

63. **(B)** When using the AEC device, it is important to select the correct ion chamber and to position the area of interest over the desired radiosensitive device. When radiographing a lateral projection of the lumbar vertebrae, the center chamber should be selected to ensure proper density in the image receptor. If the right and left chambers were selected, even with proper collimation to the area of interest, the patient would produce scatter sufficient to expose the side cell and to cause the AEC device to shut off prematurely. This happens because in an asthenic patient who is positioned properly to the center of the image receptor, very little anatomy will cover the right or left chambers. When struck by scatter, the ion chamber detects this as a sufficient amount of radiation and will terminate the exposure. The result is an underexposed radiograph with insufficient density because the timer was interrupted before proper exposure of the anatomic part could be achieved.

Carlton and McKenna-Adler, "Automatic Exposure Controls," pp 507–510; Carroll, "Evaluating Radiographs: Density," 1998, pp 248–249; Cullinan, "Basic Components of an X-Ray Generating System," p 22; Thompson et al., "Equipment and Accessory Malfunctions or Misapplications," pp 383–384.

64. **(D)** When films come out of the automatic processor damp or tacky, the most common problem is the dryer temperature. Sometimes when several large films are processed, one right after the other, there can be moisture buildup on the dryer rollers, which can stick to the last films in the group. However, other problems that may lead to damp films usually point to inadequate hardener (glutaraldehyde) in the developer. Problems with the fixer may also lead to damp films. A test should be done on the fixer to determine if it is the problem. If not, the dryer temperature should be checked. The recommended temperature is approximately 120°F. The developing tank should be checked and drained and filled with fresh chemicals if necessary.

Bushong, "Processing the Latent Image," p 186; Carlton and McKenna-Adler, "Radiographic Processing," p 304; McKinney, "The Electromechanical Systems," pp 114–115.

65. **(C)** The patient history of possible pathology should be of particular interest to radiographers prior to taking an exposure because technical factors may have to be adjusted accordingly. Radiographic pathology can be divided into two broad categories that will affect the image: (1) additive pathology and (2) destructive pathology. *Additive pathology* is a disease process that increases the density of tissue and requires an increase in technical factors. *Destructive pathology,* on the other hand, is a disease process that decreases the density of tissue and therefore requires a decrease in technical factors. Osteolytic lesions are categorized as destructive pathology, along with osteoporosis and emphysema. All of these would require a decrease in kilovolts (peak) because the tissue is easier to penetrate. Only hemothorax, a type of pleural effusion, is considered an additive

pathology because it increases the tissue density in the chest cavity and requires an increase in technical factors.

Bushong, "Radiographic Technique," pp 259–260; Carlton and McKenna-Adler, "The Pathology Problem," pp 254–263; Carroll, "Pathology and Casts," 1998, pp 166–167; Wallace, "Radiographic Techniques," pp 212–213.

66. **(A)** A good screen phosphor should be able to readily absorb x rays. Most screen phosphors can absorb about 30 to 50 percent of the x rays that strike them. A screen phosphor should also have the ability to convert those x rays into light. In a calcium tungstate screen, only about 5 percent of the x rays that are absorbed are converted into light. Rare earth phosphors, such as gadolinium and lanthanum, have much higher conversion efficiency. They convert about 15 to 20 percent of the absorbed x rays into light. Although all screen phosphors should have the ability to luminesce, or give off light, none should exhibit "afterglow," or phosphorescence. Phosphorescence is an unwanted effect in a screen phosphor because the continuation of light emission after the exposure has terminated will lead to image blur or a loss of resolution.

Bushong, "Intensifying Screens," pp 191–200; Carlton and McKenna-Adler, "Intensifying Screens," p 331; Carroll, "Intensifying Screens," 1998, pp 200, 208–209, 217; Wallace, "Intensifying Screens," pp 159–165.

67. **(D)** A large space charge may result in an increase in x-ray photons produced at the target, which will increase the intensity of the beam. It will not increase the recorded detail. A strong positive anode will increase the potential difference, or kilovoltage, in the x-ray tube. This will increase the average energy of x rays that are created at the target. It will not affect recorded detail. A thick phosphor crystal in the image receptor will increase screen speed and decrease recorded detail. Only the use of a small focal spot will result in an increase in recorded detail.

Carlton and McKenna-Adler, "Recorded Detail," pp 405–413; Cullinan, "Radiographic Quality," p 123; Wallace, "Geometric Factors Affecting Recorded Detail," p 131.

68. **(A)** The only one of the four factors listed that will have a noticeable effect on radiographic contrast is kilovolts (peak). The other technical factors of milliamperes, exposure time, and FSS have a negligible effect on contrast. Milliamperage-seconds may affect contrast if it causes excessive or insufficient radiographic density. In all of the choices given, the 15 percent difference in kilovolts (peak) is compensated by either in-

creasing or decreasing the milliamperage-seconds. The lowest kilovolts (peak) would give the highest contrast—choice A. Other controllable factors affecting contrast include (1) OID because of the "air-gap" technique, (2) grid ratio, (3) screen versus direct exposure film, (4) filtration, (5) beam restriction, (6) off-focus radiation, (7) compression of the body part, and (8) processing time and chemistry.

Carlton and McKenna-Adler, "Contrast," pp 397–401; Carroll, "Exercise No. 24," p 545; Cullinan, "Radiographic Quality," pp 120–123; Wallace, "Relationship of the Four Radiographic Qualities," p 178.

69. **(A)** Whenever distance is changed from one radiograph to another, the milliamperage-seconds should be adjusted, rather than the kilovolts (peak). To solve this problem, use the milliamperage-seconds square formula. First solve for mAs: 400 mA × 0.25 s = 100 mAs

$$\frac{mAs_1}{mAs_2} = \frac{D_1^2}{D_2^2}$$

$$\frac{100}{x} = \frac{72^2}{40^2}; \ x = \frac{100(40^2)}{(72^2)}; \ x = \frac{100(1600)}{5184};$$

$$x = 100 \times 0.3086;$$

$$x = 30 \ mAs; \ \frac{30}{400} = 0.075 \ s$$

Carlton and McKenna-Adler, "Exposure Conversion Problems," p 514; Carroll, "Source-Image Receptor Distance," 1998, pp 256–258; Dennis and Eisenberg, "Radiographic Calculations," p 65.

70. **(B)** The quantity, or number of photons, reaching the patient is dependent on many factors, including (1) milliamperage-seconds, (2) kilovolts (peak), (3) filtration, and (4) SSD. Because milliamperage-seconds is directly proportional to the quantity of photons produced, milliamperage-seconds is the technical factor of choice for regulating the intensity.

Bushong, "X-Ray Emission," p 140; Carlton and McKenna-Adler, "Minimizing Patient Dose," p 210; Carroll, "Milliampere-Seconds," 1998, p 69; Wallace, "mAs and Reciprocity," p 54.

71. **(C)** To solve this problem, use the following formula:

$$\frac{Image \ size}{Object \ size} = \frac{SID}{SOD}$$

$$\frac{15 \ in.}{x} = \frac{40 \ in.}{30 \ in.}; \ x = 15 \times \frac{30}{40}; \ x = 15 \times 0.75;$$

$$x = 11.25 \ in.$$

Bushong, "Alternative Film Procedures," p 290; Carlton and McKenna-Adler, "Distortion," p 420;

Dennis and Eisenberg, "Radiographic Calculations," p 111; Wallace, "Size Distortion," p 31.

72. **(A)** The reciprocity law states that two separate techniques using varying milliamperes and time should provide equivalent total milliamperage-seconds. To find which choices (numbers 1 to 4) are equivalent, solve for milliamperage-seconds:
    1. 200×0.05 s $= 10$ mAs*
    2. 400×0.03 s $= 12$ mAs
    3. 500×0.02 s $= 10$ mAs*
    4. 600×0.05 s $= 30$ mAs

*Numbers 1 and 3 have the same milliamperage-seconds. The reciprocity law related to linearity states that all radiographic equipment should be calibrated so that the use of varying milliampere and time settings with equivalent milliamperage-seconds should result in similar optical density readings on the radiograph. In fact, according to federal guidelines, the density should not vary by more than 10 percent from one radiograph to another.

Bushong, "Designing for Radiation Protection," p 511; Carlton and McKenna-Adler, "Density," p 370; Carroll, "Milliampere-Seconds," 1998, p 70; Wallace, "mAs and Reciprocity," p 56.

73. **(D)** Compensating filters are used to compensate for varying thickness of anatomy. A wedge filter is beneficial for anatomy that is thin at one end and thick at the other. Examples of radiographic examinations that would benefit from the use of a wedge filter include a dorsoplantar projection of the foot, AP projection of the thoracic vertebrae, and AP projection of the femur. For thoracic vertebrae and femur projections, the use of the anode heel effect is usually sufficient because the heel effect is more pronounced with large films (14×17 in.) such as those used for this anatomy. In any case, the thick end of the wedge should be placed over the thinner anatomy. For the dorsoplantar projection of the foot, the thick end of the filter should be placed over the toes.

Carlton and McKenna-Adler, "Filtration," p 173; Carroll, "Beam Filtration," 1998, pp 127–128; Cullinan, "Basic Operation of an X-Ray Tube," pp 40–42; Wallace, "Methods to Control Scatter," p 122.

74. **(C)** A contrast medium is added to the patient's body to better delineate soft-tissue anatomy. Two broad categories of contrast media exist: (1) positive and (2) negative. A positive contrast medium usually has a higher atomic number than that of the soft tissue and absorbs more radiation when introduced. Examples are barium and water-based and oil-based iodine. A negative contrast medium decreases the average tissue density because it does not absorb radiation

as easily as soft tissue. Some examples of negative contrast media include air and carbon dioxide.

Bushong, "X-Ray Interaction with Matter," p 160; Carroll, "Patient Status and Contrast Agents," 1998, pp 151–154; Cullinan, "Technical Factor Selection," pp 141–145; Wallace, "Radiographic Contrast," p 80.

75. **(B)** To answer this question, categorize the technical factors from those providing the least density to those providing the greatest density. Then summarize each set of factors as follows:

	mA	Exposure Time	kVp	Screen Speed
A.	400^3	0.01^2	94^3	$100^2 = 10$
B.	500^4	0.008^1	94^3	$200^3 = 11$
C.	200^2	0.04^4	90^2	$50^1 = 9$
D.	100^1	0.02^3	80^1	$200^3 = 8$

The combination of factors that would result in the greatest radiographic density between the choices given would be choice B.

Carlton and McKenna-Adler, "Density," pp 368–369; Carroll, "Exercise No. 24," 1998, p 545; Wallace, "The Relationship of the Four Radiographic Qualities," pp 176–177.

76. **(B)** A focused grid is intended to be used at a specific distance from the radiation source. It takes advantage of the divergence of the x-ray beam, and the lead strips should be set at a specific angle to work effectively at that particular distance. The lead strips in the center of the grid are not angled because the central ray will strike the beam in a straight line. At the edges of the grid, the strips are progressively slanted at steeper angles to correctly match the divergence of the beam. If the grid is used at the improper distance, the edges on both sides of the image will demonstrate reduced optical density because of grid cutoff.

Carroll, "Grids," 1998, pp 189–193; Cullinan, "Control of Scatter Radiation," p 82; Wallace, "Grids and the Bucky," pp 107–108.

77. **(C)** While Roentgen was working with vacuum tubes in his laboratory on November 8, 1895, he accidentally discovered x rays. A plate coated with phosphorescent barium platinocyanide on the opposite side of the room glowed whenever there was a current flowing through the tube. Today, phosphors find many uses in radiography. Calcium tungstate was first used by Thomas Edison in image intensifiers and later in intensifying screens. Sodium and cesium iodides are now used in the input phosphor of the image intensifier and as the scintillation detector in nuclear medicine gamma cameras. The output phosphor in the image intensifier is made of zinc cadmium sulfide. Lithium fluoride is a crystal that is used for the detection of radiation for personnel monitoring in the TLD badge.

Bushong, "Basic Concepts of Radiation Science," p 6; Carlton and McKenna-Adler, "Radiation Concepts," p 34; Dowd and Tilson, "Introduction to Biologic Effects: From Cells to Organs," p 69.

78. **(A)** *Radiographic contrast* is defined as the difference in gray tones between adjacent structures. The greater the difference, the higher the contrast. High contrast, also called "short-scale contrast," appears as a stark difference in adjacent structures that appear more black and white. High contrast is usually produced with a lower-kilovolt (peak) setting but may be affected by many factors. Low contrast, also called "long-scale contrast," appears as many shades of varying gray tones with very little difference between adjacent structures in the image. Low contrast is generally produced from higher-kilovolt (peak) settings and allows the radiographer greater latitude when selecting technical factors.

    Carlton and McKenna-Adler, "Contrast," pp 385–387; Carroll, "Kilovoltage-Peak," 1998, p 91; Cullinan, "Radiographic Contrast," pp 120–121; Wallace, "The Four Radiographic Qualities," pp 4, 74–76.

79. **(D)** The *grid ratio* is defined as the height of the lead strips in a grid divided by the distance between them: r = h/d. The *grid frequency* is the number of grid lines per inch, usually between 80 and 100 lines per inch. The unit of *line-pairs per millimeter* is a measurement of the resolution of an image and can be measured using a special quality control test tool.

    Carlton and McKenna-Adler, "The Grid," p 268; Carroll, "Grids," 1998, p 185; Cullinan, "Technical Formulas and Related Data," p 291; Wallace, "Grids and the Bucky," p 107.

80. **(B)** Recorded detail is affected by SID, OID, FSS, and screen speed. Although the technical factors of kilovolts (peak) and milliamperage-seconds affect visibility of detail, they have little effect on recorded detail. To solve this problem, calculate unsharpness for each combination of factors. The combination with the least unsharpness and the lowest screen speed will have the greatest recorded detail. To calculate unsharpness, the formula is as follows:

    $$\text{Unsharpness} = \frac{\text{OID}}{\text{SOD}} \times \text{FSS}$$

	Unsharpness	*Screen Speed*
A. 10/90 × 0.6 =	0.067 mm	200
B. 10/170 × 0.6 =	0.035 mm	100
C. 20/160 × 0.6 =	0.075 mm	200
D. 20/80 × 1.2 =	0.30 mm	100

    Choice B has the least unsharpness and the slowest screen speed of all of the choices and therefore has the best recorded detail.

Carlton and McKenna-Adler, "Recorded Detail," pp 405–414; Cullinan, "Total Unsharpness," pp 123–130; Dennis and Eisenberg, "Radiographic Calculations," p 103; Selman, "Radiographic Quality," p 321; Wallace, "The Relationship of the Four Radiographic Qualities," p 180.

81. **(B)** A sensitometer and densitometer are two key instruments in the quality control of an automatic processor. The densitometer and the penetrometer may also be used to calibrate x-ray equipment, although there are much more sophisticated test tools available. A sensitometer "sensitizes" or exposes the x-ray film to a predetermined level of light. The resultant radiograph exhibits an optical step wedge on it. The densitometer is then used to *measure* the optical *density* of each step on the wedge and to measure the background density (base-plus-fog). A penetrometer may be used instead of a sensitometer, but it is not as accurate. The penetrometer is more often referred to as an aluminum step wedge. The oscilloscope is another quality control test tool that may be used to test the accuracy of the timer in 3-phase and high-frequency x-ray equipment.

    Carlton and McKenna-Adler, "Sensitometry," pp 316–319; Thompson et al., "Quality Control," pp 398–401; Wallace, "mAs and Reciprocity," p 48.

82. **(C)** The film emulsion is the part of the film that contains the photosensitive silver halides. Silver halides can be either (1) silver bromide (about 90 to 99 percent) or (2) silver iodide (about 1 to 10 percent). The silver halides are suspended in a gelatin that is spread out onto the film base. The gelatin is a clear protein that is made from the hides and hoofs of animals. Some of this natural gelatin was found to contain minor traces of sulfur ingested from eating foods with mustard. The sulfur made the film emulsion more sensitive. Many manufacturers now artificially add mustard oil or sulfur to the emulsion to make the film more sensitive.

    Carroll, "Image Receptor Systems," 1998, p 222; Selman, "X-Ray Film, Film Holders, and Intensifying Screens," p 271; Thompson et al., "Radiographic Film," p 239.

83. **(B)** There are two main factors that aid the visibility of detail in an image: (1) contrast and (2) density. A third factor, which may detract from the visibility of detail, is *noise*, defined as undesirable information in the image (artifacts, motion, or fog). Visibility of detail is different from recorded detail, which is a measure of the resolving capability of the imaging system, rather than the ability to see the image.

    Burns, "Radiographic Definition and Distortion," pp 120–123; Carlton and McKenna-Adler, "Density," p 367, and "Contrast," p 385; Carroll, "Qualities of the Radiographic Image," 1998, p 30; Wallace, "Recorded Detail," p 130.

84. **(C)** Geometric unsharpness is poor resolution caused by geometric factors such as the SID, OID, and FSS. Shape distortion is caused by angulation of the tube, anatomic part, or image receptor that may produce either elongation or foreshortening of the image. Radiographic parallax is an undesirable effect seen in some double-emulsion films in which the image on one side of the emulsion is slightly offset from the image on the other side because of the thickness of the base. Motion unsharpness is specifically caused from movement during the exposure. This movement could be from the patient, the tube, or the film. Methods to eliminate motion include shorter exposure times, suspended respiration, careful immobilization, properly functioning equipment, and good communication skills.

Carroll, "Motion," 1998, pp 288–289; Selman, "Radiographic Quality," p 327.

85. **(B)** Noise may be described as any unnecessary information that interferes with the visibility of the area of interest. By far, the most common form of noise results from fogging of the image receptor by random radiation known as "scatter." Other types of noise include artifacts and motion unsharpness. An increase in kilovolts (peak) has a direct effect on increasing scatter that reaches the film due to an increase in the Compton effect. A decrease in kilovolts (peak) results in a decrease in noise. A change in milliamperes has very little effect on the noise. A decrease in milliamperes may result in an increase in noise if the decrease results in insufficient milliamperage-seconds, leading to quantum mottle in fast-speed imaging systems. Use of a slower-speed screen will decrease noise because a higher–milliamperage-second value is required which reduces the chance of quantum mottle. Slower-speed screens also offer better recorded detail because of their smaller crystals, thereby reducing image noise.

Bushong, "Intensifying Screens," p 193; Carroll, 1998, "Qualities of the Radiographic Image," p 30, and "Analyzing the Radiographic Image," pp 301–302; Cullinan, "Conventional Recording Media," pp 100–101.

86. **(B)** To calculate time when the milliamperage-seconds is known, simply divide the total milliamperage-seconds by the selected milliamperes: mAs/mA = Time; 60/400 = 0.15 s, or 150 ms.

Carlton and McKenna-Adler, "Exposure Conversion Problems," p 514; Dennis and Eisenberg, "Radi-

ographic Calculations" pp 57–59; Wallace, "mAs and Reciprocity," pp 53, 56.

87. **(A)** A positive contrast medium increases the average density of tissue because it attenuates more radiation because of the high atomic number of the medium (barium and iodine). A negative contrast medium decreases the average tissue density because it attenuates less radiation (air or carbon dioxide).

Bushong, "X-Ray Interaction with Matter," p 160; Carroll, "Patient Status and Contrast Agents," 1998, pp 157–159; Cullinan, "Technical Factor Selection," pp 141–145; Wallace, "Radiographic Contrast," p 80.

88. **(D)** The main purpose of using the line focus principle in an x-ray tube is to decrease the effective FSS, which will result in better spatial resolution in the image while using the higher combinations of kilovolt (peak), milliampere, and time settings. The heat capacity of the anode will also increase because larger milliampere stations may be used to produce the resultant high-resolution images. When using a steeper anode angle to achieve the smaller effective focal spot, the unfortunate side effect may be an increase in the anode heel effect. The radiographer should be cautious when positioning large body parts with wide differences in tissue density and/or thickness from one end to the other (femur and thoracic vertebrae) when steeper anode angles are used (5° to 15°).

Burns, "The X-Ray Tube," p 11; Bushong, "The X-Ray Tube," pp 116–117; Carlton and McKenna-Adler, "The X-Ray Tube," pp 118–120; Carroll, "The Anode Bevel," 1998, pp 241–242.

89. **(B)** To solve this problem, simply calculate milliamperage-seconds by multiplying the milliamperes by exposure time:

mA	Exposure Time	mAs
A. 200	$\frac{1}{10}$ s	20 mAs
B. 400	$\frac{1}{40}$ s	10 mAs
C. 300	$\frac{1}{20}$ s	15 mAs
D. 100	$\frac{1}{3}$ s	33.33 mAs

The combination with the lowest total milliamperage-seconds will produce the least optical density on the radiograph, all other factors remaining the same.

Carlton and McKenna-Adler, "Density," pp 368–369; Carroll, "Exercise No. 24," 1998, p 545; Wallace, "The Relationship of the Four Radiographic Qualities," pp 176–177.

90. **(C)** Simply take the object size and multiply by the MF to solve this problem:

$$\frac{\text{Image size}}{\text{Object size}} = \frac{\text{SID}}{\text{SOD}}; \text{[SID/SOD = MF]}$$

Image size = (SID/SOD) × Object size

Image size = 2 × 10 in.; Image size = 20 inches

Bushong, "Alternative Film Procedures," p 290; Carlton and McKenna-Adler, "Distortion," p 420; Dennis and Eisenberg, "Radiographic Calculations," p 111; Wallace, "Size Distortion," p 31.

91. **(C)** A compression band is used in radiography for two reasons: (1) as a restraining device for un-cooperative or unconscious patients and (2) as a compression device for abdominal radiography to produce a more uniform tissue thickness. When using the device for abdominal radiography on cooperative patients, the band improves radiographic contrast by reducing the thickness of the abdomen and by reducing scatter produced in the patient.
Carlton and McKenna-Adler, "X-Ray Equipment," p 88; Cullinan, "Radiographic Quality," p 122; Wallace, "Methods to Control Scatter," p 125.

92. **(B)** A wire-mesh test is used to determine film-screen contact. A Wisconsin test cassette and an Adran and Crookes cassette may be used to test the accuracy of the kilovolt (peak) settings. The most accurate method of testing the kilovolts (peak) is with a dosimeter connected to a digital computer. The star test pattern is the device most often used to measure FSS. A resolution bar pattern or pinhole camera may also be used.
Bushong, "Quality Assurance and Quality Control," p 410; Carlton and McKenna-Adler, "Quality Control," p 446; Carroll, "Quality Control," 1998, pp 400–403; Thompson et al., "Quality Control," p, 406.

93. **(D)** Grids are useful for examinations in which large amounts of scatter may be produced. Scatter produces unwanted "noise" in the image. When scatter is excessive, the use of a grid is highly recommended. Scatter in the diagnostic range is caused mainly by the Compton effect, which is more common in a higher-energy x-ray beam (greater than 70 kVp) and in tissues with low atomic numbers, such as fat, water, or muscle. Because scatter may be produced both by high-kilovolt (peak) settings as well as thick body parts, the thickness of the anatomic part should also be a consideration. Any body part that exceeds 10 to 12 cm should require the use of a grid. A rule of thumb is that any time the body thickness exceeds 10 cm or requires the use of 70 kVp or greater, a grid will be beneficial. For kilovolt (peak) settings higher than 90 kVp, a grid ratio of at least 8:1 is required.
Burns, "Control of Scatter Radiation: Grids and Air Gap," p 161; Carlton, "The Grid," p 265; Carroll, "Grids," p 184; Wallace, "Grid Selection," p 112.

94. **(D)** To calculate the MF, simply follow this formula: SID/(SID − OID), or SID/SOD = MF
A. 40-in. SID, 5-in. OID; *40/35 = 1.14×*
B. 60-in. SID, 10-in. OID; *60/50 = 1.2×*
C. 72-in. SID, 25-in. OID; *72/47 = 1.53×*
D. 80-in. SID, 30-in. OID; *80/50 = 1.6×*

Bushong, "Alternative Film Procedures," p 290; Carlton and McKenna-Adler, "Distortion," p 420; Dennis and Eisenberg, "Radiographic Calculations," p 111; Wallace, "Size Distortion," p 31.

95. **(B)** Sensitometry should be performed each morning to ensure proper functioning of the automatic processor. The same type of film should be used each time to ensure that the density, contrast, and inherent fog on the film stay consistent from day to day. Three factors should be measured on the sensitometric film each time the film is processed: (1) base-plus-fog, (2) median density, and (3) density difference. The base-plus-fog measures the inherent fog contributed by the film base and automatic developer. This step should not vary by more than ±0.05 optical density points from one film to another. The median density measures the speed of the film. The step that measures film speed is the step that comes closest to 1 optical density point above base-plus-fog. The density difference is also known as the average gradient of the film. The density difference can be found by subtracting the step that measures closest to the 0.25 optical density point above base-plus-fog from the step that measures closest to 2 optical density points above base-plus-fog. The difference between the greatest useful density, or darkest acceptable region of the film, and the least useful density, or the lightest acceptable region of the film (usually between 0.25 to 2.5), is the film's inherent contrast. In a sensitometry strip, both the speed and contrast of the film should not vary by more than ±0.1 optical density point from one film to another.
Carlton and McKenna-Adler, "Sensitometry," pp 323–325; Carroll, "Sensitometry & Darkroom Quality Control," 1998, p 532; McKinney, "Sensitometry," p 33.

96. **(A)** Radiographic contrast is defined as the difference in optical density between adjacent structures. The greater is the difference, the greater the contrast. A high-contrast image with a large difference in optical densities between tissues is also called short-scale contrast because it consists mainly of black and white shades with very few shades of gray. On the other hand, long-scale contrast, also called low contrast, is seen in an image

where there are many shades of gray with very little difference in optical density between adjacent structures. Contrast can be controlled in the radiographic image by adjusting the kilovolts (peak). An increase in kilovolts (peak) will decrease contrast because more of the x-ray photons will penetrate the part and expose the image receptor, creating more shades of gray with little difference in appearance between adjacent structures. Conversely, low kilovolts (peak) results in high contrast because the high-density tissues such as bone will be more likely to totally absorb the incident photons through photoelectric interaction.

Burns, "Radiographic Contrast," pp 102–105; Carlton and McKenna-Adler, "Contrast," p 385; Carroll, "Qualities of the Radiographic Image," 1998, pp 34–40; Wallace, "Radiographic Contrast," pp 75, 85.

97. **(B)** Radiographic pathology can be divided into two broad categories: (1) additive and (2) destructive. Additive pathology is a disease process that increases the density of tissue and thus requires an increase in technical factors. Destructive pathology, on the other hand, is a disease process that decreases the density of tissue and therefore requires a decrease in technical factors. Atrophy is an example of a destructive pathology because the tissue has decreased in density. Osteolytic lesions are also categorized as destructive pathology. A metastatic lesion is an example of destructive pathology because the lesion destroys surrounding healthy tissue and makes it more radiolucent. Advanced destructive pathologies usually require an adjustment in the kilovolts (peak) because the tissue is easier to penetrate.

Bushong, "Radiographic Technique," pp 259–260; Carlton and McKenna-Adler, "The Pathology Problem," pp 254–263; Carroll, "Pathology and Casts," 1998, pp 166–167; Wallace, "Radiographic Techniques," pp 212–213.

98. **(B)** There are four basic factors that affect x-ray quantity or intensity: (1) milliamperage-seconds, which is directly proportional to quantity in that a doubling of the milliamperage-seconds will result in a doubling of the x-ray quantity; (2) kilovolts (peak), which is exponentially proportional; (3) filtration, which is inversely proportional; and (4) distance, which has an inverse-square proportionality to x-ray quantity.

Bushong, "X-Ray Emission," p 140; Carlton and McKenna-Adler, "The Prime Factors," p 182; Carroll, "Milliampere-Seconds," 1998, pp 69–70; Dowd, "Protecting the Patient in Radiography," p 178.

99. **(D)** The use of a smaller focal spot will increase the resolution or recorded detail of the image. The heat capacity of the x-ray tube will decrease

with the use of a small focal spot because the anode will not be able to handle as many electrons striking it in a smaller area on the target. Therefore, there is a limit to the amount of milliamperes that may be used with small focal spots. X-ray production in the diagnostic range is a very inefficient method of producing desirable energy. Less than 1 percent of the kinetic energy of the electrons will be converted to x rays. The rest of the energy will be converted to heat or thermal radiation. The only sure way to increase x-ray production is to increase the kilovolts (peak) to energy levels that far exceed the normal useful range of diagnostic energies (greater than 150 kVp). These energy levels, however, would be inappropriate for imaging purposes.

Bushong, "The X-Ray Tube," p 112; Carlton and McKenna-Adler, "Recorded Detail," pp 406–407; Carroll, "Focal Spot Size," 1998, p 233; Selman, "Radiographic Quality," p 319.

100. **(C)** When a change in x-ray quantity is desired, the technical factor of choice is usually not kilovolts (peak), because altering the kilovolts will alter the scale of contrast. Kilovolts (peak) affects the scale of contrast because the differential attenuation of tissues is altered. In some instances, a change in the scale of contrast is desirable, and the kilovolts (peak) would be the best method to accomplish this. Adjusting the kilovolts (peak) has nothing to do with magnification. The magnification of an image, known as "size distortion," is controlled mainly by the OID and is only slightly affected by the SID. *Bremsstrahlung*, or braking radiation, can occur throughout the diagnostic range of energies. As kilovolts (peak) is increased, the percentage of Bremsstrahlung radiation in the beam decreases as the production of characteristic x rays increases.

Burns, "Radiographic Contrast," pp 102–105; Carlton and McKenna-Adler, "Contrast" p 385; Carroll, "Kilovoltage-Peak," 1998, p 91; Wallace, "Radiographic Contrast," pp 75, 85.

101. **(C)** The spinning top test is used to test the accuracy of single-phase timers. The step wedge, or penetrometer, may be used to test milliamperage-seconds linearity and reproducibility. It also may be used to check the function of the automatic processor. The star test pattern is a test tool used for measuring FSS. The HVL is the only true measure of beam quality or penetrability. The *HVL* is defined as the thickness of absorbing material that is necessary to reduce the intensity of the beam to one-half of its original intensity. The HVL changes with the penetrability of the beam, or the average energy, which is altered by either a change in kilovolts (peak) or a change in alu-

minum filtration. The HVL of a particular x-ray beam may be measured by using one of two test tools: (1) the Wisconsin kilovolt (peak) test cassette, which is also used for assessing kilovolt (peak) accuracy, or (2) a pocket ionization chamber with sleeve filters or larger ionization chambers (cutie pie) with several sheets of aluminum filters.

Carlton and McKenna-Adler, "Quality Control," p 445; Carroll, "Quality Control," 1998, pp 395–396; Cullinan, "Basic Quality Assurance Test Procedures," p 253; Selman, "X-Rays (Roentgen Rays)," p 171.

102. **(B)** The average temperature of the developer should fall somewhere between 92° and 96°F. The average temperature should not vary by more than ± 3°F. If the temperature exceeds the normal average, the result will be excess chemical fog. A temperature difference of only 0.5°F will be enough to cause a visible change in the optical density on the image. This chemical fog is due to the increased activity of the reducing agents in the developer, which will inadvertently develop unexposed silver halide as well as exposed crystals.

Carlton and McKenna-Adler, "Sensitometry," p 322; Cullinan, "Recorded Detail," pp 122–123; Wallace, "Radiographic Film & Development," p 144.

103. **(D)** SID is one of the geometric factors affecting the radiograph. An increase in SID will result in reduced magnification and increased recorded detail. Without any compensation of technical factors, an increase in the SID will cause a decrease in patient dose inverse to the square of the distance. The kilovolts (peak) usually does not need to be adjusted for changes in the SID. The milliamperage-seconds are usually adjusted.

Carlton and McKenna-Adler, "Recorded Detail," pp 405–414; Cullinan, "Total Unsharpness," pp 123–130; Selman, "Radiographic Quality," p 321; Wallace, "The Relationship of the Four Radiographic Qualities," p 180.

104. **(B)** The formation of the latent image in the film is due to the interactions of light or x rays with the atoms of silver halide crystals in the emulsion. Silver halide atoms primarily consist of silver bromide (approximately 95 percent) and silver iodide (approximately 5 percent). These silver halide crystals are suspended in a gelatin solution to evenly distribute them on the film's base. Most modern screen-type film is "duplitized," meaning that it has an active emulsion layer on both sides of the base. Once the silver halide crystals have been ionized they then migrate to the sensitivity specks. The sensitivity specks are areas of imperfection (mainly sulfur,

in the form of mustard oil, that has been added by the manufacturer to make the film more sensitive to radiation or light exposure). These areas neutralize the surface of the crystal lattice, which normally possesses a negative charge prior to exposure, thus allowing the electrons in the developer to seep through and to create the black metallic silver manifest image.

Bushong, "Radiographic Film," p 168; Carlton and McKenna-Adler, "Radiographic Film," p 285; Carroll, "Image Receptor Systems," pp 223–225; Thompson et al., "Radiographic Film," p 239.

105. **(C)** There are two main interactions of x rays with matter that occur in the diagnostic range: (1) Compton effect and (2) photoelectric effect. The photoelectric effect occurs most often with tissues of high atomic numbers, such as bone, and with incident photon energies below 70 keV. Compton scattering is more likely to occur in tissues with low atomic numbers, such as fat, muscle, or water, and when the incident photon energy is greater than 70 keV. With higher-energy photons, the beam is more penetrating and more likely to expose the film and increase the density. Conversely, when the energy of the beam is lower, the x rays are more likely to be absorbed in the patient and not expose the film.

Bushong, "X-Ray Interaction with Matter," pp 151–154; Carlton and McKenna-Adler, "X-Ray Interactions," p 194; Dowd and Tilson, "Interactions of Radiation with Matter," pp 53–54.

106. **(A)** The intensity or quantity of photons in the beam is affected by many factors but is most easily controlled by the milliamperage-seconds (mAs) because there is a direct proportional relationship between the two. As milliamperage-seconds is doubled, the x-ray quantity will be doubled. The quality of the x-ray beam is only influenced by three factors: (1) kilovolts (peak), (2) filtration, and (3) type of generator (single-phase versus 3-phase). Although milliamperage-seconds directly influences x-ray quantity, the effect to optical density on the film is much more complicated. In most instances, when milliamperage-seconds is increased, the optical density on the radiograph will also increase.

Bushong, "X-Ray Emission," p 140; Carlton and McKenna-Adler, "The Prime Factors," p 182; Carroll, "Milliampere-Seconds," 1998, pp 69–70; Dowd and Tilson, "Protecting the Patient in Radiography," p 178.

107. **(D)** An aperture diaphragm is a special type of beam-restricting device that is designed to delimit the beam in such a way that the x-ray beam will be projected slightly smaller than the image receptor. In other words, when the diaphragm is

used, an unexposed border should be visible on each edge of the radiograph. The proper SID should be used with the specified diaphragm. To solve this equation, it is easiest to use the following formula:

$$\frac{D_1}{D_2} = \frac{F_1}{F_2} \; or \; \frac{D_1}{F_1} = \frac{D_2}{F_2}$$

D_1 = The distance closest to the source

D_2 = The distance farthest from the source

F_1 = Field size at closest distance

F_2 = Field size at farthest distance

$$\frac{10}{16 \times 8} = \frac{40}{x}; \; 10x = (16 \times 8) \times 40;$$

$$x = \frac{(16 \times 8) \times 40}{10}; \; x = (16 \times 8) \times 4;$$

$$x = 64 \times 32$$

Bushong, "Scatter Radiation and Beam-Restricting Devices," p 209; Carlton and McKenna-Adler, "Beam-Restriction," p 240; Carroll, "Field Size Limitation," 1998, pp 143–144; Selman, "Devices for Improving Radiographic Quality," p 392.

108. **(C)** The size of the field has an effect on patient dose because the larger the field size, the more scatter that will be produced in the patient. Therefore, the smallest field size would be used to protect the patient from excessive radiation. To calculate the field size for each of the following, calculate the area of each field. For squares and rectangles, area may be found by multiplying length and width. For circles, area is found by multiplying πr^2 (π = 3.14 and r = $\frac{1}{2}$ diameter).
A. 15-cm diameter circular field = 3.14 $\times$ 7.5^2 = 176.63 cm^2
B. 12 $\times$ 12 cm square field = 12 $\times$ 12 = 144 cm^2
C. 14 $\times$ 10 cm rectangular field = 14 $\times$ 10 = 140 cm^2
D. 12 $\times$ 13 cm rectangular field = 12 $\times$ 13 = 156 cm^2

Carroll, "Minimizing Patient Exposure," 1998, p 374; Dennis and Eisenberg, "Basic Mathematical Concepts," pp 25, 33, 35, 37; Dowd and Tilson, "Appendix A," p 324; Selman, "Physics and the Units of Measurements," p 30.

109. **(B)** In computed radiography, the image is displayed on a CRT, which is similar to a television monitor. With this type of imaging system, the density and contrast of the image are controlled by the window level and window width. The window level adjusts the brightness or the density of the image. The window width controls the number of gray shades or contrast in the image.

The resolution, or recorded detail, is controlled by the matrix, which designates the number of pixels (bits of information in the image). The matrix is usually indicated by its length and width. For instance, 128 $\times$ 128 and 256 $\times$ 256 are common matrixes.

Bushong, "Digital X-Ray Imaging," p 361; Carlton and McKenna-Adler, "Digital Image Processing," p 627; Curry et al., "Digital Radiography," p 401;. Wolbarst, "Digital Representation of an Image," p 306.

110. **(D)** Although other types of film (multiformat camera film) may be used with digital or computerized images, laser film is gaining popularity for several reasons. It has excellent resolution. It has exceptional consistency in image quality. It is available in most modern imaging departments. A distinct advantage of the laser printer is that it can be interfaced with several imaging systems (CT, magnetic resonance imaging [MRI], and digital radiography) in the same department. Periapical and occlusal films are special types of film used for oral and dental radiography. Roll film is typically coupled to the output phosphor to obtain direct images from the image intensifier. Roll film is common in routine fluoroscopy. Cineradiography-type roll film is used for cardiac catheterization procedures.

Bushong, "Radiographic Film," p 172; Carlton and McKenna-Adler, "Digital Image Processing," p 634; Cullinan, "Recording Media for Specialized Imaging," pp 230–231.

SECTION IV: RADIOGRAPHIC PROCEDURES AND RELATED ANATOMY

111. **(B)** To overcome the magnification of the heart and to obtain sharper outlines of the delicate lung structures, a long SID should be used during chest radiography. An SID of at least 72 in. (6 ft) is usually recommended.

Ballinger, Vol 1, p 444; Bontrager, p 66; Eisenberg et al., "Chest," p 27.

112. **(C)** The routine radiographic procedure for nasal bones is generally a parietoacanthial projection, a PA projection, and both lateral projections. The lateral projections best demonstrate the nasal bones for anterior and posterior displacement. Both the parietoacanthial and the PA projections demonstrate the nasal septum. Sometimes a special view is ordered if there is particular interest in medial or lateral displacement of the nasal bones. The projection that best demonstrates lateral or medial displacement of the nasal bones is the inferosuperior axial projection.

Ballinger, Vol 2, p 317; Bontrager, pp 367–368.

113. **(C)** Because of the natural kyphotic curvature of the sacrum, it is necessary to angle the central ray so that the sacral foramina will be properly demonstrated. The necessary angulation for the routine AP projection is 15° cephalad. If the patient is prone, the angulation should be 15° caudal. Whenever possible, the sacrum should be radiographed with the AP projection to minimize the OID.

Ballinger, Vol 1, p 387; Bontrager, p 299; Eisenberg et al., "Sacrum," p 199.

114. **(A)** To properly demonstrate the apophyseal joints of the thoracic vertebrae, rotate the patient 20° from the lateral position toward the side of interest. The midcoronal plane of the patient should form a 70° angle with the plane of the film. The RAO and LAO positions demonstrate the apophyseal joints closer to the film. The RPO and LPO positions demonstrate the joints farther from the film.

Ballinger, Vol 1, p 362; Bontrager, p 277; Eisenberg et al., "Thoracic Spine," p 185.

115. **(D)** The proper central ray centering point for an AP projection of the hand is the third metacarpophalangeal joint or at the head of the third metacarpal joint.

Ballinger, Vol 1, p 74; Bontrager, p 121; Eisenberg et al., "Hand," p 50.

116. **(C)** To properly demonstrate the calcaneus or os calcis, it is necessary to angle the central ray 40° cephalic along the long axis of the foot. The central ray should enter the plantar surface of the foot at the base of the third metatarsal joint.

Ballinger, Vol 1, p 215; Bontrager, p 197; Eisenberg et al., "Calcaneus," p 112.

117. **(A)** This radiograph demonstrates a hysterosalpingogram. A hysterosalpingogram is performed to demonstrate the uterus and fallopian tubes in the female reproductive system. It is specifically performed to evaluate the patency of the oviducts in suspected cases of infertility. In some instances, the procedure is actually therapeutic in that it may clear the obstruction and open the oviduct.

Ballinger, Vol 2, p 200; Eisenberg et al., p 354; Tortorici, "Hysterosalpingography," 1995, p 58.

118. **(C)** To best demonstrate a pneumothorax, a horizontal central ray is essential. The best projections to demonstrate a pneumothorax are either an erect PA projection on expiration or a lateral decubitus projection. Small amounts of free air might be obscured in the full inhalation radiograph. When a pneumothorax is suspected, the physician or radiologist will usually request two

PA projections: one on inspiration and one on expiration. A ventral decubitus projection would be a lateral projection and would be of little value in comparing both lung cavities.

Ballinger, Vol 1, p 444; Bontrager, p 66; Eisenberg et al., pp 25, 27, 34, 53; Laudicina, "Respiratory System," p 29; Linn-Watson, "Respiratory System," p 209.

119. **(D)** There are three different methods for demonstrating the intercondyloid fossa: (1) the Holmblad method, with the patient on all four extremities on the radiographic table; (2) the Be-Clere method, using the curved cassette; and (3) the Camp-Coventry method, in which the patient is prone and the lower leg is elevated off the table. In all three cases, it is necessary to ensure that the central ray remains perpendicular to the lower leg. Also, in all three projections the knee should be flexed slightly, but should not be flexed a full 90°.

Ballinger, Vol 1, pp 251, 252, 254; Bontrager, p 210.

120. **(A)** When performing abdominal and GI radiography, it is essential to understand the different types of body habitus. There are four categories of body types: (1) sthenic, which is the average build (about 50 percent of the population); (2) hypersthenic, which is a very large build (about 5 percent of the population); (3) hyposthenic, which is slightly smaller than average build (about 35 percent of the population); and (4) asthenic, which is less common (about 10 percent of the population) and is an extremely slender build. The hypersthenic build tends to have all of the abdominal organs high and transverse across the body. To the other extreme, the asthenic individual tends to have abdominal organs that lie very low and vertical. The stomach in an asthenic person is said to be "J"-shaped.

Ballinger, Vol 1, p 42; Bontrager, p 420; Eisenberg et al., p 21.

121. **(D)** The aorta is the main artery in the body and is responsible for delivering oxygenated blood from the heart. It arises from the superior portion of the left ventricle through the semilunar (aortic) valve. It then arches around the left side of the heart and passes along the thoracic vertebrae to the level of the fourth lumbar vertebra, where it divides into the left and right common iliac arteries.

Ballinger, Vol 2, p 516; Mallett, "The Circulatory System," pp 133–134; Tortora and Grabowski, "The Cardiovascular System," p 598.

122. **(A)** There are many variations of evaluating the esophagus radiographically. Some radiologists prefer to have the patient start erect, whereas

others prefer the patient to start in the RAO recumbent position. But, when the swallowing function is the specific physiologic function of interest, it is always best to place the patient in the erect position, either lateral or oblique, to best demonstrate deglutition. Usually the radiographer will be responsible for taking overheads with the patient recumbent while swallowing barium so that the entire esophagus can be seen filled with barium.

Ballinger, Vol 2, p 93; Bontrager, p 428.

123. **(B)** The malleus, incus, and stapes are three small bones found in the middle ear that are responsible for transmitting sound waves to the cochlea in the inner ear. The inner ear has two important functions. Aside from hearing, the inner ear is also responsible for balance, or equilibrium, which is accomplished by the semicircular canals.

Gylys and Wedding, "Special Senses," pp 346–347; Tortora and Grabowski, "The Special Senses," p 496.

124. **(C)** The aorta is the largest blood vessel in the body, having a typical diameter in an adult of about 1 inch. The superior and inferior vena cavae are also very large. The longest vessel in the body is the great saphenous vein found in the lower extremities. Because of its great length, this vein is commonly used to replace damaged coronary arteries in bypass surgeries.

Memmler and Wood, "Blood Vessels and Blood Circulation," p 211; Spence, "Anatomy of the Vascular System," pp 322, 329; Tortora and Grabowski, "The Cardiovascular System," p 668.

125. **(D)** The OML is the line that is drawn from the outer canthus of the eye to the external auditory meatus (EAM). The OML is the most commonly used baseline. The glabellomeatal line is the line drawn from the glabella to the EAM. When positioning a PA axial projection (Caldwell) for the facial bones, the radiographer may position the patient so that the OML is perpendicular to the plane of the film. In this instance, the central ray would need to be directed caudally 15° to exit the nasion to properly demonstrate the facial structures. If the patient is positioned so that the glabellomeatal line is perpendicular to the plane of the film, it is then necessary to angle the central ray 23° caudad—a difference of 8°.

Ballinger, Vol 2, p 233; Bontrager, p 345.

126. **(B)** In any traumatic injury to an extremity, it is essential to always obtain two projections, preferably at 90° apart from each other. In the case of a fracture, the orthopedic surgeon will be able to accurately assess any possible displacement of the long bones. In almost all cases of extremity radiography, the AP projection will best demonstrate

medial or lateral displacement of the bones. The lateral projection will demonstrate any anterior or posterior displacement of the bones.

Bontrager, pp 50–51; Eisenberg et al., p 98.

127. **(A)** Before injecting a contrast medium into the lymphatic vessels for a lymphangiogram, it is usually necessary to inject a blue-staining dye. Some brands use the color indigo or a mixture of blue-violet and sky blue. Normally, the lymph vessels are colorless and very difficult to find. Prior to attempting to locate a lymph vessel, the blue dye is injected into the webbing of the toes. To promote uptake of the dye, the patient should be instructed to wiggle the toes for several minutes. The dye should visualize the lymphatic vessels within 20 minutes. The actual contrast medium that is used for the procedure is ethiodized oil, which should be warmed prior to administration to reduce its viscosity.

Ballinger, Vol 2, p 574; Eisenberg et al., p 354; Tortorici, "Pedal Lymphography," p 67.

128. **(C)** To better demonstrate the intervertebral foramina of the cervical vertebrae, the patient should be rotated 45° and the central ray is angled 15° and centered to C4. For the anterior oblique positions (RAO and LAO), the central ray angulation is caudad. For the posterior oblique positions (RPO and LPO), the central ray angulation is cephalad.

Ballinger, Vol 1, pp 340–343; Bontrager, p 267; Eisenberg et al., p 175.

129. **(A)** In the lateral projection of the thoracic vertebrae, the structures best demonstrated are the intervertebral foramina, the intervertebral disk spaces, the vertebral bodies, and the spinous processes. The apophyseal joints are seen best in the oblique projection.

Ballinger, Vol 1, p 360; Bontrager, p 276; Eisenberg et al., p 183.

130. **(C)** As the ascending colon arises, it passes by the liver and curves at an angle called the right colic (hepatic) flexure, where it then joins the transverse colon. The splenic flexure is located on the left side of the patient's body as the transverse colon passes by the spleen and curves downward into the descending colon. The ileocecal valve is the junction between the distal part of the small bowel and the proximal part of the large intestine. The sigmoid is the most distal "S"-shaped portion of the colon.

Ballinger, Vol 2, p 87; Bontrager, p 448; Eisenberg et al., p 209.

131. **(A)** For the routine PA projection of the clavicle, it is not necessary to angle the central ray. However, a second projection (axial projection) with

a 15° to 25° caudal angulation is usually desirable to demonstrate the apices of the lung below the clavicle.

Ballinger, Vol 1, p 159; Bontrager, p 165.

132. **(A)** The nephron is the functional unit of the kidney. There are believed to be over 1 million nephrons in each kidney. There are two main parts to the nephron: (1) the *renal corpuscle,* which filters the blood, and (2) the *renal tubule,* which is responsible for the expulsion of waste in the form of urine. The renal corpuscle consists of a C-shaped structure called Bowman's capsule, which surrounds a tuft of capillaries called the glomerulus. The glomerulus receives blood from the afferent arteriole and empties filtered blood into the circulatory system through the efferent arteriole.

Ballinger, Vol 2, pp 153–154; Bontrager, p 507; Scanlon and Sanders, "The Urinary System," pp 419–420; Spence, "Anatomy of the Kidneys," pp 572–574.

133. **(B)** In almost all instances of cholecystography, the patient should be positioned in the prone position. This will reduce OID because of the more anterior location of the gallbladder. A PA projection in the erect position is especially significant for two reasons: (1) to demonstrate stratification of gallstones, and (2) to better visualize the gallbladder because of the movement of abdominal organs that ordinarily would obstruct the gallbladder. The LAO projection is often performed as well as the PA projection to project the gallbladder away from the vertebral column.

Ballinger, Vol 2, pp 34, 66; Bontrager, p 500.

134. **(A)** The tangential projection is performed specifically to demonstrate the parotid gland. The right and left lateral projections are performed to demonstrate both the parotid and submandibular glands. The axial projection using an intraoral periapical film is the best method used to demonstrate the entire sublingual gland free of superimposition.

Ballinger, Vol 2, pp 4–10.

135. **(D)** To best demonstrate the pharynx and larynx in the AP projection, the central ray should be directed to the laryngeal prominence, which is just inferior to the thyroid cartilage. This is approximately the level of T1. The mandibular rami, the C3–4 level, and the thyroid cartilage are all too superior for correct positioning.

Ballinger, Vol 2, p 27; Bontrager, p 82.

136. **(B)** There are two basic projections for radiographing the humerus: the AP and the lateral. The anatomic landmarks that should be used for positioning are the epicondyles. For the AP projection, the epicondyles should be placed parallel to the plane of the film to demonstrate the greater tuberosity in profile. For the lateral projection, the epicondyles should be placed perpendicular to the plane of the film. This position will project the epicondyles superimposed on each other on the image and will place the lesser tuberosity in profile.

Ballinger, Vol 1, p 115; Bontrager, pp 143–145; Eisenberg et al., p 76.

137. **(D)** The term *lateral* is used to refer to anatomic parts that are away from the median plane of the body. *Abduction* refers to the movement of an anatomic part away from the midline of the body. *Ipsilateral* refers to anatomy on the same side of the body, which is the opposite of *contralateral,* or on opposite sides of the body.

Ballinger, Vol 1, p 49; Bontrager, p 22; Tortora and Grabowski, "The Spinal Cord and Spinal Nerves," p 387.

138. **(C)** For either the lateromedial or mediolateral projection of the foot, the central ray should be directed to the base of the third metatarsal joint. Bontrager said to center to the first (medial) cuneiform, which is approximately at the same level as the base of the third metatarsal joint. Eisenberg said to center to the bases of the metatarsal joints. The base of the fifth metatarsal joint is more proximal than all of the other metatarsal joints and is not used as a centering point. The head of the fifth metatarsal joint is too distal for proper centering. The longitudinal arch is the soft-tissue section on the plantar surface and is too inferior for proper centering. The calcaneus is too proximal for proper centering.

Ballinger, Vol 1, pp 205–206; Bontrager, p 195; Eisenberg et al., p 108.

139. **(A)** The medial oblique projection of the knee is specifically performed to demonstrate the proximal tibiofibular articulation. It also projects the patella over the medial condyle of the femur.

Ballinger, Vol, 1, p 247; Bontrager, p 207; Eisenberg et al., p 125.

140. **(C)** The AP axial projection is often requested for routine radiography of the mandible for demonstrating the temporomandibular joints (TMJs). It is the preferred method for demonstrating the condyles as well as the mandibular rami. Some institutions prefer this view be taken prone for a PA projection with a 30° cephalic angle. To demonstrate the body, symphysis, and angles of the mandible, various axiolateral projections may also be requested.

Ballinger, Vol 2, pp 356–357; Bontrager, p 375; Eisenberg et al., p 306.

141. **(B)** To properly locate foreign bodies, it is important to limit motion during the exposure. Compression should not be used to limit motion because it will reduce tissue thickness, which in turn results in imprecise depth measurements. Therefore, reducing the exposure time is probably the best method to reduce motion for foreign body localization.
Ballinger, Vol 1, p 505.

142. **(D)** Trauma patients who are referred to the radiology department for imaging are usually not able to move or be positioned in a routine manner. Often, trauma patients have experienced some type of spinal injury and should be moved cautiously, if at all, until the initial vertebral radiographs have been "cleared." Splints or any immobilization devices also should *not* be removed by the radiographer unless he or she is instructed to do so by the physician. Remember, the quality of the radiographs may have to be sacrificed for the safety of the patient. If the patient is conscious and alert, the radiographer should explain exactly what is going to be done *before* starting the examination. This explanation will result in better image quality as well as in enhanced safety and comfort for the patient.
Ballinger, Vol 1, p 519; Eisenberg et al., pp 333–334; Torres, "Care of Patients with Special Problems," p 120.

143. **(D)** Arthrography is a special radiographic examination performed specifically to examine diarthrodial joints. This examination has been replaced for the most part by MRI because it is noninvasive and offers superior soft-tissue resolution. During arthrography, a contrast medium is injected into the synovial space. The contrast medium usually consists of an iodinated contrast medium mixed with air. Although many structures of the joint may be examined during contrast arthrography, such as the menisci, ligaments, cartilage, and bursae, the most common radiographic finding is a torn meniscus. Other less common findings include ligament tears; capsular tears; popliteal, or Baker's, cysts; and loose bodies.
Eisenberg and Dennis, "Skeletal System," p 93; Tortorici, "Knee Arthrography," 1995, pp 39–44.

144. **(B)** For all AP or PA projections of the chest (including the lordotic and lateral decubitus projections), the MSP should be perpendicular to the image receptor. This placement ensures that there is no rotation of the thorax. For the lateral projection, however, the patient should be positioned so that the MSP is aligned parallel with the image receptor so that there is no rotation of the body part.

Ballinger, Vol 1, p 456; Bontrager, p 74; Eisenberg et al., p 28.

145. **(C)** To ensure that the entire set of ribs above the diaphragm (usually 1 to 10) is included on the AP projection radiograph, the cassette should be placed so that the top border is $1\frac{1}{2}$ inches above the patient's shoulders.
Ballinger, Vol 1, p 426; Bontrager, pp 318–319; Eisenberg et al., p 158.

146. **(B)** The articulating facets, or demifacets, are found only on the thoracic vertebrae. They are located on each side of the vertebral bodies, at both the superior and inferior borders. They serve as articulations for the head of the ribs. Because there are 12 pairs of ribs, there are also 12 thoracic vertebrae. Neither the cervical nor the lumbar vertebral bodies contain these demifacets.
Ballinger, Vol 1, p 318; Bontrager, p 254; Eisenberg et al., p 166.

147. **(C)** The ischial rami project anteriorly and medially to their junction with the rami of the pubic bone. This union on either side of the pelvis forms the largest foramen in the body—the obturator foramen.
Ballinger, Vol, p 272; Bontrager, p 224; Eisenberg et al., p 99; Tortora and Grabowski, "The Skeletal System: The Appendicular Skeleton," p 205.

148. **(D)** The central ray should be directed to the center of the cassette when radiographing a pelvis. The center of the cassette should be placed at the level of the soft-tissue depression just superior to the level of the greater trochanter. The greater trochanter is easily palpated when the patient medially rotates the foot. Centering 3 inches above the symphysis pubis or at the level of the iliac crest is too superior. Centering 2 inches inferior to the greater trochanter is too inferior. Both Bontrager and Ballinger said to center 2 inches superior to the symphysis pubis or about 2 inches inferior to the anterosuperior iliac spine, which are both approximately at the level of the soft-tissue depression above the greater trochanter.
Ballinger, Vol 1, p 276; Bontrager, p 234; Eisenberg et al., p 142.

149. **(C)** The joints that form the union between the wrist bones (carpals) and the hand bones (metacarpals) are called the carpometacarpal joints. The joints that are found between the small bones of the digits (phalanges) are the interphalangeal joints. The joints that are often referred to as the "knuckles" are formed between the bones of the hand (metacarpals) and the bones of the fingers (phalanges) and are referred to as metacarpophalangeal joints.

Ballinger, Vol 1, p 63; Bontrager, p 103; Eisenberg et al., p 37.

150. **(B)** The AP semiaxial (Grashey-Towne) projection is the best method for examining the occipital bone of the skull. If the frontal bone is of primary interest, the modified PA axial (Caldwell) projection is usually performed. The submentovertical projection is the best method for demonstrating the basilar area of the skull, particularly the petrous portion of the temporal bone and the sphenoid bones. The lateral projection is used to demonstrate the sella turcica and the squamous portions of the parietal and temporal bones.

Ballinger, Vol 2, pp 246–248; Bontrager, p 349; Eisenberg et al., p 274.

151. **(C)** A Baker's cyst is a common finding on knee arthrograms as well as on MRI evaluation of the knee. A Baker's cyst is found in the popliteal area, a soft-tissue region behind the knee. Baker's cysts are so called because they are benign tumors that may arise as a result of standing for long periods.

Linn-Watson, "Skeletal System," p 29; Mosby's Medical, Nursing and Allied Health Dictionary, p 165; Tortorici, "Knee Arthrography," 1995, p 35.

152. **(D)** In conventional lumbar myelography, AP or PA projection radiographs are usually performed during fluoroscopy with the spot film device. Once the physician has removed the spinal needle, the radiographer obtains a cross-table lateral projection with the patient in the prone position. Requests for additional projections are usually not necessary because these images have already been obtained under fluoroscopy.

Ballinger, Vol 2, p 502; Tortorici, "Myelography," 1995, p 81.

153. **(D)** The most superior portion of the lungs is the apex, which is located just above the clavicles. The mediastinum is the center portion of the thorax where the esophagus and trachea are located. The costophrenic angle is the lower outer margin of the lungs. *Costo* is the medical term for ribs, and *phrenic* means diaphragm. Where the ribs and diaphragm meet are the costophrenic angles.

Ballinger, Vol 1, pp 438, 454; Bontrager, p 62; Eisenberg et al., p 24.

154. **(D)** The most anterior portion of the tibia is a projection called the tibial tuberosity, which is usually palpable on the superior aspect of the tibia just below the apex of the patella. It serves as an attachment to the patellar ligament.

Ballinger, Vol 1, p 182; Bontrager, p 178; Eisenberg et al., p 97; Tortora and Grabowski, "The Skeletal System: The Appendicular Skeleton," p 208.

155. **(A)** Because of the anode heel effect—by which the heel of the anode absorbs a large percentage of radiation produced at the target—the thinner body part should be placed under the anode and the thicker part under the cathode end of the x-ray tube. The anode heel effect is most pronounced with short SIDs, with large image receptors, and in areas with large differences in tissue density from one end of the film to the other. All of these are factors when radiographing either the thoracic vertebrae or the femur. In the AP projection of the thoracic vertebrae, the thinner body part (T1–6) is placed under the anode and the thicker part (T7–12) under the cathode. When radiographing the patient in the lateral position for the thoracic vertebrae, the thicker part is now the upper thoracic spine (T-spine [T1–6]) because of the superimposition of the shoulders, and the thinner part is the lower T-spine because the waist is much narrower than the shoulders. The AP projection of the femur would use the anode heel effect if the hip joint were placed under the cathode and the knee joint under the anode. Therefore, if it is desirable to take advantage of the anode heel effect for the AP projection of the femur or the lateral projection of the thoracic vertebrae, the patient's head may need to be placed at the foot end of the table. The lumbar vertebrae are not as affected by the anode heel effect because there is not a great variation in tissue thickness from L1–5.

Ballinger, Vol 1, p 357; Carlton and McKenna-Adler, "Density", p 375.

156. **(A)** The AP open-mouth projection and the AP projection (Judd method) are both performed to demonstrate the odontoid process. To properly demonstrate this joint, it is usually not necessary to angle the central ray, and in fact, angulation may lead to distortion of the part. For anterior oblique projections of the cervical vertebrae, when angulation is necessary, the central ray should be directed caudally. Only the routine AP axial projection of the cervical vertebrae requires a 15–20° cephalad angulation of the central ray.

Ballinger, Vol 1, p 334; Bontrager, p 266; Eisenberg et al., "Cervical Spine," p 168.

157. **(B)** The fovea capitis is a depression located at the center of the femoral head. It serves as an attachment for a ligament for better stabilization of the hip joint.

Bontrager, p 222; Mallett, "The Lower Limb: Bones and Joints," p 59; Spence, "Appendicular Skeleton," p 140.

158. **(C)** The "dorsoplantar projection" is the preferred term used for the AP projection of the foot.

With the entire plantar surface of the foot flat on the cassette, the foot is not in a true anatomic position when it is correctly positioned for a dorsoplantar projection. The dorsoplantar projection denotes that the central ray enters on the dorsal surface of the foot and exits the plantar surface.

Ballinger, Vol 1; Bontrager, p 193; Eisenberg et al., p 106.

159. **(D)** The lateral border of the scapula may also be termed the "axillary border" because it is located near the axilla or armpit. The medial border is also known as the "vertebral border" because it is closer to the vertebral column. The superior border extends from the medial angle to the coracoid process.

Ballinger, Vol 1, pp 122–123; Bontrager, p 150; Eisenberg et al., p 40.

160. **(A)** This is a lateral projection of the wrist with incorrect positioning. The patient's hand is pronated, causing rotation. Pronation projects the head of the ulna slightly posterior to the radius, giving the appearance of a dislocated ulna. There is no pathology on this radiograph.

Carroll, "Evaluating Radiographs: Upper Extremities," 1993, p 158.

161. **(A)** For a proper demonstration of the scapular "Y," the patient should be placed prone and then rotated toward the side of interest until the lateral and medial borders of the scapula are superimposed over the shaft of the humerus. To demonstrate the right scapula in a PA projection (scapular Y), the patient should be in the right anterior oblique position. This view can be obtained with an AP projection as well, but the OID is excessive, and thus recorded detail is decreased.

Ballinger, Vol 1, p 142; Bontrager, p 169.

162. **(D)** Throughout the GI tract, each section has variations of mucosal folds for specific functions of digestion. The stomach has folds called *rugae* to help break down solid pieces of food. The small intestine has folds that contain the *crypts of Lieberkühn,* which function to absorb nutrients from digested food. The colon has large mucosal folds called *haustra* to absorb any excess fluids from the remaining waste.

Ballinger, Vol 2, p 87; Bontrager, p 449; Tortora and Grabowski, "The Digestive System," p 808.

163. **(A)** With the head in the true lateral position, many anatomic areas may be clearly demonstrated. To ensure proper demonstration, correct centering is essential. When the sinuses are of primary interest, the central ray should enter ½ to 1 inch posterior to the outer canthus. When the sella turcica is of main interest, the central ray

should enter ¾ inch anterior and ¾ inch superior to the EAM. For the facial bones, the central ray should enter at approximately midzygoma.

Ballinger, Vol 2; Bontrager, p 363; Eisenberg et al., p 299.

164 and 165. **(B)** and **(C)** Referring to Figure 3–8, the structure labeled number 1 is the renal pelvis, 2 the renal artery, 3 the renal vein, 4 the ureter, 5 the renal medulla (pyramids), 6 the papilla of the pyramid, 7 the renal cortex, and 8 the major calyx.

Ballinger, Vol 2, p 153; Bontrager, p 507; Mallett, "The Urinary System," p 188; Scanlon and Sanders, "The Urinary System," p 418; Spence, "The Urinary System," p 571; Tortora and Grabowski, "The Urinary System," p 867.

166. **(B)** Spina bifida is a congenital disorder in which the posterior laminae fail to fuse, leaving a gap in the spinal canal. This disease can manifest with several degrees of severity. The most common, spina bifida occulta, is also the least severe. In this case, it is usually only the last two or three lumbar vertebrae that fail to fuse posteriorly and therefore leave a gap in the spinal canal. Because the spinal cord ends at approximately the first lumbar vertebra, there is usually no external protrusion of tissue through this opening. However, if spina bifida occurs higher up in the vertebral column, the meningeal tissue and the spinal cord itself may also herniate through the opening (meningocele or myelomeningocele), causing severe deformities and possible paralysis. Spina bifida occulta is usually diagnosed on an AP projection of the lumbar vertebrae.

Eisenberg and Dennis, pp 66–67; Linn-Watson, "Nervous System," p 263; Mace and Kowalczyk, "The Skeletal System," p 21; Tortora and Grabowski, "The Skeletal System: The Axial Skeleton," p 195.

167. **(C)** *Digestion* is the medical term for the mechanical and chemical breakdown of food into a fuel source for the body. Peristalsis, mastication, and deglutition are all parts of the mechanical function of digestion. *Peristalsis* is the medical term for wavelike muscular contractions of the GI tract that propel digested materials through the tubular canal. *Mastication* is the medical term for chewing. *Deglutition* is the medical term for swallowing.

Gylys and Wedding, "Gastrointestinal System," pp 88, 101; Spence, "The Digestive System," pp 555–557; Tortora and Grabowski, "The Digestive System," pp 775–776.

168. **(D)** In conventional tomography, structures that are not of interest are blurred through the process of motion unsharpness. The motion is caused by movement of the tube and film during the expo-

sure. The anatomic structures of primary interest should be set at a focal point where there is relatively little motion throughout the exposure. This focal plane is also called the objective plane and should be at the level of the fulcrum.

Ballinger, Vol 3, p 52; Carlton and McKenna-Adler, "Tomography," p 558; Curry et al., "Body Section Radiography," p 243; Eisenberg et al.," p 362.

169. **(D)** The "dens" is another medical term for the odontoid process, which projects superiorly from the second cervical vertebra or the axis. The first cervical vertebra, called the "atlas," is also an atypical vertebra because it has very few projections. It has a large foramen in the center for articulation with the dens and passage of the spinal cord.

Ballinger, Vol 1, p 315; Eisenberg et al., pp 164–165; Mallett, "The Vertebral Column: Bones and Joints," p 73; Tortora and Grabowski, "The Skeletal System: The Axial Skeleton," pp 187–188.

170. **(A)** For the AP projection of the shoulder with the humerus in external rotation, the humerus should be positioned so that the coronal plane of the epicondyles is parallel with the image receptor. The structure of interest in this position is the greater tuberosity seen in profile.

Ballinger, Vol 1, p 126; Bontrager; Eisenberg et al., p 82.

SECTION V: PATIENT CARE

171. **(D)** Hypertension is indicated by either a systolic pressure that consistently exceeds 140 mm Hg or a diastolic pressure that consistently exceeds 90 mm Hg.

Adler and Carlton, "Vital Signs and Oxygen," p 187; Ehrlich and McCloskey, "Patient Care and Assessment," p 127; Kowalczyk, "Patient Assessment and Assistance," p 112; Torres, "Vital Signs and Oxygen Administration," p 137.

172. **(B)** Isolation is used for patients whenever there may be a risk of either the patient or medical personnel contracting infections. Most forms of isolation are used to restrict the patient's infectious disease process from being transmitted to other patients or medical personnel. This is accomplished with some type of barrier, such as a private room. When transporting an infectious patient, a gown, gloves, and mask should be worn by the patient and any medical personnel involved with his or her care. Protective isolation is specifically designed to protect the immunosuppressed patient from contracting infections. Examples of these types of patients would be burn victims, those with an active HIV infection, those undergoing chemotherapy, or high-risk infants. For protective isolation, the same procedure as for strict isolation should be followed.

Adler and Carlton, "Infection Control," p 210; Ehrlich and McCloskey, "Infection Control," pp 163, 165; Kowalczyk, "Infection Control and Aseptic Technique," p 88; Torres, "Infection Control and Institutional Safety," pp 60–61.

173. **(D)** Fainting, or syncope, is usually caused by a lack of blood supply to the brain. Heart disease, emotional shock, hunger, and poor ventilation are all causes of syncope. If the patient feels faint, the radiographer should assist the patient into a recumbent position. If the patient is already recumbent, it is not advisable to sit the patient up. It may be helpful to place the patient in the Trendelenburg position so that the head is lower than the feet. This position should help to increase blood flow to the brain. The Fowler's position places the head higher than the feet.

Adler and Carlton, "Medical Emergencies," p 269, and "Aseptic Techniques," p 217; Bontrager, "Terminology," p 17; Ehrlich and McCloskey, "Dealing with Acute Situations," p 239, and "Safety, Transfer and Positioning," p 93; Kowalczyk, "Patient Care in Critical Situations," p 210; Torres, "Medical Emergencies in Diagnostic Imaging," p 166, and "Basic Patient Care and Safety in Radiographic Imaging," pp 85–86.

174. **(C)** Although most arthrographic procedures are uneventful, the most common complication to an arthrogram is a postprocedural infection either at the puncture site or within the joint itself.

Tortorici, "Knee Arthrography," 1995, p 39.

175. **(C)** Prior to injecting a contrast medium for myelography, it is usually routine to aspirate some CSF at the injection site. This fluid is then sent to the laboratory for analysis. Although the laboratory tests ordered may vary from one physician to another, one of the more common laboratory tests performed on the CSF is the VDRL test, which can be used to diagnose syphilis.

Sheldon, "Bacterial Infections," pp 215, 621–623; Tamparo and Lewis, "Reproductive System Diseases," p 111; Tortorici, "Myelography," 1995, p 79.

176. **(C)** To maintain the proper flow rate and to ensure that the patency of the IV line is not compromised, all IV solutions should be kept at least 18 to 20 inches above the injection site. If the solution is placed below the level of the vein, blood will flow back into the tubing, clot, and cause the cessation of fluid flow. Aside from poor patency of the catheter line, there may be other reasons for a slow flow rate, including a dislodged needle

or catheter, or extravasation, in which the fluid leaks outside the vein.

Ehrlich and McCloskey, "Medications and Their Administration," p 211; Torres, "Methods of Drug Administration," p 293; Springhouse, "Maintaining I.V. Therapy," p 215.

177. **(D)** The medical term *asepsis* denotes the reduction of the spread of microorganisms. There are two main types of asepsis: (1) *surgical asepsis,* which is defined as the complete removal of all microorganisms (necessary for surgical procedures), and (2) *medical asepsis,* which limits the number and prevents the spread of infectious microorganisms. Medical asepsis is performed prior to an IV injection and for routine cleaning of the environment between patient procedures.

Adler and Carlton, "Aseptic Techniques," p 217; Kowalczyk, "Infection Control and Aseptic Technique," p 79; Torres, "Surgical Asepsis," p 104.

178. **(B)** Universal precautions were first instituted in 1985 by the CDC because of public concern over transmitting HIV or hepatitis B virus (HBV) infections. The CDC has now adopted the new term "standard precautions," which is more sweeping in its scope and includes using protective apparel, especially gloves, for all patients, not just patients with blood and body fluid secretions. According to the latest CDC report, all soiled linen should be handled in exactly the same manner—with standard precautions. Health-care personnel should treat all patients—and, therefore, all linens—as if the patient had an infectious disease. The CDC's standard precautions state that a gown and gloves should be worn when handling all linens because these may be soiled with blood or body fluids. Any linen used by patients should be handled as little as possible. To prevent airborne contamination, the edges should be folded in toward the middle. All linens should be placed in a moisture-tight container and washed in very hot water. There is no reason to selectively separate linens for specific types of diseases. In fact, this practice can be considered counterproductive because of the added time and expense involved.

Centers for Disease Control and Prevention; Kowalczyk, "Infection Control and Aseptic Technique," p 86; Torres, "Infection Control and Institutional Safety," p 51.

179. **(C)** The use of a PEG tube is sometimes necessary for patients who are having difficulty swallowing and are therefore lacking in nutrition. PEG tubes are a much safer and faster alternative for providing nutrients than a nasogastric tube. The radiographer may be asked to insert barium sulfate into a PEG tube for an upper gastrointestinal examination.

Kowalczyk, "Tubes, Catheters & Vascular Access Lines," p 150.

180. **(B)** Edema is characterized by abnormal amounts of fluid in the intercellular tissue spaces or body cavities. It can be localized as a result of trauma or generalized with swelling throughout the body. Overall body edema is most often seen in patients with congestive heart failure, cirrhosis of the liver, and renal failure. A common treatment for generalized edema is to administer a diuretic such as furosemide (Lasix).

Adler and Carlton, "Pharmacology," pp 273, 284; Eisenberg and Dennis, "Introduction to Pathology," p 4; Scanlon and Sanders, "Fluid-Electrolyte and Acid-Base Balance," p 439.

181. **(D)** Soapsuds enemas are very common in some radiology departments and may even be a routine procedure prior to beginning the barium enema examination. Castile soap is an excellent preparation for promoting peristalsis and defecation and is also much less irritating than other types of soap. Castile soap is slightly irritating to the bowel of some patients and should only be used under the direction of a physician.

Adler and Carlton, "Nonaseptic Techniques," pp 246–247; Ehrlich and McCloskey, "Preparation & Examination of the Gastrointestinal Tract," p 246; Torres, "Patient Care during Imaging Examinations of the Gastrointestinal System," p 203.

182. **(A)** The grieving process may occur as a result of the loss of a loved one, the loss of a body part, or the loss of a body function. It is important for radiographers to understand this process so that they can better empathize with what the patient is experiencing. The grieving process occurs in five stages: (1) denial, (2) anger, (3) bargaining, (4) depression, and (5) acceptance (DABDA).

Kowalczyk, "Communication," p 37; Ehrlich and McCloskey, "Professional Communications," p 77; Torres, "The Patient in Radiographic Imaging," pp 32–33.

183. **(D)** Airway obstructions that require suctioning may include such signs and symptoms as gurgling sounds, drooling, gastric secretions from the mouth, and ineffective coughing that is unable to clear secretions, resulting in gag reflexes. Although it is preferable to have the patient forcefully cough to clear secretions, some patients are physically unable to do so, making suction necessary.

Ehrlich and McCloskey, "Dealing with Acute Situations," pp 223–224; Kowalczyk, "Patient Care in Critical Situations," p 204; Torres, "Caring for Patients Needing Alternative Medical Treatments," p 226.

184. **(C)** Anaphylactic reactions occur as a result of an allergic reaction to an antigen that was previously

introduced to the patient's body. Radiographers should be aware of the early signs and symptoms of anaphylaxis because this condition can occur as the result of exposure to an iodinated contrast medium. Recognizing the early warning signs can prevent life-threatening outcomes. The first signs of anaphylaxis are usually mild and may include any or all of the following: apprehensiveness, tightness in the chest, itching at the site of medication, nasal congestion, sneezing or coughing, nausea, and vomiting.

Adler and Carlton, "Medical Emergencies," p 261; Kowalczyk, "Patient Care in Critical Situations," p 213; Torres, "Medical Emergencies in Radiographic Imaging," p 155.

185. **(D)** All patients have legal rights regarding their health care, and radiographers should be acutely aware of these rights as well as of their own ethical and moral responsibilities to care for the patient. Performing a radiological procedure on a patient who refuses treatment is considered a form of battery. If a patient refuses medical treatment, continuing to coerce the patient into completing the procedure is considered a type of assault. *Assault* is defined as willfully attempting or threatening to harm someone. *Battery* is defined as intentionally touching another individual without their consent. An injury does not have to occur for the individual to report either assault or battery. If the patient is restrained against his or her will to complete the examination, the healthcare worker may also be guilty of false imprisonment. If a patient refuses an examination, the radiographer must respect the patient's rights and stop the procedure. When a procedure has been halted at the request of the patient, the referring physician should be notified immediately.

Adler and Carlton, "Medical Law," p 348; Kowalczyk, "Medical Ethics and Legalities," pp 68–69; Obergfell, "Civil Liability," p 44; Wilson, "Basic Concepts of Medical Law," p 145.

186. **(D).** When producing radiographs of the skull or vertebral column on a patient with spinal trauma, great skill and patience are required because this type of injury may result in either paralysis or death. Many times, routine radiographs cannot be achieved in the usual manner. The patient should be moved as little as possible to reduce the chance of causing further damage. When moving the patient with spinal trauma from the stretcher to the examining table, at least four people should assist and the log-rolling method should be used. The radiographer should exercise great care to achieve the best-quality images with the least movement of the patient.

Adler and Carlton, "Immobilization Devices," pp 168–169; Ballinger, Vol 1, p 519; Kowalczyk, "Emergency Medicine," p 223; Torres, "Basic Patient Care and Safety in Radiographic Imaging," pp 78–79.

187. **(C)** If a postoperative patient is brought to the radiology department for orthopedic radiographs and begins to complain of symptoms such as chest pain, dyspnea, apprehension, syncope, or hemoptysis, the radiographer may anticipate that this is a medical emergency signaling a possible pulmonary embolus. A pulmonary embolus is caused by a thrombic (blood clot or fatty plaque) blockage of the pulmonary artery. This thrombus usually originates in the venous system and can occur following illness, surgery, or trauma to the long bones. It is important for the radiographer to become aware of this possible complication. Other vital signs that may signal a pulmonary embolus are rapid and weak pulse, diaphoresis, shock, tachypnea, and eventually coma.

Laudicina, "Respiratory System," p 33; Torres, "Medical Emergencies in Radiographic Imaging," p 157.

188. **(D)** A systolic blood pressure reading of 120 mm Hg and a diastolic reading of 80 mm Hg are in the normal range and usually indicate that the patient is stable. Shock is usually indicated by a systolic reading lower than 90 mm Hg. Hypotension usually accompanies shock and indicates a loss of blood volume in the circulating blood, which may result from hemorrhage, severe burns, dehydration, or heat exhaustion.

Adler and Carlton, "Vital Signs and Oxygen," p 187; Ehrlich and McCloskey, "Dealing with Acute Situations," p 239; Kowalczyk, "Patient Assessment & Assistance," p 112; Torres, "Medical Emergencies in Radiographic Imaging," p 153.

189. **(C)** The normal pulse rate for the average adult is usually between 60 to 80 beats per minute. A pulse that exceeds 100 beats per minute is called *tachycardia* and is considered abnormal. Tachycardia may accompany certain medical conditions such as shock, overexertion, or a damaged heart. *Bradycardia* is a slower than normal heart rate, usually less than 60 beats per minute. Bradycardia may be perfectly normal in certain individuals, such as athletes.

Ehrlich and McCloskey, "Dealing with Acute Situations," p 239; Kowalczyk, "Patient Assessment and Assistance," p 112; Torres, "Medical Emergencies in Radiographic Imaging," p 153.

190. **(A)** For the contrast medium to fill the colon at the appropriate flow rate without causing damage, the enema bag should be placed about 30 inches above the level of the table (approxi-

mately 18 to 24 inches above the level of the patient's hip). Raising the enema bag any higher may cause severe cramping and may even cause a diverticulum to rupture.

Adler and Carlton, "Non-Aseptic Techniques," p 251–252; Ehrlich and McCloskey, "Preparation & Examination of the Gastrointestinal Tract," p 251; Torres, "Patient Care during Imaging Examinations of the Gastrointestinal System," p 206.

191. **(B)** The normal adult respiratory rate is between 12 to 20 breaths per minute. The normal rate for children under the age of 10 is between 20 and 30 breaths per minute. Infants under 1 year old breathe at a rate of 30 to 60 breaths per minute. *Tachypnea* is a term used to describe a higher-than-normal respiratory rate of more than 20 breaths per minute in an adult. *Bradypnea* is a slower-than-normal respiratory rate. *Dyspnea* is difficulty in breathing, and *apnea* is cessation of breathing.

Adler and Carlton, "Vital Signs and Oxygen," p 183; Kowalczyk, "Patient Assessment and Assistance," p 112; Torres, "Vital Signs and Oxygen Administration," p 136.

192. **(B)** In patients of over age 65, the greatest cause of trauma or injury is due to falls. Part of the natural aging process includes a loss of mobility, agility, and balance. There is also a loss of bone density that makes bony tissue in older adults more brittle and susceptible to fracture. Poor blood circulation may also lead to vertigo or fainting. Even a minor fall for an elderly patient may be disastrous. The radiographer should take special care when moving an elderly patient. Back injuries are the most common cause of injury for health-care workers.

Adler and Carlton, "Immobilization Techniques," p 175; Kowalczyk, "Age-Related Considerations," p 54.

193. **(B)** Oxygen therapy delivered through a nasal cannula is usually indicated for patients whose breathing rate and depth are normal and even. When oxygen is administered in this matter, it usually requires a rate of delivery between 1 to 5 L/min. If a higher rate is necessary, a plastic mask is usually the means by which to deliver oxygen.

Adler and Carlton, "Vital Signs and Oxygen," p 188; Kowalczyk, "Patient Care in Critical Situations," p 201; Torres, "Vital Signs and Oxygen Administration," pp 142–143.

194. **(B)** As mentioned in question 186, the patient who has a possible spinal injury should be moved very carefully, if at all. Spinal cord injuries are very serious and may result in either paralysis or death. If it is necessary to move the patient, at least four people should assist and the log-rolling method should be used to prevent further damage to the patient's spinal cord.

Adler and Carlton, "Immobilization Devices," pp 168–169; Ballinger, Vol 1, p 519; Kowalczyk, "Emergency Medicine," p 223; Torres, "Basic Patient Care and Safety in Radiographic Imaging," pp 78–79.

195. **(A)** A pulse oximeter is a device that is used to determine the percentage of oxygen circulating in the arterial blood. The pulse oximeter is a noninvasive device that is usually attached to the finger or toe of an individual in a critical care setting (trauma, postoperative, or sedated patients in MRI and in cardiac catheterization laboratory) to continuously monitor the oxygen saturation in the blood.

Adler and Carlton, "Vital Signs & Oxygen," p 184; Torres, "Vital Signs and Oxygen Administration," p 140.

196. **(B)** Radiographers should be familiar with how to monitor a patient's vital signs to properly assess a patient's condition while the patient is in the imaging department. There are typically four major vital signs that are important for the health-care worker to know: (1) pulse, (2) temperature, (3) blood pressure, and (4) respiration. Pulse may be monitored by palpating the patient's radial artery and using a watch with a second hand. Respiration may be monitored by simple observation and also with a watch with a second hand. Blood pressure is monitored with a sphygmomanometer and a stethoscope. Temperature is monitored with a thermometer. A tongue depressor is not necessary for monitoring a patient's vital signs.

Adler and Carlton, "Vital Signs and Oxygen," p 180; Ehrlich and McCloskey, "Patient Care and Assessment," p 120; Kowalczyk, "Patient Assessment and Assistance," p 112; Torres, "Vital Signs and Oxygen Administration," p 145.

197. **(C)** Sterilization is a very important aspect of surgical asepsis for invasive procedures. One of the most common means of sterilization uses a method of high-pressure steam to completely destroy microorganisms. This method is convenient, fast, and economical. The most common way to apply this high-pressure steam is inside a chamber called an autoclave.

Adler and Carlton, "Infection Control," p 208; Ehrlich and McCloskey, "Infection Control," p 166; Kowalczyk, "Infection Control & Aseptic Technique," p 90; Torres, "Surgical Asepsis," p 106.

198. **(A)** There are several means by which an infectious microorganism may be transmitted. Some microbes may be transmitted by several routes, whereas others may be transmitted only by cer-

tain modes. These different routes include: (1) airborne contamination, (2) direct contact, (3) fomites, and (4) vector transmission. A vector transmission means that the infection is transported from one human host to another by way of an arthropod such as a flea, tick, or mosquito. The vector takes a meal of blood from one human from whom it also ingests the infectious microbe, and as it goes on to its next meal, it transmits the disease to another human host, thereby infecting the second individual. Infections such as malaria and Lyme disease are two good examples of microbes transmitted by vector contamination. The HIV infection can be transmitted only through the direct contact route, specifically through contact with blood or body fluids.

Adler and Carlton, "Infection Control," p 203; Ehrlich and McCloskey, "Infection Control," p 146; Kowalczyk, "Infection Control and Aseptic Technique," pp 81–83; Torres, "Infection Control & Institutional Safety," p 46.

199. **(D)** When the threat of HIV and HBV first became acute in the early 1980s, patients diagnosed with acquired immunodeficiency syndrome (AIDS) were severely restricted and placed in special isolation rooms. In the 1990s, with the advent of many new privacy laws, health-care workers were not made aware of a patient's HIV status. Therefore, the CDC now recommends that health-care workers use standard precautions (more widespread practice of protection than the original "universal" precautions) on *all* patients who are receiving care. Standard precautions focus more on the use of barriers as a means of protection than on isolating patients with a diagnosed disease. One of the most important recommendations is the frequent use of hand washing between patient encounters and proper disposal and handling of all linens, needles, and syringes. Standard precautions protect not only the health-care workers, but also the immunosuppressed patients, from contracting other diseases.

Ehrlich and McCloskey, "Infection Control," p 152; Kowalczyk, "Infection Control and Aseptic Technique," p 86; Torres, "Infection Control," p 30.

200. **(A)** A patient with diabetes who is insulin dependent has to be very cautious of his or her food intake, because this could affect blood glucose levels. A patient who is using insulin therapy may have various reactions associated with low blood sugar, or hypoglycemia. Hypoglycemia may result from (1) insulin overdose, (2) inadequate food intake, (3) increased exercise, and (4) nutritional and fluid imbalances. Hypoglycemia, if not treated, may lead to insulin shock. The symptoms

of hypoglycemia, or the possible onset of insulin shock, are diaphoresis, confusion, difficulty talking, weakness or shakiness, blurred or double vision, and tachycardia. If a patient describes any of these symptoms, assist the patient into a recumbent position and offer orange juice, hard candy, or anything containing sugar. Immediate action is necessary to prevent the patient from lapsing into a coma.

Adler and Carlton, "Medical Emergencies," p 261; Ehrlich and McCloskey, "Dealing with Acute Situations," p 235; Kowalczyk, "Patient Care in Critical Situations," p 216; Torres, "Medical Emergencies in Radiographic Imaging," p 158.

BIBLIOGRAPHY

Adler, AM and Carlton, RR: Introduction to Radiography and Patient Care. WB Saunders, Philadelphia, 1993.

American Heart Association: Basic Life Support for Healthcare Providers. AHA, Dallas, TX, 1997.

Ballinger, PW: Merrill's Atlas of Radiographic Positions and Radiological Procedures, ed 8, 3 vols. Mosby–Year Book, St Louis, 1995.

Bontrager, KL: Textbook of Radiographic Positioning and Related Anatomy, ed 4. Mosby–Year Book, St Louis, 1997.

Burns, EF: Radiographic Imaging: A Guide to Producing Quality Radiographs. WB Saunders, Philadelphia, 1992.

Bushong, S: Radiological Science for Technologists: Physics, Biology and Protection. Mosby–Year Book, St Louis, 1997.

Carlton, R, and McKenna-Adler, A: Principles of Radiographic Imaging: An Art and a Science, ed 2. Delmar, Albany, NY, 1996.

Carroll, QB: Evaluating Radiographs. Charles C Thomas, Springfield, IL, 1993.

Carroll, QB: Fuchs's Radiographic Exposure, Processing and Quality Control, ed 6. Charles C Thomas, Springfield, IL, 1998.

Centers for Disease Control and Prevention: Infection Control Standards & Guidelines for Healthcare Workers. CDC: Atlanta, GA, 1997.

Cullinan, AM: Producing Quality Radiographs, ed 2. Lippincott, Philadelphia, 1994.

Curry, TS, et al: Christensen's Physics of Diagnostic Radiology, ed 4. Lea & Febiger, Philadelphia, 1990.

Dennis, CA, and Eisenberg, RL: Applied Radiographic Calculations. WB Saunders, Philadelphia, 1993.

Dowd, SB, and Tilson, ER: Practical Radiation Protection and Applied Radiobiology, ed 2. WB Saunders, Philadelphia, 1999.

Ehrlich, RA, and McCloskey, ED: Patient Care in Radiography, ed 5. Mosby, St Louis, 1999.

Eisenberg, RL, and Dennis, CA: Comprehensive Radiographic Pathology, ed 2. Mosby, St Louis, 1995.

Eisenberg, RL, et al: Radiographic Positioning. Little, Brown & Co, Boston, 1989.

Gray, JE, et al: Quality Control in Diagnostic Imaging. University Park Press, Baltimore, 1983.

Gurley, LT, and Callaway, WJ: Introduction to Radiological Technology, ed 4. Mosby, St Louis, 1996.

Gylys, BA, and Wedding, ME: Medical Terminology: A Systems Approach, ed 4. FA Davis, Philadelphia, 1999.

Hendee, WR: Medical Radiation Physics: Roentgenology, Nuclear Medicine and Ultrasound, ed 2. Year Book Medical Publishers, Chicago, 1979.

Hiss, SS: Understanding Radiography, ed 3. Charles C Thomas, Springfield, IL, 1993.

Ireland, SJ: Integrated Mathematics of Radiographic Exposure. Mosby, St Louis, 1994.

Kowalczyk, N: Integrated Patient Care for the Imaging Professional. Mosby, St Louis, 1996.

Laudicina, P: Applied Pathology for Radiographers. WB Saunders, Philadelphia, 1989.

Linn-Watson: Radiographic Pathology. WB Saunders, Philadelphia, 1996.

Mace, JD, and Kowalczyk, N: Radiographic Pathology, ed 2. Mosby–Year Book, St Louis, 1994.

Mallett, M: Anatomy and Physiology for Students of Medical Radiation Technology. Burnell, Mankato, MN, 1981.

Malott, JC, and Fodor, J: The Art and Science of Medical Radiography, ed 7. Mosby, St Louis, 1993.

McKinney, WEJ: Radiographic Processing and Quality Control. Lippincott, Philadelphia, 1988.

McQuillen-Martensen, K: Radiographic Critique. WB Saunders, Philadelphia, 1996.

Memmler, RL, and Wood, DL: The Human Body in Health & Disease, ed 5. Lippincott, Philadelphia, 1983.

Mosby's Medical, Nursing and Allied Health Dictionary, ed 3. Mosby, St Louis, 1993.

National Council on Radiation Protection and Measurements (NCRP): Limitation of Exposure to Ionizing Radiation, Report No. 116. Author, Bethesda, MD, 1993.

NCRP: Medical X-Ray Electron Beam and Gamma-Ray Protection for Energies up to 50 MeV (Equipment Design, Performance and Use), Report No. 102. Author, Bethesda, MD, 1989.

NCRP: Quality Assurance for Diagnostic Imaging, Report No. 99. Author, Bethesda, MD, 1988.

NCRP: Radiation Protection for Medical and Allied Health Personnel, Report No.105. Author, Bethesda, MD, 1989.

Obergfell, AM: Law and Ethics in Diagnostic Imaging and Therapeutic Radiology. WB Saunders, Philadelphia, 1995.

Papp, J: Quality Management in the Radiological Sciences. Mosby, St Louis, 1998.

Scanlon, VC, and Sanders, T: Essentials of Anatomy and Physiology, ed 3. FA Davis, Philadelphia, 1999.

Selman, J: The Fundamentals of X-Ray and Radium Physics, ed 8. Springfield, IL, Charles C Thomas, Springfield, IL, 1994.

Sheldon, H: Boyd's Introduction to the Study of Disease, ed 10. Lea & Febiger, Philadelphia, 1988.

Snopek, AM: Fundamentals of Special Radiographic Procedures, ed 3. WB Saunders, Philadelphia, 1992.

Spence, AP: Basic Human Anatomy, ed 3. Benjamin/Cummings, Redwood City, CA, 1990.

Springhouse Medication Administration & I.V. Therapy Manual: Process & Procedures Springhouse Corp, Springhouse, PA, 1988.

Statkiewicz-Sherer, MA, et al: Radiation Protection in Medical Radiography, ed 3. Mosby, St Louis, 1998.

Sweeney, RJ: Radiographic Artifacts: Their Cause and Control. Lippincott, Philadelphia, 1983.

Taber's Cyclopedic Medical Dictionary, ed 18. FA Davis, Philadelphia, 1996.

Tamparo, CD, and Lewis, MA: Diseases of the Human Body, ed 2. FA Davis, Philadelphia, 1995.

Thompson, MA, et al: Principles of Imaging Science and Protection. WB Saunders, Philadelphia, 1994.

Torres, LS: Basic Medical Techniques and Patient Care in Imaging Technology, ed 5. Lippincott, Philadelphia, 1997.

Tortora, GJ, and Grabowski, SR: Principles of Anatomy and Physiology, ed 7. HarperCollins, New York, 1993.

Tortorici, MR: Concepts in Medical Radiographic Imaging: Circuitry, Exposure and Quality Control. WB Saunders, Philadelphia, 1992.

Tortorici, MR, and Apfel, PJ: Advanced Radiographic and Angiographic Procedures. FA Davis, Philadelphia, 1995.

Travis, EL: Primer of Medical Radiobiology, ed 2. Year Book, Chicago, 1989.

Wallace, JE: Radiographic Exposure: Principles and Practice. FA Davis, Philadelphia, 1995.

Wilson, BG: Ethics and Basic Law for Medical Imaging Professionals. FA Davis, Philadelphia, 1997.

Wolbarst, AB: Physics of Radiology. Norwalk, CT, Appleton & Lange, 1993.

SIMULATION TEST #3

NAME_____

        Last   First   Middle

ADDRESS _____

          Street

_____

          City   State   Zip

. . . .

MAKE
ERASURES
COMPLETE

PLEASE USE NO. 2 PENCIL ONLY.

↓ BEGIN HERE

Radiation Protection and Radiobiology

01 Ⓐ Ⓑ Ⓒ Ⓓ	21 Ⓐ Ⓑ Ⓒ Ⓓ	41 Ⓐ Ⓑ Ⓒ Ⓓ	61 Ⓐ Ⓑ Ⓒ Ⓓ
02 Ⓐ Ⓑ Ⓒ Ⓓ	22 Ⓐ Ⓑ Ⓒ Ⓓ	42 Ⓐ Ⓑ Ⓒ Ⓓ	62 Ⓐ Ⓑ Ⓒ Ⓓ
03 Ⓐ Ⓑ Ⓒ Ⓓ	23 Ⓐ Ⓑ Ⓒ Ⓓ	43 Ⓐ Ⓑ Ⓒ Ⓓ	63 Ⓐ Ⓑ Ⓒ Ⓓ
04 Ⓐ Ⓑ Ⓒ Ⓓ	24 Ⓐ Ⓑ Ⓒ Ⓓ	44 Ⓐ Ⓑ Ⓒ Ⓓ	64 Ⓐ Ⓑ Ⓒ Ⓓ
05 Ⓐ Ⓑ Ⓒ Ⓓ	25 Ⓐ Ⓑ Ⓒ Ⓓ	45 Ⓐ Ⓑ Ⓒ Ⓓ	65 Ⓐ Ⓑ Ⓒ Ⓓ
06 Ⓐ Ⓑ Ⓒ Ⓓ	26 Ⓐ Ⓑ Ⓒ Ⓓ	46 Ⓐ Ⓑ Ⓒ Ⓓ	66 Ⓐ Ⓑ Ⓒ Ⓓ
07 Ⓐ Ⓑ Ⓒ Ⓓ	27 Ⓐ Ⓑ Ⓒ Ⓓ	47 Ⓐ Ⓑ Ⓒ Ⓓ	67 Ⓐ Ⓑ Ⓒ Ⓓ
08 Ⓐ Ⓑ Ⓒ Ⓓ	28 Ⓐ Ⓑ Ⓒ Ⓓ	48 Ⓐ Ⓑ Ⓒ Ⓓ	68 Ⓐ Ⓑ Ⓒ Ⓓ
09 Ⓐ Ⓑ Ⓒ Ⓓ	29 Ⓐ Ⓑ Ⓒ Ⓓ	49 Ⓐ Ⓑ Ⓒ Ⓓ	69 Ⓐ Ⓑ Ⓒ Ⓓ
10 Ⓐ Ⓑ Ⓒ Ⓓ	30 Ⓐ Ⓑ Ⓒ Ⓓ	50 Ⓐ Ⓑ Ⓒ Ⓓ	70 Ⓐ Ⓑ Ⓒ Ⓓ
11 Ⓐ Ⓑ Ⓒ Ⓓ	31 Ⓐ Ⓑ Ⓒ Ⓓ	51 Ⓐ Ⓑ Ⓒ Ⓓ	71 Ⓐ Ⓑ Ⓒ Ⓓ
12 Ⓐ Ⓑ Ⓒ Ⓓ	32 Ⓐ Ⓑ Ⓒ Ⓓ	52 Ⓐ Ⓑ Ⓒ Ⓓ	72 Ⓐ Ⓑ Ⓒ Ⓓ
13 Ⓐ Ⓑ Ⓒ Ⓓ	33 Ⓐ Ⓑ Ⓒ Ⓓ	53 Ⓐ Ⓑ Ⓒ Ⓓ	73 Ⓐ Ⓑ Ⓒ Ⓓ
14 Ⓐ Ⓑ Ⓒ Ⓓ	34 Ⓐ Ⓑ Ⓒ Ⓓ	54 Ⓐ Ⓑ Ⓒ Ⓓ	74 Ⓐ Ⓑ Ⓒ Ⓓ
15 Ⓐ Ⓑ Ⓒ Ⓓ	35 Ⓐ Ⓑ Ⓒ Ⓓ	55 Ⓐ Ⓑ Ⓒ Ⓓ	75 Ⓐ Ⓑ Ⓒ Ⓓ
16 Ⓐ Ⓑ Ⓒ Ⓓ	36 Ⓐ Ⓑ Ⓒ Ⓓ	56 Ⓐ Ⓑ Ⓒ Ⓓ	76 Ⓐ Ⓑ Ⓒ Ⓓ
17 Ⓐ Ⓑ Ⓒ Ⓓ	37 Ⓐ Ⓑ Ⓒ Ⓓ	57 Ⓐ Ⓑ Ⓒ Ⓓ	77 Ⓐ Ⓑ Ⓒ Ⓓ
18 Ⓐ Ⓑ Ⓒ Ⓓ	38 Ⓐ Ⓑ Ⓒ Ⓓ	58 Ⓐ Ⓑ Ⓒ Ⓓ	78 Ⓐ Ⓑ Ⓒ Ⓓ
19 Ⓐ Ⓑ Ⓒ Ⓓ	39 Ⓐ Ⓑ Ⓒ Ⓓ	59 Ⓐ Ⓑ Ⓒ Ⓓ	79 Ⓐ Ⓑ Ⓒ Ⓓ
20 Ⓐ Ⓑ Ⓒ Ⓓ	40 Ⓐ Ⓑ Ⓒ Ⓓ	60 Ⓐ Ⓑ Ⓒ Ⓓ	80 Ⓐ Ⓑ Ⓒ Ⓓ

Equipment Operation and Maintenance (section begins at 31)

Image Production and Evaluation (section begins at 61)

081 (A) (B) (C) (D)

Radiographic Procedures and Related Anatomy

111 (A) (B) (C) (D)

141 (A) (B) (C) (D)

Patient Care

171 (A) (B) (C) (D)

082 (A) (B) (C) (D)

112 (A) (B) (C) (D)

142 (A) (B) (C) (D)

172 (A) (B) (C) (D)

083 (A) (B) (C) (D)

113 (A) (B) (C) (D)

143 (A) (B) (C) (D)

173 (A) (B) (C) (D)

084 (A) (B) (C) (D)

114 (A) (B) (C) (D)

144 (A) (B) (C) (D)

174 (A) (B) (C) (D)

085 (A) (B) (C) (D)

115 (A) (B) (C) (D)

145 (A) (B) (C) (D)

175 (A) (B) (C) (D)

086 (A) (B) (C) (D)

116 (A) (B) (C) (D)

146 (A) (B) (C) (D)

176 (A) (B) (C) (D)

087 (A) (B) (C) (D)

117 (A) (B) (C) (D)

147 (A) (B) (C) (D)

177 (A) (B) (C) (D)

088 (A) (B) (C) (D)

118 (A) (B) (C) (D)

148 (A) (B) (C) (D)

178 (A) (B) (C) (D)

089 (A) (B) (C) (D)

119 (A) (B) (C) (D)

149 (A) (B) (C) (D)

179 (A) (B) (C) (D)

090 (A) (B) (C) (D)

120 (A) (B) (C) (D)

150 (A) (B) (C) (D)

180 (A) (B) (C) (D)

091 (A) (B) (C) (D)

121 (A) (B) (C) (D)

151 (A) (B) (C) (D)

181 (A) (B) (C) (D)

092 (A) (B) (C) (D)

122 (A) (B) (C) (D)

152 (A) (B) (C) (D)

182 (A) (B) (C) (D)

093 (A) (B) (C) (D)

123 (A) (B) (C) (D)

153 (A) (B) (C) (D)

183 (A) (B) (C) (D)

094 (A) (B) (C) (D)

124 (A) (B) (C) (D)

154 (A) (B) (C) (D)

184 (A) (B) (C) (D)

095 (A) (B) (C) (D)

125 (A) (B) (C) (D)

155 (A) (B) (C) (D)

185 (A) (B) (C) (D)

096 (A) (B) (C) (D)

126 (A) (B) (C) (D)

156 (A) (B) (C) (D)

186 (A) (B) (C) (D)

097 (A) (B) (C) (D)

127 (A) (B) (C) (D)

157 (A) (B) (C) (D)

187 (A) (B) (C) (D)

098 (A) (B) (C) (D)

128 (A) (B) (C) (D)

158 (A) (B) (C) (D)

188 (A) (B) (C) (D)

099 (A) (B) (C) (D)

129 (A) (B) (C) (D)

159 (A) (B) (C) (D)

189 (A) (B) (C) (D)

100 (A) (B) (C) (D)

130 (A) (B) (C) (D)

160 (A) (B) (C) (D)

190 (A) (B) (C) (D)

101 (A) (B) (C) (D)

131 (A) (B) (C) (D)

161 (A) (B) (C) (D)

191 (A) (B) (C) (D)

102 (A) (B) (C) (D)

132 (A) (B) (C) (D)

162 (A) (B) (C) (D)

192 (A) (B) (C) (D)

103 (A) (B) (C) (D)

133 (A) (B) (C) (D)

163 (A) (B) (C) (D)

193 (A) (B) (C) (D)

104 (A) (B) (C) (D)

134 (A) (B) (C) (D)

164 (A) (B) (C) (D)

194 (A) (B) (C) (D)

105 (A) (B) (C) (D)

135 (A) (B) (C) (D)

165 (A) (B) (C) (D)

195 (A) (B) (C) (D)

106 (A) (B) (C) (D)

136 (A) (B) (C) (D)

166 (A) (B) (C) (D)

196 (A) (B) (C) (D)

107 (A) (B) (C) (D)

137 (A) (B) (C) (D)

167 (A) (B) (C) (D)

197 (A) (B) (C) (D)

108 (A) (B) (C) (D)

138 (A) (B) (C) (D)

168 (A) (B) (C) (D)

198 (A) (B) (C) (D)

109 (A) (B) (C) (D)

139 (A) (B) (C) (D)

169 (A) (B) (C) (D)

199 (A) (B) (C) (D)

110 (A) (B) (C) (D)

140 (A) (B) (C) (D)

170 (A) (B) (C) (D)

200 (A) (B) (C) (D)

SIMULATION EXAMINATION 4

Questions

Directions: (Questions 1 to 200) For each of the following items, select the best answer among the four possible choices (A, B, C, or D). For ease of scoring, it is suggested that you use the bubble sheet provided in the back of this examination. Make sure to answer all questions. You should allow yourself a maximum of 3 hours to take this examination.

Refer to the scale in the back of the book to determine a passing score in each section. It is not necessary that you pass each section, but you must receive a total "scaled" score of 75 to pass the examination.

SECTION I: RADIATION PROTECTION AND RADIOBIOLOGY

1. When radiographing a pregnant patient for a posteroanterior (PA) view of the chest, where should the lead barrier be placed to best protect from backscatter?
   A. The lead barrier should be placed on the patient's posterior side facing the primary beam.
   B. A shadow shield should be used attached to the collimator.
   C. An apron should be worn that completely surrounds the patient's abdomen.
   D. No shield should be used because this would interfere with the ability to visualize the structures of interest.

2. The roentgen is the principal unit used to measure the "in air" dose and can be used in the measurement of:
   1. X- and gamma radiation
   2. Beta radiation
   3. Alpha radiation
   A. 1 only
   B. 1 and 2 only
   C. 2 and 3 only
   D. 1, 2, and 3

3. If the exposure factors of milliamperes, time, and kilovolts (peak) (kVp) remain the same, a change in which of the other listed factors would affect the dose received by the patient?
   A. Focal spot size (FSS)
   B. Source-image receptor-distance (SID)
   C. Screen speed
   D. Grid ratio

4. What is the most radiosensitive cell of those listed below?
   A. Erythrocyte
   B. Osteocyte
   C. Neuroblast
   D. Spermatozoa

5. What percentage of the gonadal dose is decreased when using a properly placed shield of 1-mm lead (Pb) equivalent over the reproductive organs of a female?
   A. 50 percent
   B. 75 percent
   C. 90 percent
   D. 99 percent

163

6. What type of radiation will produce the greatest amount of biologic damage in human tissue?
   A. High linear energy transfer (LET)
   B. Low LET
   C. Low quality factor
   D. Highly penetrating

7. Death by radiation as a result of the hemopoietic syndrome is characterized by:
   1. Severe infection
   2. Electrolyte imbalance
   3. Bowel obstruction

   A. 1 and 2 only
   B. 1 and 3 only
   C. 2 and 3 only
   D. 1, 2, and 3

8. The ALARA concept was initiated by the National Council on Radiation Protection and Measurement (NCRP) to ensure that radiation levels are:
   A. Always monitored in children
   B. Kept at dose-equivalent limits
   C. Monitored for fetal doses
   D. Kept as low as reasonably achievable

9. A therapy patient receives a dose of 50 mGy (5 rad) of neutrons having a quality factor of 10. This patient's dose equivalent is:
   A. 50 mSv (5 rem)
   B. 500 mSv (50 rem)
   C. 1.5 mSv (150 mrem)
   D. 15 mSv (1.5 rem)

   [handwritten: 50 mGy × 10 = 500]

10. When exposed to a 70–kiloelectron-volt (keV) beam, the human tissue that will attenuate the least amount of radiation is:
    A. Tooth enamel
    B. Liver
    C. Skeletal muscle
    D. Bowel gas

11. Which of the following effects have been observed in fetuses exposed in utero to radiation?
    1. Growth malformations
    2. Neonatal death
    3. Spontaneous abortion

    A. 1 and 2 only
    B. 1 and 3 only
    C. 2 and 3 only
    D. 1, 2, and 3

12. What is the minimum amount of Pb required in the x-ray tube housing to keep leakage at or below acceptable levels?
    A. 0.25-mm Pb
    B. 0.50-mm Pb
    C. 1.5-mm Pb
    D. 2.0-mm Pb

13. All x-ray switches that maintain current flow by the application of continuous pressure are called:
    A. Relay switches
    B. Circuit breakers
    C. Dead-man switches
    D. Microswitches

14. Which of the following materials would offer the best protection from a 250-keV gamma source?
    A. Wood
    B. Concrete
    C. Aluminum
    D. Lead

15. Gamma rays can be described as having:
    1. Very little mass
    2. Negative charge
    3. Low LET

    A. 1 only
    B. 1 and 2 only
    C. 3 only
    D. 1, 2, and 3

16. How many neutrons are in one atom of an isotope of $^{132}_{-56}Ba$? *[handwritten: 132 - 56 = 76]*
    A. 188
    B. 132
    C. 76
    D. 56

17. A film badge monitor will normally contain filters to:
    A. Intercept harmful radiation
    B. Differentiate between various energies
    C. Prevent exposure from particulate radiation
    D. Act as a mechanical support for the film

18. Approximately what percentage of the public's annual exposure to ionizing radiation is attributed to medical and dental radiographic procedures?
    A. 12 percent
    B. 25 percent
    C. 50 percent
    D. 85 percent

19. The amount of time that x rays are being directed toward a particular wall or barrier is referred to as:
    A. Workload
    B. Use factor
    C. Occupancy factor
    D. Distance factor

20. In which of the following ways can a radiographer reduce the amount of scatter produced?
    1. Tight beam restriction
    2. Use of a small focal spot
    3. Use of lower kilovolts (peak)

    A. 1 and 2 only
    B. 1 and 3 only

C. 2 and 3 only
D. 1, 2, and 3

21. If the intensity of radiation at 3 m from a source is 27 R/min, what will the intensity be at 9 m from the source?
    A. 3 R/min
    B. 9 R/min
    C. 81 R/min
    D. 243 R/min

22. Which of the following examinations, in combination, may cause the highest occupational exposure to radiographers?
    A. Fluoroscopy, special procedures, and extremity radiography
    B. Mobile radiography, chest radiography, and fluoroscopy
    C. Fluoroscopy, mobile radiography, and special procedures
    D. Special procedures, fluoroscopy, and skull radiography

23. Which of the following sets of radiographic exposure factors will produce the lowest absorbed dose for an anteroposterior (AP) projection of the female abdomen?
    A. 50 kVp, 300 mAs
    B. 60 kVp, 200 mAs
    C. 70 kVp, 100 mAs
    D. 80 kVp, 50 mAs

24. Which of the following are considered the target organs for radiation-induced leukemia?
    A. Breasts
    B. Gonads
    C. Bone marrow
    D. White blood cells

25. Cleaved or broken chromosomes are a consequence of ionizing radiation striking and breaking:
    A. The center of the sugar-phosphate molecular chain on one side of a DNA macromolecule
    B. Two different areas of the sugar-phosphate molecular chain of a DNA macromolecule that are remote from one another
    C. Two opposite areas of the sugar-phosphate molecular chain of a DNA macromolecule that lie within the same rung
    D. A single area of the sugar-phosphate molecular chain of a DNA macromolecule on either the upper or the lower end

26. Which of the following will help to reduce the absorbed dose equivalent for the radiographer?
    1. The use of high-speed image receptor systems
    2. The proper use of beam limitation devices
    3. Ensuring proper radiographic processing techniques

A. 1 and 2 only
B. 1 and 3 only
C. 2 and 3 only
D. 1, 2, and 3

27. During a radiographic examination, the probability of biologic damage to the patient increases as:
    A. Less energy is absorbed by body atoms
    B. More energy is absorbed by body atoms
    C. Normally aerated cells become deoxygenated
    D. Protein synthesis increases in the ribosomes

28. When should the radiographer be exposed to the primary beam?
    A. Not under any circumstances
    B. When performing fluoroscopic procedures on an infant
    C. When holding the cassette for a "shoot-through" lateral projection
    D. When restraining a combative patient for a trauma series

29. Carcinogenesis, cataractogenesis, and lymphocytic leukemia are all examples of:
    A. Genetic defects
    B. Short-term somatic effects
    C. Acute radiation syndrome
    D. Long-term somatic effects

30. The lowest intensity of radiation from the patient is scattered:
    A. Toward the head of the table
    B. Toward the foot of the table
    C. At a 90° angle from the patient
    D. At a 45° angle from the patient

SECTION II: EQUIPMENT OPERATION AND MAINTENANCE

31. What device must be adjusted to change the voltage flowing to the primary side of the step-up transformer in an x-ray generating circuit?
    A. Choke coil
    B. Rectifier
    C. Autotransformer
    D. Rheostat

32. The image on the output phosphor of the intensifier tube is:
    1. Brighter than the image at the input phosphor
    2. Dimmer than the image at the input phosphor
    3. Larger than the image at the input phosphor

A. 1 only
B. 2 only
C. 3 only
D. 1 and 3 only

33. The property of an electric circuit that allows the electrons to move along the surface of the conductor is known as:
    A. Current
    B. Electromotive force
    C. Resistance
    D. Inductance

34. Unlike cassettes used for conventional radiography, cassettes used with automatic exposure control (AEC) devices are constructed:
    A. With an additional layer of thick lead
    B. With a radiolucent back
    C. Without intensifying screens
    D. Without a radiolucent front

35. An area of blurring on a radiograph of a wire-mesh device would indicate:
    A. Quantum mottle
    B. Phosphorescence
    C. Modulation transfer function
    D. Poor screen-film contact

36. In a full-wave rectification circuit, the
    A. Negative wave of AC is suppressed
    B. Positive wave of AC is suppressed
    C. Negative wave of AC is changed into a second positive wave
    D. Positive wave of AC is changed into a second negative wave

37. Ion chambers used in AEC devices contain a gas that is usually:
    A. Free air
    B. Neon
    C. Freon
    D. Hydrogen

38. Static images may be recorded directly from the output phosphor of the image intensifier by using:

    1. Direct or conventional spot filming
    2. 70-mm photospot camera
    3. VCR recorder

    A. 1 only
    B. 2 only
    C. 3 only
    D. 1, 2, and 3

39. The reduction of voltage and production of high amperage by a step-down (Coolidge) transformer occurs in the _____ of the x-ray circuit.
    A. X-ray tube
    B. Primary section
    C. Secondary section
    D. Filament portion

40. Most computers operate on a dual-number system consisting of only the digits 0 and 1. This is referred to as the
    A. Binary system
    B. Voxel system
    C. Byte system
    D. Pixel system

41. Figure 4–1 demonstrates which of the following target interactions between electrons and tungsten atoms:
    A. Bremsstrahlung
    B. Characteristic radiation
    C. Photoelectric effect
    D. Compton scattering

42. During fluoroscopic procedures, the automatic brightness control (ABC) functions to:
    A. Increase resolution in the image
    B. Decrease noise in the image
    C. Compensate for changes in patient part/thickness
    D. Change the focal point, thus magnifying the image

43. What effect does the diameter of the rotating anode disk have on the operation of the x-ray tube?
    A. Larger diameters increase heat-loading capabilities
    B. Larger diameters decrease image resolution
    C. Smaller diameters have smaller FSSs
    D. Smaller diameters possess higher rotational speeds

44. What is the power rating of a generator capable of operating at 500 mA and 110 kVp?
    A. 22 millijoules
    B. 55,000 electron volts (eV)
    C. 22 mHz
    D. 55 kW

45. If an x-ray beam is created using exposure factors of 70 kVp, 500 mA, and 45 milliseconds and produces an exposure output of 340 mR, what is the milliroentgen per milliamperage-seconds?
    A. 7650 mR/mAs
    B. 15 mR/mAs
    C. 4.6 mR/mAs
    D. 2.1 mR/mAs

46. A properly operating AEC device is not able to automatically compensate for changes in:
    A. SID
    B. Kilovolts (peak)
    C. Tissue density
    D. Screen speed

47. A transformer with 20 turns on the primary coil and 1000 turns on the secondary coil and an input voltage of 220 V would have an output voltage of:
    A. 4.4 V
    B. 4.4 kV
    C. 11 V
    D. 11 kV

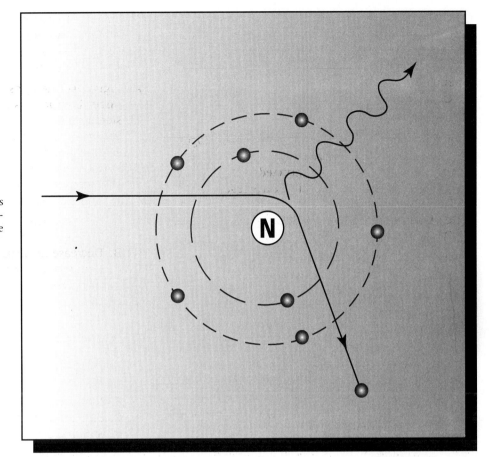

FIGURE 4–1. An electron approaches the nucleus of an atom and alters direction and speed, resulting in the production of an x ray.

48. What type of components are used as rectifiers in most modern radiographic units?
    A. n-Type and p-type semiconductors
    B. Rheostats
    C. Choke coils
    D. Valve tubes

49. The smallest particle of a compound that retains the characteristics of the compound is a (an):
    A. Atom
    B. Molecule
    C. Electron
    D. Element

50. The force that keeps electrons in their orbit about the nucleus is referred to as:
    A. Nuclear force
    B. Electrostatic force
    C. Binding force
    D. Electron-binding energy

51. The proper care of lead apparel includes the following procedures:
    1. Check for cracks with fluoroscopy.
    2. Hang on appropriate racks.
    3. Neatly fold aprons when not in use.
    A. 1 and 2 only
    B. 1 and 3 only

C. 2 and 3 only
D. 1, 2, and 3

52. The life of an x-ray tube may be extended by:
    1. Using low–milliamperage-seconds and high-kilovolt (peak) exposure factors
    2. Avoiding lengthy preparation or boost times
    3. Avoiding exposures to a cold anode
    A. 1 and 2 only
    B. 1 and 3 only
    C. 2 and 3 only
    D. 1, 2, and 3

53. The device that converts electrical energy into mechanical energy is called a(an)
    A. Motor
    B. Battery
    C. Generator
    D. Dynamo

54. What is the device that may be used to direct the light emitted from the image intensifier to various viewing and imaging apparatuses?
    A. Photocathode
    B. Beam splitter
    C. Photomultiplier tube
    D. Cathode-ray tube (CRT)

55. Radiation that passes through the tube housing in directions other than through the port window is termed:
    A. Off-focus radiation
    B. Scatter radiation
    C. Leakage radiation
    D. Remnant radiation

56. The material of choice for the construction of the focusing cup is:
    A. Lead
    B. Aluminum
    C. Tungsten
    D. Nickel

    filament – tungsten

57. The brightness gain in an image intensifier may be determined by:
    A. The intensification factor
    B. The penumbra formula
    C. The product of minification gain and flux gain
    D. (Input phosphor size/output phosphor size)^2

58. The waveform produced by a battery-operated mobile x-ray unit most closely resembles that of a:
    A. Single-phase, half-wave rectified generator
    B. Single-phase, full-wave rectified generator
    C. Capacitor discharge generator
    D. High-frequency generator

59. Which of the following components make up the emulsion of the radiographic film?
    1. Silver halide crystals
    2. Polyester
    3. Gelatin

    A. 1 and 2 only
    B. 1 and 3 only
    C. 2 and 3 only
    D. 1, 2, and 3

60. What would be the best selection of technical factors for the initial warm-up procedure of an x-ray tube?

	mA	Exposure Time	kVp	FSS
A.	100	1 second	110	1 mm
B.	200	2 seconds	90	0.6 mm
C.	100	1 second	75	1 mm
D.	500	0.2 second	70	2 mm

SECTION III: IMAGE PRODUCTION AND EVALUATION

61. When using an AEC device, inadequate collimation can result in:
    A. Overexposed radiograph
    B. Underexposed radiograph
    C. Increased image blur
    D. Excessive contrast

62. Which of the following processing artifacts runs opposite the direction the film travels?
    A. Pi lines
    B. Guide-shoe marks
    C. Wet-pressure sensitization
    D. Crescent marks

63. The most common method of designating screen speed is:
    A. Medium density
    B. Intensification factor
    C. Relative speed
    D. Spectral matching

64. When all technical factors (kilovolts [peak], milliamperage-seconds, and time) remain the same, the radiation intensity should not vary by more than _____ between each exposure.
    A. 5 percent
    B. 10 percent
    C. 15 percent
    D. 20 percent

65. The density (mass per unit volume) of the patient's anatomy can affect:
    1. Radiographic density
    2. Radiographic contrast
    3. Differential absorption

    A. 1 and 2 only
    B. 1 and 3 only
    C. 2 and 3 only
    D. 1, 2, and 3

66. A radiograph is produced at 800 mA, 250 milliseconds with a 100-speed imaging system. What new milliamperage-seconds is required to maintain radiographic density if a 400-speed imaging system is used?
    A. 12.5 mAs
    B. 50 mAs
    C. 200 mAs
    D. 800 mAs

67. The main purpose of radiographic grids is to:
    A. Decrease the exposure to the patient
    B. Increase radiographic density
    C. Decrease radiographic contrast
    D. Absorb scatter radiation from the exit beam

68. Which of the following chemicals retards oxidation in the automatic processor?
    A. Sodium sulfite
    B. Glutaraldehyde
    C. Hydroquinone
    D. Ammonium thiosulfate

69. What percentage of silver from the film's emulsion is normally dissolved in the fixer during film processing?

A. 15 percent
B. 30 percent
C. 50 percent
D. 80 percent

70. Which of the following advanced pathologies would require an increase in penetration of the x-ray beam?
A. Aseptic necrosis
B. Hemothorax
C. Emphysema
D. Osteoporosis

71. If the developer temperature is excessive on an automatic processor, one can expect to see:
A. A decrease in contrast in the manifest image
B. An increase in contrast in the manifest image
C. An increase in contrast in the latent image
D. A reduction in radiographic density

72. Using an AEC unit, a decrease in exposure time can be accomplished by:
1. Decreasing SID
2. Increasing kilovolts (peak)
3. Decreasing the backup time

A. 1 and 2 only
B. 1 and 3 only
C. 2 and 3 only
D. 1, 2, and 3

73. An object is radiographed measuring 18 inches in diameter and lies 8 inches above the image receptor. The SID is 40 inches. What is the percentage of magnification of this radiographic image?
A. 25 percent
B. 50 percent
C. 100 percent
D. 125 percent

74. What is the smallest percentage of increase in milliamperage-seconds that will produce a noticeable change in radiographic density?
A. 10 percent
B. 30 percent
C. 50 percent
D. 100 percent

75. A diagnostic image is produced with a 40-inch SID, 80 kVp, and 20 mAs. What new milliamperage-seconds should be used to maintain radiographic density if a 72-inch SID is now used?
A. 40 mAs
B. 65 mAs
C. 130 mAs
D. 150 mAs

76. What is the most probable cause of a finished radiograph that emerges from the processor with regularly spaced scratches?

A. Dirt deposits on the rollers
B. Improperly mixed chemicals
C. Improperly seated guide shoes
D. Excessively worn gears and sprockets

77. Orthochromatic film emulsions are most sensitive to:
A. All colors of the light spectrum
B. Red light only
C. All of the light spectrum except red
D. Blue-green light only

78. An image with short-scale contrast exhibits:
A. Small differences between two areas of radiographic density in the image
B. Great differences between two areas of radiographic density in the image
C. Many shades of gray and black with few white areas
D. Few black areas with mostly white and gray areas

79. A radiograph is produced with an 8:1 grid and 20 mAs. What new milliamperage-seconds should be used if a 16:1 grid is used instead?
A. 30 mAs
B. 40 mAs
C. 80 mAs
D. 120 mAs

80. Which of the following techniques would produce the greatest amount of recorded detail?

	mAs	kVp	SID	OID	FSS
A.	100	70	36 in.	10 in.	1 mm
B.	200	80	40 in.	8 in.	2 mm
C.	300	70	60 in.	6 in.	2 mm
D.	400	90	72 in.	4 in.	1 mm

81. The test tool in Figure 4–2 demonstrates line-pairs per millimeter and is used to express:
A. Radiographic distortion
B. Intensifying screen resolution
C. Film-screen contact
D. Amount of photoelectric absorption

82. To apply the 15% kilovolts (peak) rule to maintain radiographic densities from one exposure to another, you should decrease the kilovolts (peak) by 15% and
A. Increase mAs by 15 percent from the original value
B. Decrease the milliamperage-seconds by 15 percent from the original value
C. Increase the milliamperage-seconds by 100 percent from the original value
D. Decrease the milliamperage-seconds by 50 percent from the original value

83. To maintain quality control (QC) of a radiographic processor, a sensitometric strip should be passed through the system to measure:

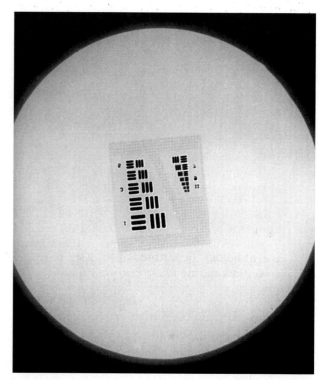

FIGURE 4–2.

A. Fog, speed, and contrast
B. Fog, temperature, and speed
C. Contrast, density, and speed
D. Density, contrast, and latitude

84. If the distance between the object and the image receptor is decreased by a factor of 2, the amount of image blur will:
    A. Increase proportionally
    B. Decrease proportionally
    C. Remain unchanged
    D. Increase by a factor of 4

85. The use of a small focal spot is useful for:
    A. Short exposure times
    B. Increased SIDs
    C. Magnification procedures
    D. High-speed rotating anodes

86. A radiograph taken with a film-screen combination possessing a wide latitude will likely exhibit:
    A. Low contrast
    B. High contrast
    C. Low recorded detail
    D. High density

87. What is the main purpose of washing in an automatic processor?
    A. Stop the fixation process
    B. Stop the action of the developer
    C. Maintain the proper solution activity
    D. Remove the clearing agent from the film

88. The grid radius may best be described as:

A. The height of the lead strips divided by the distance between them
B. The number of grid lines per inch
C. The grid-focusing distance
D. The size of the grid (10 × 12; 14 × 17, etc.)

89. As the screen speed increases in an imaging system, the
    A. Radiographic contrast will decrease
    B. Latitude will increase
    C. Resolution will increase
    D. Radiographic density will increase

Refer to Figure 4–3 to answer questions 90 and 91:

90. Which area of the Hurter and Driffield (H & D) curve in Figure 4–3 is represented by the letter B?
    A. Base-plus-fog
    B. D-max
    C. Straight-line portion
    D. Shoulder

91. Which area of the H & D curve in Figure 4–3 is represented by the letter E?
    A. Base-plus-fog
    B. Optical density
    C. Log relative exposure
    D. Straight-line portion

92. The proper developer action will occur only in a(an) _____ solution.
    A. Ionic
    B. Colloidal
    C. Acidic
    D. Alkaline

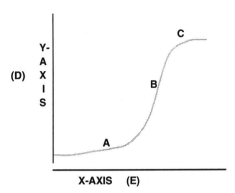

FIGURE 4–3. Hurter and Driffield (H & D) curve.

93. If a radiology department processes a total of 1240 films during a 2-week period and 165 are repeated, the department's repeat rate is:
A. 1.33 percent
B. 7.5 percent
C. 13.3 percent
D. 14.5 percent

94. The ability of a substance to emit light only during excitation is termed:
A. Fluorescence
B. Phosphorescence
C. Incandescence
D. Effervescence

95. The smell of ammonia from which part of the processor would indicate a problem?
A. Developer tank
B. Fixer tank
C. Wash tank
D. Dryer tank

96. What is the primary factor that controls the quantity of x-ray photons being created at the target?
A. Milliamperage-seconds
B. Kilovolts (peak)
C. SID
D. Anode bevel

97. Which of the radiographs in Figure 4–4 would be considered unacceptable because of excessive radiographic contrast?
A. Film A
B. Film B
C. Both films A and B
D. Both are acceptable

98. Which of the QC tests should be included in a routine annual calibration of radiographic equipment?
1. Reproducibility
2. Reciprocity
3. Filtration test

A. 1 and 2 only
B. 1 and 3 only
C. 2 and 3 only
D. 1, 2, and 3

99. An exposure was made at a 40-inch SID using technical factors of 100 mA, 0.25 second, and 75 kVp a 400-speed screen and a 12:1 grid. If it is necessary to repeat the radiograph to improve recorded detail using a 48-inch SID and a 100-speed screen at 0.18 second, what new milliampere station should be used to maintain radiographic density?
A. 300 mA
B. 400 mA
C. 600 mA
D. 800 mA

100. When a radiograph appears with sufficient radiographic density in the center of the image and insufficient radiographic density at the perimeter, possible causes could be:
1. An upside-down grid
2. Insufficient SID with a focused grid
3. Lateral decentering of the grid

FIGURE 4–4. Two skull radiographs for contrast. (From Wallace, JE: Radiographic Exposure: Principles and Practice. FA Davis, Philadelphia, 1995, p 90, with permission.)

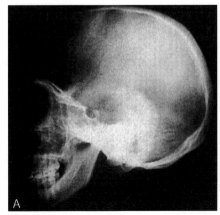
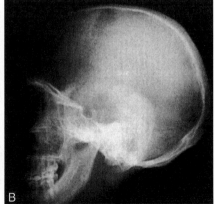

A. 1 and 2 only
B. 1 and 3 only
C. 2 and 3 only
D. 1, 2, and 3

101. The base-plus-fog density on a radiograph may be due to which of these?

    1. Blue-tinted base
    2. X-radiation fog
    3. Chemical development

    A. 1 and 2 only
    B. 1 and 3 only
    C. 2 and 3 only
    D. 1, 2, and 3

102. When all other technical factors remain the same, an increase in grid ratio will result in:
    A. Decreased blur
    B. Decreased recorded detail
    C. Decreased radiographic density
    D. Decreased radiographic contrast

103. In which of the following parts of the processor is the thermostat usually set at 120°F?
    A. Developer tank
    B. Fixer tank
    C. Wash tank
    D. Dryer tank

104. A lateral radiograph of the thoracic spine was made using a 400-speed screen with an AEC device and had adequate density but insufficient recorded detail. If the radiograph were repeated using a 200-speed screen, the result would be:
    A. Quantum mottle
    B. Excessive radiographic contrast
    C. Insufficient radiographic density
    D. Excessive radiographic density

105. When performing a portable radiograph on a fractured hip, the cassette was misaligned with the central ray. The resultant image would display:
    A. Size distortion
    B. Shape distortion
    C. Magnification
    D. Anode heel effect

106. If the timer was set at 25 milliseconds for a particular exposure, what milliampere station should be used to produce 30 mAs?
    A. 120 mA
    B. 600 mA
    C. 833 mA
    D. 1200 mA

107. An adequate exposure was made using 6 mAs at 61 kVp. If the degree of penetration needed to be increased by changing the kilovolts (peak) to 70, what new milliamperage-seconds should be used?

A. 3 mAs
B. 4.5 mAs
C. 12 mAs
D. 18 mAs

108. If a particular grid has 100 lead strips per inch that are 0.30 mm thick, 4 mm high, and 0.25 mm apart, what is its grid ratio?
    A. 6:1
    B. 8:1
    C. 12:1
    D. 16:1

109. Radiographic cassettes are often manufactured with a lead-foil backing that serves to:
    A. Improve resolution
    B. Increase screen speed
    C. Improve conversion efficiency
    D. Absorb backscatter

110. When an anatomic structure appears on the radiograph as shorter than its actual size, this best describes:
    A. Elongation
    B. Foreshortening
    C. Size distortion
    D. Magnification

SECTION IV: RADIOGRAPHIC PROCEDURES AND RELATED ANATOMY

111. A plane passing through the body perpendicular to the longitudinal axis is termed:
    A. Oblique
    B. Sagittal
    C. Coronal
    D. Horizontal

112. Which of the following best describes the hypersthenic body habitus?
    A. Heart is long and narrow.
    B. Lungs are short and broad at the base.
    C. Stomach is vertical and near midline.
    D. Build comprises 50 percent of the population.

113. Which of the following principles is correct regarding trauma radiography?
    A. Any two projections that can be obtained are adequate for an accurate diagnosis.
    B. A full routine series is essential for a trauma examination.
    C. Only one good image is required for a severely traumatized patient.
    D. Two projections taken 90° apart are required for an accurate diagnosis.

114. Where should the compression be applied during an intravenous urogram?

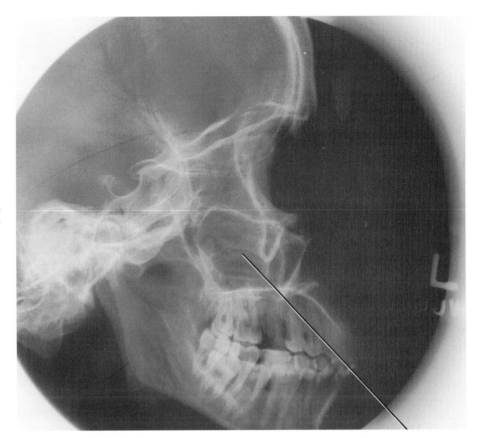

FIGURE 4–5. Lateral projection of the sinuses. (Courtesy of JRMC Radiology Department.)

A. Over the kidneys
B. At distal ends of the ureters
C. At middle portion of the ureters
D. Over the bladder

115. Which paranasal sinus is identified in Figure 4–5?
    A. Maxillary
    B. Anterior ethmoid
    C. Posterior ethmoid
    D. Sphenoid

116. When performing an AP projection of the acromioclavicular (AC) joints, how many pounds of weight should be affixed to each wrist?
    A. 1 lb
    B. 2 lb
    C. 3 to 4 lb
    D. 5 to 8 lb

For questions 117 and 118, refer to Figure 4–6:

117. In Figure 4–6, the anatomic part referenced by the number 2 is:
    A. Navicular bone
    B. Cuboid bone
    C. Second cuneiform bone
    D. Talus

118. In Figure 4–6, the anatomic part referenced by the number 5 is:

A. Middle cuneiform bone
B. Cuboid bone
C. Navicular bone
D. Fourth metatarsal

119. The site of the duodenojejunal flexure is held tightly in position by a fibrous connective band of tissue called the
    A. Taeniae coli
    B. Falciform ligament
    C. Ligament of Treitz
    D. Crypt of Lieberkühn

120. If a breathing technique cannot be used for the transthoracic lateral projection of the shoulder, the exposure should be made on:
    A. Full expiration
    B. Full inspiration
    C. Second full inspiration
    D. Suspended breathing

121. The head of the radius articulates on the medial side with the
    A. Coronoid process
    B. Trochlear notch
    C. Ulnar styloid process
    D. Radial notch of the ulna

122. The part of the lung that extends above the clavicle is termed the

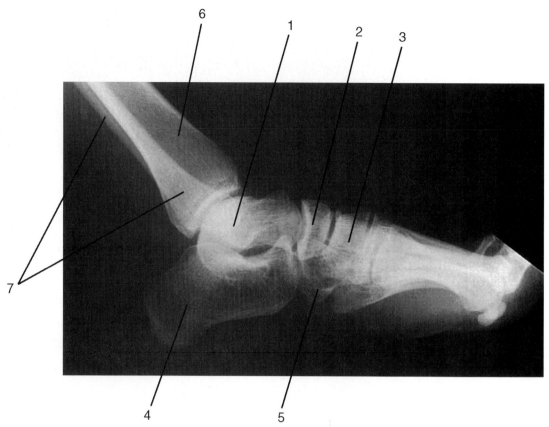

FIGURE 4–6. Lateral projection of the foot. (Adapted from McKinnis, LN: Fundamentals of Orthopedic Radiology. FA Davis, Philadelphia, 1997, p 297, with permission.)

A. Base
B. Hilum
C. Apex
D. Mediastinum

123. Long-bone measurement most frequently requires radiography of the
    A. Hands and feet
    B. Upper limbs only
    C. Lower limbs only
    D. Femurs only

124. Which of the following should be centered to the cassette for a PA projection of the mandibular rami?
    A. Inferior alveolar process
    B. Mental point
    C. Nasion
    D. Lips

125. The degree of obliquity for a PA projection of the stomach will vary with the patient's body habitus. Which body habitus will require the greatest degree of obliquity?
    A. Asthenic
    B. Sthenic
    C. Hyposthenic
    D. Hypersthenic

126. On a parietoacanthial (Waters) projection of the sinuses, the petrous ridges should:
    A. Be projected just below the maxillary sinuses
    B. Be projected in the lower third of the orbits
    C. Completely fill the orbits
    D. Not be demonstrated

127. For the lateral projection of the knee, the knee should be flexed how many degrees?
    A. 20°–30°
    B. 35°
    C. 45°
    D. 90°

128. The radiograph in Figure 4–7 demonstrates a common pathology of the vertebral column called:
    A. Spondylolysis
    B. Spondylolisthesis
    C. Spina bifida
    D. Herniated nucleus pulposus

129. When the gallbladder is stimulated to secrete bile, the bile first passes through the
    A. Common bile duct
    B. Ampulla of Vater
    C. Cystic duct
    D. Duct of Santorini

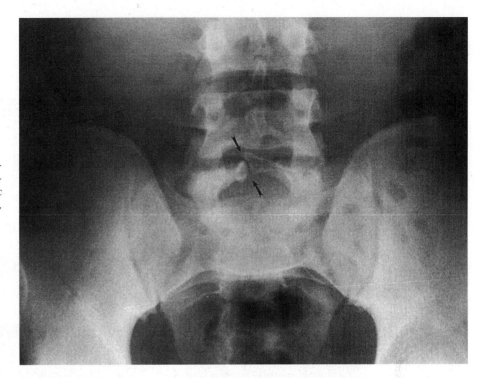

FIGURE 4–7. Anteroposterior projection of a lumbar spine. (From McKinnis, LN: Fundamentals of Orthopedic Radiology. FA Davis, Philadelphia, 1997, p 205, with permission.)

130. Which of the following positions would best demonstrate a left pneumothorax?
    A. Recumbent left lateral projection of the chest with full expiration
    B. Left lateral decubitus projection of the chest with full inspiration
    C. Supine AP projection of the chest with full inspiration
    D. Erect PA projection of the chest with full expiration

131. Which of the following sets of technical factors would most likely eliminate motion on a kidney-ureter-bladder (KUB) image?
    A. 74 kVp, 600 mA, 0.04 second
    B. 74 kVp, 150 mA, 0.16 second
    C. 85 kVp, 300 mA, 0.04 second
    D. 85 kVp, 600 mA, 0.02 second

132. A small-bowel series is considered complete when the column of barium sulfate enters the
    A. Cecum
    B. Jejunum
    C. Transverse colon
    D. Rectum

133. Coarctation of the aorta means:
    A. Enlarging of the aorta
    B. Narrowing of the aorta
    C. Striation of the aorta
    D. Widening of the aorta

134. Which of the following radiographic examinations would most likely demonstrate a rupture of the lateral ligament of the ankle?

A. Composite study
B. AP projection with eversion stress
C. AP projection with inversion stress
D. Weight-bearing study

135. A lateral radiograph of the skull demonstrates the presence of a curvilinear area with overlapping fragments in the parietal region. These radiographic indications are commonly seen in:
    A. Blowout fractures resulting from impact
    B. Depressed fractures resulting from blunt trauma
    C. Linear fractures resulting from a fall
    D. Multilinear fractures resulting from a bump on the head

136. The submentovertex (SMV) projection of the cranium best demonstrates the
    A. Frontal and ethmoid sinuses
    B. Ethmoid and maxillary sinuses
    C. Maxillary and frontal sinuses
    D. Sphenoid and ethmoid sinuses

137. When the patient takes in a deep breath during chest radiography, the diaphragm:
    A. Contracts and the dome moves downward
    B. Relaxes and the dome moves upward
    C. Contracts and the dome moves upward
    D. Relaxes and the dome moves downward

138. For an AP projection of the coccyx, the central ray should be directed:
    A. 10° cephalic
    B. 10° caudal

C. 25° cephalic
D. 25° caudal

139. For myelography, the contrast medium is introduced into the
A. Dura mater
B. Cauda equina
C. Spinal cord
D. Subarachnoid space

140. The most anterior part of a typical vertebra is the
A. Body
B. Lamina
C. Pedicle
D. Transverse process

141. Which of the following facilitates arterial communication between the anterior and posterior circulation along the base of the brain?
A. Basilar artery
B. Carotid artery
C. Circle of Willis
D. Vertebral artery

142. For the Camp-Coventry method of demonstrating the intercondyloid fossa, the knee should be flexed _____ if the central ray is angled 40° caudad.
A. 30°
B. 35°
C. 40°
D. 45°

143. To adequately demonstrate the zygapophyseal articulations of the lumbar vertebrae, the _____ position should be used.
A. Lateral
B. Supine
C. 45° oblique
D. Decubitus

144. What type of fracture is characterized by separation of the bone into numerous fragments at the midshaft?
A. Compound
B. Comminuted
C. Impacted
D. Torus

145. What is the function of the falciform ligament?
A. Attaches the kidneys to the posterior abdominal wall
B. Interconnects the basilar artery with the vertebral artery
C. Maintains the position of the carpal bones
D. Separates the right lobe of the liver from the left lobe

146. Which structure is *not* found in the mediastinum?
A. Esophagus
B. Lungs

C. Superior vena cava
D. Thymus gland

147. Which of the following structures of the stomach is the most proximal?
A. Pylorus
B. Body
C. Fundus
D. Cardia

148. Lumbar lordosis can be reduced for the AP projection by:
A. Extending the legs and arching the back
B. Flexing both hips and knees
C. Slightly flexing one hip and one knee
D. Placing the patient in the erect position

149. What is it called when the fifth lumbar vertebra slips forward on the sacrum?
A. Spondylolysis
B. Spondylosis
C. Spondylolisthesis
D. Ankylosing spondylitis

150. The olecranon process is a part of the
A. Humerus
B. Scapula
C. Radius
D. Ulna

151. Which of the following is a type of pathology sometimes seen in acquired immunodeficiency syndrome (AIDS) patients?
A. Pneumoconiosis
B. Ewing's sarcoma
C. Anthracosis
D. *Pneumocystis carinii* pneumonia

152. Which of the following positions of the elbow should clearly demonstrate the coronoid process of the ulna?
A. Supination
B. Lateral oblique
C. Lateral
D. Medial oblique

153. The zygomatic arch is formed by part of which bone?
A. Temporal
B. Frontal
C. Parietal
D. Sphenoid

154. Cephalopelvic disproportion (CPD) in a primigravid patient can be diagnosed using which of the following?

1. Sonography
2. Hysterosalpingography
3. Pelvimetry (Colcher-Sussman method)

A. 1 and 2 only
B. 1 and 3 only

C. 2 and 3 only
D. 1, 2, and 3

155. How much should the body be rotated for the AP oblique projection of the urinary bladder during cystography?
A. 25°
B. 35°
C. 40°–60°
D. 65°–80°

156. What will be demonstrated if the patient places the hand in an extended lateral position, and the central ray enters the first metacarpophalangeal joint?
A. Lateral projection of the hand
B. Foreign bodies of the hand
C. Oblique projection of the thumb
D. PA projection of the thumb

157. The neck of the "Scottie dog" seen on the oblique projections of the lumbar spine series is formed by:
A. Pars interarticularis
B. Pedicle
C. Laminae
D. Superior articulating process

158. Arthrography is usually performed on what type of joints?
A. Synarthrodial
B. Diarthrodial
C. Amphiarthrodial
D. Cartilaginous

159. The first sacral vertebra (S1) is located at the level of the
A. Inferior margin of the rib cage
B. Level of the umbilicus
C. Superior aspect of the iliac crest
D. Anterior superior iliac spine (ASIS)

160. Which projection of the paranasal sinuses best demonstrates the maxillary sinus?
A. PA (Caldwell) projection
B. Parietoacanthial (Waters) projection
C. Lateral projection
D. SMV projection

161. Which position or projection of the elbow is done specifically for the demonstration of elevated fat pads?
A. Lateral
B. Medial oblique
C. Lateral oblique
D. AP

162. Which position or projection best demonstrates an open hepatic flexure during a barium enema?
A. AP
B. PA

C. Right posterior oblique
D. Left posterior oblique

163. The largest bone in the proximal row of carpals is the
A. Hamate
B. Scaphoid
C. Lunate
D. Capitate

164. Blood leaving the right ventricle of the heart will enter the
A. Right atrium
B. Superior vena cava
C. Pulmonary artery
D. Aortic arch

165. When radiographing the proximal humerus using the transthoracic (Lawrence) method, the plane of the epicondyles should be _____ to the plane of the cassette.
A. At a 45° angle
B. Perpendicular
C. Parallel
D. At a 30° angle

166. The movement of a structure toward the central axis of the body is termed:
A. Adduction
B. Abduction
C. Eversion
D. Supination

167. The aspect of the kidney on which the renal hilum is located is the
A. Superior
B. Inferior
C. Lateral
D. Medial

168. A correctly positioned parieto-orbital oblique (Rhese) projection should demonstrate the optic canal in the
A. Upper outer quadrant
B. Upper medial quadrant
C. Lower outer quadrant
D. Lower medial quadrant

169. A colon that has not been properly prepared for a barium enema examination may cause retained fecal material to resemble:
A. Diverticulitis
B. Polyposis
C. Ulcerative colitis
D. Crohn's disease

170. What breathing instructions should be given to a patient for a lateral projection of the sternum?
A. Tell the patient to breathe quietly.
B. Respiration should be suspended on full inspiration.

C. Respiration should be suspended on full expiration.

D. Breathing instructions are not necessary for a lateral sternum.

SECTION V: PATIENT CARE

171. What type of shock is associated with pooling of blood in the peripheral vessels?
    A. Cardiogenic
    B. Neurogenic
    C. Hypovolemic
    D. Septic

172. What is the proper method of administering rescue breathing to an adult who is suffering from respiratory arrest?
    A. One breath every 2 seconds
    B. One breath every 3 seconds
    C. One breath every 4 seconds
    D. One breath every 5 seconds

173. If the oral temperature is consistently below _____, the patient is said to be suffering from hypothermia.
    A. 95°F
    B. 90°F
    C. 85°F
    D. 80°F

174. If a patient's blood pressure is 120/70 mm Hg, the systolic pressure is:
    A. 50 mm Hg
    B. 70 mm Hg
    C. 120 mm Hg
    D. 190 mm Hg

175. Which of the following should be the first step when a victim has a foreign body lodged in the airway?
    A. Heimlich maneuver
    B. Modified Valsalva's maneuver
    C. Valsalva's maneuver
    D. Insertion of an endotracheal (ET) tube

176. A patient with epistaxis is suffering from:
    A. Earache
    B. Infection
    C. Laceration
    D. Nosebleed

177. What is the main consideration when radiographing an unconscious patient who has suffered a head injury?
    A. Keeping an open airway
    B. Maintaining a normal pulse
    C. Maintaining normal respiration
    D. Preventing hemorrhage

178. The average rate of respiration in the adult is:
    A. 8 to 12 breaths per minute
    B. 16 to 20 breaths per minute
    C. 21 to 25 breaths per minute
    D. 26 to 30 breaths per minute

179. Which of the following are true statements regarding the use of barium sulfate as a contrast medium?
    1. It dissolves when mixed with water.
    2. It forms a suspension when combined with water.
    3. It is radiopaque.

    A. 1 and 2 only
    B. 1 and 3 only
    C. 2 and 3 only
    D. 1, 2, and 3

180. When taken orally, the normal body temperature is:
    A. 96.6°F
    B. 97.6°F
    C. 98.6°F
    D. 99.6°F

181. Which of the following statements is (are) true regarding precautions for body substances?
    1. Used needles should be recapped before placing them in the disposable container.
    2. Latex gloves need not be worn when wiping up blood spills.
    3. Protective mask and/or eye shield should be worn whenever the face could be splashed with body fluids.

    A. 1 only
    B. 2 only
    C. 3 only
    D. 1, 2, and 3

182. Freely discussing a patient's confidential medical information with an unauthorized person is known as:
    A. Defamation of character
    B. Misconduct
    C. Negligence
    D. Invasion of privacy

183. The proper patient care procedure for extravasation of a contrast medium is to:
    A. Continue the injection and tell the patient the burning sensation will subside
    B. Remove the needle and hold pressure on the vein until the bleeding stops
    C. Remove the needle, repuncture the same vein, and continue the injection
    D. Place a warm compress above the site of the injection and continue administering the contrast

184. If a radiographer performs an IVU on a patient who was supposed to have had a lumbar spine series, the radiographer may be charged with:
    A. Negligence
    B. Assault
    C. Battery
    D. Confidentiality breech

185. A patient with pulmonary emphysema is having difficulty breathing and is in need of oxygen. The correct flow rate through the nasal cannula should be:
    A. 2 to 3 L/min
    B. 4 to 5 L/min
    C. 6 to 7 L/min
    D. 8 to 10 L/min

186. Patient preparation for an upper gastrointestinal (UGI) series should include:
    1. NPO after midnight prior to the examination
    2. No gum chewing
    3. No smoking

    A. 1 and 2 only
    B. 1 and 3 only
    C. 2 and 3 only
    D. 1, 2, and 3

187. What action should a radiographer take to reduce the occurrence of postural hypotension?
    A. Place the patient in the Trendelenburg position.
    B. Sit the patient up slowly from a recumbent position.
    C. Elevate the patient's legs with pillows.
    D. Give the patient something sweet to eat.

188. What unit is used to measure pulse rate?
    A. mm Hg
    B. beats per minute
    C. °F
    D. systole/diastole

189. By what mode of transmission are respiratory diseases usually spread?
    A. Direct contact
    B. Droplet
    C. Fomites
    D. Vector

190. Isopropyl alcohol and povidone-iodine (Betadine) are two common agents that may be used for:
    A. Surgical asepsis
    B. Topical anesthetic
    C. Disinfecting the skin
    D. Lubricating enema tips

191. A stat portable chest radiograph has been ordered on a patient in the intensive care unit for placement of an infusion port. An infusion port is a(an)

    A. Chest drainage tube
    B. Angiocatheter
    C. Pacemaker lead
    D. Arteriovenous shunt

192. An emetic is used to:
    A. Stimulate defecation
    B. Induce vomiting
    C. Increase urine output
    D. Suppress coughing

193. The advantages of using nonionic, water-soluble contrast media may include:
    1. Low osmolality
    2. Low toxicity
    3. Cost effectiveness

    A. 1 and 2 only
    B. 1 and 3 only
    C. 2 and 3 only
    D. 1, 2, and 3

194. An inanimate object that has been exposed to an infectious microorganism is considered what type of carrier of that infection?
    A. Host
    B. Reservoir
    C. Vector
    D. Fomites

195. Which of the following is an effective method of reducing the viscosity of contrast media?
    A. Refrigerating prior to administration
    B. Warming prior to administration
    C. Shaking vigorously prior to administration
    D. Storing at room temperature at low humidity at all times

196. Which of the following conditions is usually indicative of a patient with emphysema?
    A. Bradycardia
    B. Orthopnea
    C. Dysphagia
    D. Epistaxis

197. To ensure proper renal function, blood urea nitrogen (BUN) levels are often checked. What is the normal BUN range?
    A. 0.6 to 1.5 mg/100 mL
    B. 2.5 to 7 mg/100 mL
    C. 8 to 23 mg/100 mL
    D. 25 to 50 mg/100 mL

198. The gauge on an IV needle indicates its
    A. Length
    B. Bevel angle
    C. Diameter
    D. Circumference

199. Which type of medical equipment is used to correct for abnormal cardiac rhythms?

A. Pulse oximeter
B. Sphygmomanometer
C. Defibrillator
D. Arrhythmia stimulator

200. Intrathecal contrast media may be administered in which of the following positions?
A. Lithotomy
B. Fowler's
C. Supine
D. Seated and bent forward

Answers and Explanations

Each rationale is followed by references to texts listed in the bibliography at the end of this chapter.

SECTION I: RADIATION PRTECTION AND RADIOBIOLOGY

1. **(C)** In most cases, the gonadal shield should be placed facing the primary beam. However, when chest radiography is performed in the PA erect position, the wall stand becomes a scattering object whereby the patient's gonads are also exposed to backscatter. Thus, some physicists recommend placing an additional shield between the patient and the wall stand. For a pregnant patient, a wraparound lead apron would afford the best protection to the fetus.
   Bontrager, "Chest," p 65.

2. **(A)** The roentgen is the most commonly used unit to express the exposure in air. The in air dose is an expression of radiation intensity, and the roentgen or milliroentgen is often used to verify that radiographic equipment is operating safely. Use of the roentgen, however, is limited to measuring only photons of less than 3 megaelectron-volts (X and gamma) and cannot be used for accurate measurements of exposure to particulate radiations such as alpha, beta, or neutrons.
   Bushong, "Radiographic Definitions and Mathematics Review," p 13; Carlton and McKenna-Adler, "Radiation Protection Concepts and Equipment," p 147; Dowd and Tilson, "Ionizing Radiation," pp 43–44; Statkiewicz-Sherer et al., "Radiation Quantities and Units," p 44.

3. **(B)** Screen speed and grid ratio would only affect patient dose if the radiographer adjusted the exposure factors of milliamperes, time, and kilovolts (peak) to compensate for a change in either screen speed or grid ratio. FSS has no effect on patient dose. If exposure factors remain the same, only changing the SID will affect the patient's dose according to the inverse-square law.

Bushong, "Radiographic Exposure," pp 252–257; Dowd and Tilson, "Appendix A," pp 320–321; Statkiewicz-Sherer et al., "Protection of the Patient during Diagnostic Radiologic Procedures," pp 161–166.

4. **(C)** Cells and tissues are usually more sensitive to radiation the more immature or highly mitotic they are. This follows the law of Bergonie and Tribondeau regarding cell sensitivity to radiation. The only exception to this law is the mature lymphocyte, which is said to be the most radiosensitive cell in the human body even though it is highly specialized and a mature end cell. The erythrocyte, osteocyte, and spermatozoa are all nondividing and mature cells that are highly specialized. The neuroblast is an embryonic cell and the only cell listed that is immature and highly mitotic, and therefore it would be the most radiosensitive.
   Bushong, "Fundamental Principles of Radiobiology," p 442; Dowd and Tilson, "Principles of Radiobiology," pp 120–121; Travis, "Tissue Radiation Biology," p 70.

5. **(A)** When used properly, a gonadal shield of 1-mm Pb equivalent placed over the female reproductive organs reduces gonadal dose by about 50 percent. When the shield is placed correctly over the male reproductive organs, the dose is reduced by 90 to 95 percent.
   Statkiewicz-Sherer et al., "Protection of the Patient during Diagnostic Radiologic Procedures," p 157.

6. **(A)** Linear energy transfer is the measurement of how much energy is deposited by a certain type of radiation as it travels through matter. In general, low LET radiation, such as x- or gamma, deposits very little energy as it travels through matter and is highly penetrating. Thus, neither are considered as potentially damaging to biologic tissue as high LET radiation, such as alpha or neutrons. X- and gamma radiation are given a quality factor of 1 when converting from rad to rem; this compares to a quality factor of 20 given to alpha radiation.
   Dowd and Tilson, "Interactions of Radiation with Matter," pp 76–78; Statkiewicz-Sherer et al., "Radiation Biology," pp 94–95; Travis, "Cell and Tissue Responses to Radiation," p 92.

7. **(A)** Death can occur from exposures to radiation following acute whole-body exposures that exceed 2 Gy (200 rad). In general, this is termed the "acute radiation syndrome" and can take three specific forms, depending on the dose. The hemopoietic syndrome occurs at the lowest doses (between 1 to 10 Gy [100 to 1000 rad]). Below 6 Gy (600 rad), it is possible for an individual to survive. Nevertheless, death from the hemopoietic syndrome is characterized by damage to the bone marrow in which all of the blood cells are

affected in some way. Signs and symptoms include nausea and vomiting in the earliest stages, followed by severe anemia, hemorrhage, dehydration causing electrolyte imbalance, and severe infection in the manifest stage. Death usually occurs in matter of weeks as a result of severe infection. Bowel obstruction is characteristic of the gastrointestinal syndrome, in which doses exceed 1000 rad.

Bushong, "Early Effects of Radiation," p 465; Dowd and Tilson, "Early Effects of Radiation," p 129; Statkiewicz-Sherer et al., "Radiation Biology," p 118.

8. **(D)** The ALARA philosophy was set up by the NCRP in the 1950s to try to minimize exposure to patients, the public, and occupational personnel working in and around the radiation industry. Maintaining occupational exposure to dose-equivalent limits is not the goal of the ALARA principle, but rather it is to encourage radiographers to always keep exposures in diagnostic radiology to as low as reasonably achievable. It should be the radiographer's goal to keep doses as low as possible, not just to maintain them at the levels limited by the NCRP.

NCRP Report No. 105, pp 15–16.

9. **(B)** The dose equivalent is measured in rems in the traditional system and sieverts in the SI system. To find the dose equivalent, you must know the absorbed dose measured in either rad or Grays and know the quality factor of the radiation that was absorbed. The formula to convert absorbed dose to dose equivalent in the traditional system is as follows: Absorbed dose (rad) × Quality factor = Dose equivalent (rems). Therefore, an absorbed dose of 50 mGy (5 rad) of radiation having a quality factor of 10 would convert to 500 mSv (50 rem).

Bushong, "Radiographic Definitions and Mathematics Review," p 13; Carlton and McKenna-Adler, "Radiation Protection Concepts and Equipment," p 147; Statkiewicz-Sherer et al., "Radiation Quantities and Units," p 45.

10. **(D)** Attenuation is the loss of x-ray photons as radiation passes through matter. The higher are the atomic number and density of the tissue, the more attenuation occurs due to the photoelectric effect. The tissue with the highest effective atomic number in the body is bone, specifically tooth enamel, because of the concentration of calcium in this type of tissue. The tissue with the least density (lowest concentration of molecules) and also a low effective atomic number would be air or gas; this type of tissue would absorb, or attenuate, the least amount of radiation when exposed to x rays.

Bushong, "Interactions of X-rays with Matter," pp 155–158; Carlton and McKenna-Adler, "The Patient as a Beam Emitter," pp 248–250; Curry et al., "Attenuation," p 79.

11. **(D)** Growth malformations have been observed in fetuses exposed to radiation in utero. Such congenital anomalies due to radiation include microcephaly, hydrocephaly, anencephaly, spina bifida, shortened limbs, and decreased growth rate. Neonatal death can also be attributed to radiation exposure in utero, usually due to the severity of the abnormality induced. Spontaneous abortion is also another effect of radiation. This effect may occur if the radiation was received during the preimplantation stage before the zygote had attached itself to the uterine wall (2 to 10 days postconception).

Bushong, "Late Effects of Radiation," pp 489–491; Dowd and Tilson, "Late Effects of Radiation," pp 121–124; Travis, "Total Body Radiation Response," p 153.

12. **(D)** The image intensifier is considered a primary protective barrier and must be lined with a minimum of 2-mm Pb equivalent to keep leakage radiation to a minimum. Another requirement is that the image intensifier must be "coupled" with the fluoroscopic x-ray tube so that the x-ray beam will not be energized if the image intensifier is pushed back into the "parked" position.

Bushong, "Designing for Radiation Protection," p 511.

13. **(C)** A dead-man switch is one that maintains current flow, or a closed circuit, only with the application of continuous pressure. Dead-man switches are most often used in radiography during fluoroscopic procedures because exposures would be excessive to both patients and radiographers if the current were allowed to flow freely with the simple flip of a switch. With the dead-man type, if the operator becomes "incapacitated," the exposure will terminate. Relay switches are electromagnetic devices that are most commonly used in radiographic equipment for the purpose of centering the x-ray tube to the Bucky or wall stand. Circuit breakers are a type of relay switch and are "tripped" when the current in a circuit exceeds the capacity of the circuit. Circuit breakers protect the circuit from overloads that may lead to electrical fires. A microswitch is used in an automatic processor to control the replenishment rate of chemicals. The microswitch is activated every time a film is run through the feed tray on the processor.

Bushong, "Designing for Radiation Protection," pp 511–512; Statkiewicz-Sherer et al., "Protection of the Patient during Diagnostic Radiologic Procedures," p 168.

14. **(D)** Materials with the highest atomic numbers offer the best protection from electromagnetic ionizing radiation such as X- or gamma rays. This is because materials with a high atomic number are more likely to absorb the radiation through the photoelectric effect. Of all these materials, lead has the highest atomic number ($Z = 82$). In fact, lead has the highest atomic number of all other elements without itself being radioactive. All elements above the atomic number of 82 are naturally radioactive and therefore would not be appropriate for radiation protection purposes. Although wood, concrete, and other building materials with low atomic numbers may also be substituted for protective shielding, their thickness *must* be comparable to the lead equivalent. For instance, 4 inches of masonry is equivalent to $\frac{1}{16}$ inch of lead.

Bushong, "X-ray Interaction with Matter," p 154, and "Designing for Radiation Protection," p 512; Dowd and Tilson, "Protecting the Radiographer and Other Workers," p 202; Hendee, "Protective Barriers for Radiation Sources," p 451; Selman, "Protection in Radiology: Health Physics," p 538.

15. **(C)** Gamma rays are just like x rays in that both are electromagnetic ionizing radiation. The only difference is their origin. X rays are produced by the sudden deceleration of electrons, whereas gamma rays are emitted from the nucleus of a radioactive atom. All electromagnetic radiation has no mass and no charge; it is simply a form of energy. Because x rays and gamma rays have relatively high energy and no mass or charge, they are highly penetrating and therefore deposit very little energy as they pass through matter. They are much more likely to pass right through tissue rather than to interact at all. This property is called "low LET." In contrast, radiation with significant mass and/or charge, such as alpha particles, is not very penetrating and therefore is more likely to deposit all of its energy at once, referred to as "high LET."

Bushong, "Electromagnetic Radiation," p 50, and "Fundamental Principles of Radiobiology," p 442; Dowd and Tilson, "Ionizing Radiation," p 43; Travis, "Basic Biologic Interactions of Radiation," p 31.

16. **(C)** An isotope is an atom with the same number of protons but with differing numbers of neutrons. Sometimes, this imbalance of protons versus neutrons in the same element can cause an element to become radioactive. All barium atoms have 56 protons in their nucleus; the subscript 56 determines the element's atomic number (Z). However, the atomic weight or mass (designated by the superscript) is determined by the number of protons plus neutrons and may vary depending on the numbers of neutrons in each nucleus. Find the number of neutrons by subtracting the atomic number (subscript) from the mass number (superscript). For this atom: $132 - 56 = 76$. There are 76 neutrons in the nucleus of this isotope of barium.

Bushong, "The Atom," pp 32–34; Selman, "The Structure of Matter," pp 43–45.

17. **(B)** A film badge monitor is one of three types of personnel monitors that may be used to estimate the radiation dose received by an occupational worker. Personnel monitors are *not* designed to protect the individual, but rather to ensure that the radiographer is practicing proper radiation protection. The filters inside of a film badge, usually made of aluminum or copper, are used for the purpose of estimating the various energy levels to which an individual may be exposed. For instance, it usually can estimate with some degree of accuracy whether the exposure came from the primary beam or whether the badge received secondary, or scatter, radiation. Finally, the filters do not support the film; the film badge holder, made of a lightweight, radiolucent material, is used for this purpose.

Bushong, "Radiation Protection Procedures," pp 532–533; Dowd and Tilson, "Ionizing Radiation," pp 50–52; Statkiewicz-Sherer et al., "Radiation Monitoring," p 218.

18. **(A)** In the United States, the majority (82 percent) of our exposure to ionizing radiation comes from natural background radiation such as radon gas found in building materials, cosmic radiation from extraterrestrial sources, terrestrial radiation, and internal sources of radioisotopes such as carbon-14. Only 18 percent of the total annual dose to the U.S. population comes from man-made sources such as nuclear power and consumer products. However, of this man-made radiation, 12 percent of the 18 percent, or about two-thirds, can be attributed to medical and dental x rays. Therefore, it is very important for all diagnostic radiographers to try to limit exposures to themselves, their patients, and the public to keep doses as low as reasonably achievable.

Bushong, "Basic Concepts of Radiation Science," p 6; Statkiewicz-Sherer et al., "Introduction to Radiation Protection," p 6; Travis, "Diagnostic Radiology and Nuclear Medicine," p 187.

19. **(B)** When considering the design of a radiographic room, there are several factors that must be considered. First, there is the *workload factor*, which takes into account the amount of radiation that is used per unit time, usually designated by either the unit milliamperage-seconds per week

or milliamperage-minutes per week. Second, there is the *distance factor*, which is based on the premise of the inverse-square law; because intensity decreases inversely to the square of the distance from a particular source, the farther the source is from the wall, the less lead is required in the wall. Third, there is the *use factor*, which is based on how often the primary beam faces a certain wall (i.e., the wall with a chest stand would have a higher designated use factor than a wall that never has the primary beam facing it). The final factor to consider is the *occupancy factor*. The occupancy factor takes into consideration how often the rooms adjacent to the x-ray walls will be occupied per unit time. That is, an office adjacent to an x-ray room will receive an occupancy factor of 1, whereas a hall or stairwell adjacent to the x-ray room will receive a fraction of that, usually a factor of ⅛ or 1/16.

Bushong, "Designing for Radiation Protection," pp 514–515; Statkiewicz-Sherer et al., "Protecting Occupationally Exposed Personnel during Diagnostic Radiologic Procedures," pp 202–204.

20. **(B)** There are several interactions that can occur when x rays travel through matter. The two most common in the diagnostic range are the photoelectric effect and the Compton scattering. The photoelectric interaction is desirable in a diagnostic x ray because it is the basis for the formation of the image and contributes to the contrast seen on the radiograph. Compton scattering, on the other hand, is not desirable and causes degradation of the radiographic image. Compton scattering is more prevalent with low atomic number of tissues (e.g., fat or muscle) and at higher radiographic energy levels (usually greater than 70 keV). Two effective ways of reducing the production of Compton scattering is to lower the kilovolt (peak) setting and to restrict the beam size, or collimate. Reducing the FSS will greatly increase the resolution of the image but will have no effect on the production of Compton scattering.

Bushong, "Scatter Radiation and Beam-Restricting Devices," pp 208–209; Carlton and McKenna-Adler, "Contrast," pp 395–398.

21. **(A)** According to the inverse-square law, as the distance increases, the intensity decreases to the square of the distance. Thus, if the distance is doubled, the intensity is reduced to one-fourth the original value. Consequently, if the distance is tripled, the intensity is reduced to one-ninth the original value. The equation is set up as follows:

$$\frac{I_1}{I_2} = \frac{(D_2)^2}{(D_1)^2};$$

$$\frac{27}{x} = \frac{9^2}{3^2};$$

$$\frac{27}{x} = \frac{81}{9};$$

$$\frac{27}{9} = x; \ x = 3 \ R/min$$

Bushong, "Electromagnetic Radiation," pp 47–48; Gurley and Callaway, "Radiation Safety and Protective Measures," pp 239–240; Statkiewicz-Sherer et al., "Protecting Occupationally Exposed Personnel during Diagnostic Radiologic Procedures," p 199.

22. **(C)** The greatest exposure to diagnostic radiographers occurs during fluoroscopic and mobile radiography. Fluoroscopic procedures include (1) dynamic procedures of the gastrointestinal (GI) tract, usually performed in the routine diagnostic imaging department, (2) dynamic procedures performed in surgery through the use of a C-arm device, and (3) dynamic procedures of the cardiovascular system, usually performed in the special procedures or cardiac catheterization suite. In comparison, routine spot films of the skull, extremities, and chest contribute very little to occupational exposure.

Bushong, "Radiation Protection Procedures," p 524; Statkiewicz-Sherer et al., "Protecting Occupationally Exposed Personnel during Diagnostic Radiologic Procedures," p 196.

23. **(D)** Increasing technical factors of both kilovolts (peak) and milliamperage-seconds will increase the intensity of the x-ray beam and thus increase exposure to the patient. However, milliamperage-seconds has a direct effect on exposure, and if milliamperage-seconds is doubled, the patient dose is doubled. In comparison, kilovolts (peak) has an exponential effect on exposure; a small increase in kilovolts (peak) has a large effect on intensity. At the same time, as kilovolts (peak) increases, the average energy of the beam increases, which means that the beam is more penetrating and thus much less likely to interact with the patient's tissue. Therefore, if it will not compromise the quality of the image, it is best to use high-kilovolt (peak), low–milliamperage-second exposure factors to minimize patient dose.

Dowd and Tilson, "Protecting the Patient in Radiography," pp 219–221; Statkiewicz-Sherer et al., "Protection of the Patient during Diagnostic Radiologic Procedures," pp 161–163.

24. **(C)** Leukemia is a malignant disease affecting the circulating blood. There are many variations of leukemia, but the one most commonly linked to radiation-induced malignancy is lymphocytic leukemia. The blood cells are formed in the red

bone marrow of the hemopoietic system. Of all of the systems in the human body, the hemopoietic system is considered the most sensitive because it can easily be damaged by radiation, even at fairly low doses. For instance, at a threshold of just 25 rad, the white blood cell count may begin to drop. Several irradiated populations have been studied, but the one that points to the bone marrow as the most obvious culprit of radiation-induced leukemia is persons who received radiation treatments for ankylosing spondylitis in the 1940s. The treatment areas focused mainly on the spines of these individuals, the tissue of which has a large concentration of active red bone marrow. Although the white blood cells, especially the lymphocytes, are very easily damaged by radiation, the stem cells, or precursor cells, in the red bone marrow are suspected of giving rise to cancer or lymphocytic leukemia because these eventually give rise to the mature lymphocytes. Because the life span of the white blood cells is so short (just a matter of hours to days), this would not be sufficient time for a malignancy to grow and affect the entire system as a precursor cell might.

Bushong, "Late Effects of Radiation," pp 483–485; Dowd and Tilson, "Late Effects of Radiation," p 144; Travis, "Late Effects of Radiation," pp 169–171.

25. **(C)** Effects of ionizing radiation to the DNA molecule inside the cell can be devastating. If a DNA molecule is struck by ionizing radiation, there are basically four things that can occur:
    1. **Base damage:** One or more of the organic bases sustains a hit. This is also called a "gene" mutation, or point mutation, because it affects only one specific area or gene. Although base damage can be life-threatening to the cell, it is not a gross abnormality in that the DNA molecule maintains its shape and appears normal.   2. **Single-strand break (SSB):** Only one side of the chain sustains a hit. SSBs are very easily repaired and usually do not result in any permanent damage.   3. **Double-strand break (DSB):** A break in both sides of the chain in the same rung may result in gross abnormalities, such as cleavage, deletion of information through breaks in the entire chain, or reattachment to another portion of the chain, also known as: 4. **Crosslinks:** The broken chain may reattach to an entirely different chromosome or to another type of structure altogether, such as a DNA-protein crosslink. Two SSBs occurring on two different areas of the chain are still considered to be very easily repaired by the DNA molecule. Examples of these were given in choices A, B, and D. Only choice C was an example of a DSB.

Bushong, "Molecular and Cellular Radiobiology," p 452; Dowd and Tilson, "Principles of Radiobiology," pp 114–117; Statkiewicz-Sherer et al., "Radiation Biology," pp 100–106.

26. **(D)** Proper radiation protection procedures should be practiced at all times for all patients. Not only do these practices protect the patient, but they also serve to protect the radiographer. A rule of thumb is that reduction of the patient dose by a factor of 2 also reduces the occupational worker's exposure by a factor of 2. Therefore, the use of a high-speed imaging system would require a lower–milliamperae-seconds setting and would therefore reduce dose to the patient and to the radiographer as well. Using proper beam restriction is not only beneficial to the patient, but is especially beneficial to the radiographer because the scatter radiation is reduced. The use of proper processing techniques through a system of sensitometric monitoring will ensure that radiographs will not have to be repeated because of poor quality, thus reducing the dose to both patient and radiographer.

Dowd and Tilson, "Radiographer and Other Workers," pp 189–199.

27. **(B)** Biologic damage will increase in tissues when those tissues have a higher oxygen content, when the tissues have been exposed to a higher LET radiation (radiations that deposit more energy as they penetrate matter), and when the intensity or amount of radiation increases. More energy will be deposited in tissues with a higher LET radiation. However, when using x-radiation, which is considered to be relatively low-LET radiation, absorption will increase in tissue with lower-energy ranges (low-kilovolt [peak] techniques) due to the increase in the photoelectric effect. This is why high-kilovolt (peak), low–milliamperage-seconds exposure factors are suggested as a form of radiation protection, but only when the image quality will not be adversely affected. For instance, it would not be wise to use 90 kilovolts (peak) when performing a urographic examination because the x rays may penetrate and "miss" being absorbed by a small kidney stone or be attenuated by iodinated contrast media in the ureters.

Dowd and Tilson, "Protecting the Patient in Radiography," pp 219–221; Statkiewicz-Sherer et al., "Protection of the Patient during Diagnostic Radiologic Procedures," pp 161–163.

28. **(A)** The radiographer should *never* be exposed to the primary beam. If it becomes necessary to restrain a patient during a procedure, such as when performing a fluoroscopic procedure on an infant, proper restraining devices should be used

first. If restraining devices are not appropriate for the examination and the radiographer is required to hold the patient, then proper shielding devices, such as lead gloves with a minimum lead thickness (0.5-mm Pb equivalent), should be worn.

Dowd and Tilson, "Radiation Safety/Protection and Health Physics," p 188. NCRP Report No. 102, p 18; Statkiewicz-Sherer et al., "Protecting Occupationally Exposed Personnel during Diagnostic Radiologic Procedures," pp 200–201.

29. **(D)** Genetic defects may occur as a result of radiation to the gonads; specifically, damage sustained by the ova or mature sperm of the irradiated individual is then passed along to future generations. To date, there are no studies on humans that give concrete evidence that such a risk exists. All of the current data on genetic effects of radiation have been performed on animals: mice, rats, and fruit flies. Acute radiation syndrome is a type of short-term somatic effect that occurs within a matter of hours to days following a total body dose of a large amount of radiation. Long-term somatic effects are those that affect the irradiated individual and usually do not occur for several years following exposure to ionizing radiation. Cataractogenesis, if induced by an acute high dose of radiation, will usually take several months to occur, but because it is also a cumulative effect, it may take several years following low-dose, long-term exposure such as that received from radiation in the diagnostic range. Most radiation-induced cancers, such as leukemia, have a latent period of 10 to 20 years or more.

Bushong, "Late Effects of Radiation," pp 478–493; Dowd and Tilson, "Late Effects of Radiation," pp 144–156; Travis, "Late Effects of Radiation," pp 164–181.

30. **(C)** The single most important scattering object in diagnostic radiology is the patient. Thus, as a matter of protection for the radiographer, it is recommended that the radiographer stand at a 90° angle to the patient, because at this angle, the scatter coming off the patient is at its lowest intensity. In fact, the radiation intensity at 1 m from the patient at a right angle to the beam is approximately 0.1 percent, or 1/1000, of the skin dose received by the patient.

Bushong, "Designing for Radiation Protection," p 513; NCRP Report No. 105, p 28.

SECTION II: EQUIPMENT OPERATION AND MAINTENANCE

31. **(C)** There are two types of devices in the x-ray circuit that may be used to select the desired milliampere setting; they are either the choke coil or the rheostat, which serve to vary the resistance in the circuit. The rectifier is used to change the alternating current into pulsating direct current and can be found between the secondary side of the step-up transformer and the x-ray tube. The autotransformer operates on the principle of self-induction and is used to select the desired kilovolt (peak) setting in most modern x-ray circuits.

Bushong, "The X-Ray Unit," pp 94–96; Carlton and McKenna-Adler, "Electromagnetism," p 76; Thompson et al., "X-Ray Machine Operation: The X-Ray Circuit," p 172.

32. **(A)** For every x-ray photon that strikes the input screen of an image intensifier, there is a corresponding light photon that is given off as a result. Consequently, for every light photon that strikes the photocathode, there is one electron that is given off as a result. This is not the case at the output phosphor, where the light intensity is greatly increased as a result of the flux gain. The flux gain is essentially a measure of the efficiency of the output phosphor to emit light in response to being stimulated by an electron. For example, if one electron strikes the phosphor and 50 light photons are produced, the phosphor has a flux gain of 50. Flux gain is not the only factor affecting the brightness of the image at the output phosphor. There is also another factor called minification gain, which takes into account the square of the ratio of the size of the input phosphor (usually about 6 or 9 inches in diameter) over the size of the output phosphor (usually about 1 inch). Because the output phosphor is much smaller than the input phosphor, there is also an increased brightness that results at the output side. The total brightness gain can be calculated as follows: Brightness gain = Minification gain × Flux gain

Bushong, "Fluoroscopy," p 325; Carlton and McKenna-Adler, "Fluoroscopy," p 539; Thompson et al.,"Fluoroscopy: Viewing Motion with X-ray," p 366.

33. **(B)** Without a potential difference between one side of the circuit and the other, the electrons will not flow through the circuit. The potential difference is usually dependent on how strong the positive charge is at one end of the circuit as compared with the negative charge at the other end. The greater the difference is, the faster the electrons will be pulled from one side to the other. The property of potential difference is also known as "electromotive force," and its unit of measurement is the volt. A circuit with high voltage has a high potential difference. The current, measured in amperes, is simply a measure of how many electrons are flowing in a wire per unit time. A

high current has a negative impact on resistance. Resistance is inherent in any conductor, with the exception of a superconductor, because the movement of electrons will tend to build up heat resisting the flow of electrons. Without a potential difference, however, current will not flow.

Bushong, "Electricity," p 61; Carlton and McKenna-Adler, "Electricity," p 47; Thompson et al., "Electricity," p 92.

34. **(B)** When using an AEC device, it is not necessary to set the exact milliamperes and exposure time because there is a radiation sensor present in the Bucky or wall mount. For the radiation sensor to function properly, it must shut off after the correct amount of radiation has been received by the image receptor. Some sensors (ion chambers) are located in front of the image receptor (cassette). However, other types of sensors (photomultiplier tubes) are located behind the cassette. In this case, the back of the cassette should be constructed of a radiolucent material to ensure that the sensor is detecting the correct amount of radiation so that neither the patient nor the image receptor receives unnecessary radiation.

Carlton and McKenna-Adler, "Intensifying Screens," p 337; Selman, "X-Ray Film, Film Holders, and Intensifying Screens," p 275.

35. **(D)** A wire-mesh test is a quality control (QC) device used to detect film-screen contact. This test should be performed routinely once a year and also when the quality of images is compromised by using certain cassettes. Poor film-screen contact will result in a localized area of poor resolution. Quantum mottle also results in poor resolution, but it is caused by insufficient milliamperage-seconds when high-speed or rare earth screens are used. Phosphorescence, or afterglow, also can affect resolution but cannot be measured accurately with a wire-mesh test. Modulation transfer function is a measure of the resolution of an imaging system, but it usually requires more specialized equipment, such as a resolution bar pattern.

Carroll, "Quality Control," p 404; Cullinan, "Basic Components of an X-Ray Generating System," p 23; Papp, "Radiographic Ancillary Equipment," pp 106–107.

36. **(C)** If a current is rectified, it only allows electrons to flow in one direction, and that is toward the positive side. If a current is half-wave rectified, the negative half of the cycle is suppressed, resulting in 60 positive pulses per second. If a current is full-wave rectified, it takes advantage of both sides of the cycle by changing the negative wave into a second positive wave per cycle, resulting in 120 positive pulses per second.

Bushong, "The X-Ray Unit," pp 101–102; Selman, "Rectification," pp 143–148; Thompson et al., "X-Ray Machine Operation: The X-Ray Circuit," pp 179–180.

37. **(A)** Ion chambers operate on the principle of x rays causing ionization (free electrons) as they come in contact with matter. These free electrons cause a charge in air that can then be measured by a positive electrode. The most common type of gas that is used in an ion chamber is free air consisting of 80 percent nitrogen and 20 percent oxygen, because these atoms tend to be easily ionized by x-radiation.

Bushong, "Designing for Radiation Protection," p 516; Thompson et al., "X-Ray Machine Operation: The X-Ray Circuit," pp 184–185; Wolbarst, "The X-Ray Beam," p 95.

38. **(B)** Static images may be obtained directly from the light image generated by the output phosphor of the image intensifier by coupling the output side with a photospot camera. There are several types of photospot cameras available, including the 70-mm and 105-mm, and the 16-and 35-mm cine photospot models. Photospot cameras have less resolution than conventional cassette-loaded spot films, because with conventional filming, the image is obtained directly from the remnant, or exit, x-ray beam. VCRs are coupled with the CRT, or television screen, and not with the output phosphor. VCR images suffer a substantial loss of resolution, but they do offer the advantage of recording dynamic images.

Bushong, "Fluoroscopy," pp 330–331; Curry et al., "Viewing and Recording the Fluoroscopic Image," pp 186–195.

39. **(D)** The step-down transformer is used in the filament circuit to "step down," or decrease, the voltage and to increase the amperage. This is needed to supply a sufficient amount of current to heat the filament during the preparation or boost stage of x-ray production. The "step-up" transformer is found in the secondary portion of the x-ray circuit, and the autotransformer is found in the primary portion of the x-ray circuit.

Curry et al., "X-Ray Generators," p 40; Hendee, "The Filament Circuit," pp 84–85; Thompson et al., "X-Ray Machine Operation: The X-Ray Circuit," pp 187–189; Tortorici, "Production of X-Rays," p 71, 1992.

40. **(A)** There are several types of number systems that are available to categorize numerical information. Among the most common is the decimal system, which uses numbers from 0 to 9. There is also the duodecimal system, which uses numbers through 12 based on the months of the year and the hours in a day. Computers operate on the simplest of all numbering systems, the binary sys-

tem, which consists of two digits—0 and 1. In this system, a single digit, 0 or 1, is called a *bit.* Bits can then be bunched into groups of eight called *bytes.* One kilobyte is equal to 1,024 bytes, and 1 megabyte is equal to 1, 048,576 bytes in the binary system.

Bushong, "Computer Science," pp 349, 350; Carlton and McKenna-Adler, "Digital Image Processing," p 620; Curry et al., "Digital Radiography," p 399; Wolbarst, "Digital Representation of an Image, and a Bit about Computers," pp 299–301.

41. **(A)** Only two types of interactions exist between electrons and the target atoms of tungsten during the production of x rays: (1) bremsstrahlung and (2) characteristic. Photoelectric and Compton interactions occur when x-ray photons interact with various atoms either in air or inside structures. *Bremsstrahlung radiation* is produced most often (about 90 percent of the time) at the tungsten target. It is created when a fast-moving electron is slowed and then changes direction when coming near the nucleus of a tungsten atom, as shown in Figure 4–1. *Characteristic radiation* is produced when an incoming electron interacts with the inner (K-shell) electron, removing it from its shell and thus causing ionization of the target atom. It is called "characteristic radiation" because the radiation that is produced from this process is characteristic of the type of element with which the electrons interacted. In other words, characteristic radiation is produced only at very specific energy ranges, about 69.5 keV, when an outer-shell electron drops down to fill the void in the K shell.

Bushong, "X-Ray Production," pp 128–130; Cullinan, "Production of X-Radiation," pp 6–8; Curry et al., "Production of X-Rays," p 30; Selman, "X-Rays (Roentgen Rays)," pp 156–158.

42. **(C)** The brightness of a fluoroscopic image is mainly dependent on anatomic thickness, kilovolts (peak), and milliamperage. The ABC in an image intensifier serves to maintain the correct level of brightness on the television monitor as the x-ray tube scans across various body structures. Thus, as patient thickness and tissue density vary, the technical factors of milliamperage and kilovolts (peak) will automatically be adjusted to maintain brightness at all times. The main disadvantage of the ABC system is that as tissue density increases, the patient dose will also be substantially increased.

Bushong, "Fluoroscopy," pp 326–327; Carlton and McKenna-Adler, "Fluoroscopy," p 540; Curry et al., "Viewing and Recording the Fluoroscopic Image," pp 185–186.

43. **(A)** The main purpose for rotating the anode disk during the production of x rays is to spread the heat over a larger area of the anode surface. In a stationary anode, only high-speed electrons strike a very small portion of the anode's surface. In comparison, a rotating anode disperses the electrons over a much wider area, based on the formula of circumference: $C = 2\pi r$. Therefore, it stands to reason that an anode disc with a larger diameter would also produce a larger circumference, resulting in greater heat dissipation. The area struck by the electron stream is not dependent on the size of the anode. It is dependent on the size of the filament, and thus the FSS and consequently the image resolution would be unaffected by the diameter size. The speed of the rotor is also not greatly affected by the diameter of the anode, although most anodes have diameters ranging from 7.5 to 12.5 cm (3 to 5 in.).

Curry et al., "Production of X-Rays," pp 14–15; Selman, "X-Ray Tubes & Rectifiers," p 211; Tortorici, "Production of X-Rays," pp 74–75, 1992; Wolbarst, "X-Ray Tubes," p 88.

44. **(D)** The power rating of an electric circuit is derived from the product of the voltage and amperage, and the unit of power is expressed in watts or kilowatts as follows:

P = IV; P = 0.5 A × 110,000 V = 55,000 W or 55 kW

Bushong, "Electricity," p 66; Carlton and McKenna-Adler, "Electricity," p 50.

45. **(B)** The mR/mAs formula is a common formula used to calibrate modern radiographic equipment. It is essential that the intensity of the x-ray beam stay within a certain limit even when a variety of technical factors are used. The intensity is usually read by a survey instrument, usually an ion chamber or cutie pie, which calculates the mR/mAs for a variety of milliampere and time settings, ensuring that the milliamperage-seconds does not vary by more than 10 percent for the same equivalent milliamperage-seconds. To find mR/mAs in this example, first calculate the milliamperage-seconds by multiplying milliamperes × Time:

500 × 0.045 second = 22.5 mAs

Next divide the milliroentgen reading by the milliamperage-seconds given:

$$\frac{340}{22.5} = 15.1 \text{ mR/mAs}$$

Carlton and McKenna Adler, "Minimizing Patient Dose," p 206.

46. **(D)** Automatic exposure control (AEC) devices are designed to be sensitive to radiation exiting

the patient, thus terminating the exposure when it perceives an optimal image has been obtained. AECs can therefore accurately adjust for changes in the following: (1) SID, (2) kilovolts (peak), and (3) tissue density, because for all three factors, the intensity of the exit beam would also vary. However, an AEC device must be calibrated for factors such as grid ratio and screen speed because the AEC cannot tell the difference between a slow-speed screen and a fast-speed screen.

Carroll, "Automatic Exposure Controls," p 352; Curry et al., "Luminescent Screens," p 131.

47. **(D)** Transformers serve to vary voltage and current, based on the principles of electromagnetic induction. This is achieved by increasing or decreasing the number of turns, or coil windings, on the secondary side of the transformer in relation to the primary side. The ratio between the number of turns and voltage is directly proportional and is known as the "turns ratio," stated in the formula: $V_s/V_p = N_s/N_p$, where V = voltage; N = number of turns (windings); s = secondary coil; and p = primary coil.

$$\frac{x}{220} = \frac{1000}{20}; x = 220 \times 50; x = 11,000 \text{ V or } 11 \text{ kV}$$

Bushong, "Electromagnetism," p 83; Carlton and McKenna-Adler, "Electromagnetism," p 74; Curry et al., "X-Ray Generators," p 38; Selman, "Production and Control of High Voltage," p 125.

48. **(A)** Most modern x-ray circuits use solid-state conductors such as n-type and p-type diodes that only allow current to flow in one direction. Solid-state conductors are generally composed of silicon or germanium. The original rectification system consisted of an elaborate connection of valve tubes that looked similar to x-ray tubes with cathode and anode ends, which were very bulky and inefficient. Rheostats and choke coils are used to vary the resistance in a circuit and are used in the filament portion of the x-ray circuit to select the milliampere setting.

Bushong, "Electromagnetism," pp 85, 100; Carlton and McKenna-Adler, "Electromagnetism," pp 77–79; Thompson et al., "X-Ray Machine Operation: The X-Ray Circuit," pp 176–177; Tortorici, "Rectification," pp 42–47, 1992.

49. **(B)** The smallest part of an element that still retains the characteristics of that element is called an *atom*. Atoms consist of neutrons and protons in the nucleus and electrons orbiting in shells around the nucleus. The smallest part of a compound that still retains the characteristics of that compound is called a *molecule*. A molecule is simply a combination of many atoms; an example would be the common water molecule (H_2O).

Carlton and McKenna-Adler, "Radiation Concepts," p 23; Selman, "The Structure of Matter," p 40.

50. **(D)** Nuclear energy gets its power from two different sources inside the nucleus: (1) the electrostatic force, which is generated by the positive charge of the protons in the nucleus, and (2) the binding force, which is generated by the neutrons. Neutrons act as the "glue" to keep the protons' natural repulsion (electrostatic force) from disrupting the balance inside the nucleus. When there is an excess or deficiency of neutrons inside the nucleus, the atom becomes unstable, or "radioactive," and must emit radiation in the form of gamma rays and other particles in order to stabilize. The electron-binding energy is exerted by the negative charge of the electron being attracted to the positive charge in the nucleus. The closer the electron to the nucleus (i.e., the K-shell electron) and the higher the atomic number of the atom is, the more "tightly" bound it is in its orbit.

Bushong, "X-Ray Interaction with Matter," p 153; Carlton and McKenna-Adler, "Radiation Concepts," p 26; Selman, "X-Rays (Roentgen Rays)," p 178.

51. **(A)** Lead aprons should be checked semiannually for cracks or tears in the lead lining with a fluoroscopic machine, more often if there is suspected damage. Lead aprons should also be properly cared for by hanging them on designated storage racks. They should never be folded; folding a lead apron may cause a rip or tear in the lead.

Papp, "Quality Control of Radiographic Equipment," p 71; Thompson et al., "Radiological Health Physics," p 466.

52. **(D)** The most common cause of tube failure is filament burnout. With this fact in mind, there are many practices that a radiographer can use to extend the life of the x-ray tube. Some of the suggested practices include (1) using proper warm-up procedures prior to beginning a busy day, (2) using high-kilovolt (peak) and low–milliampere-seconds techniques because the milliampere-seconds has the greatest effect on the life of the filament, and (3) avoiding lengthy preparation or boost times, which can lead to overheating of the filament.

Bushong, "The X-Ray Tube," pp 120–121; Carlton and McKenna-Adler, "The X-Ray Tube," pp 112–114, 128–129; Selman, "X-Ray Tubes and Rectifiers," pp 222–223.

53. **(A)** The generator, sometimes referred to as the "dynamo," is a device that converts mechanical energy into electrical energy. The generator forms the basis for most electrical power plants. Whether the mechanical energy comes in the

form of falling water (waterfall), pressurized steam (nuclear power producing heat), or from the motion of a windmill, the mechanical motion of a rotating magnet induces a current in a coil of wire. This electrical energy can then be stored for future use to homes throughout a specific region. A battery converts chemical energy to electrical energy. A motor converts electrical energy into mechanical energy. An example is the induction motor of the X ray used to rotate the anode.

Bushong, "Electromagnetism," p 81; Selman, "Electric Generators and Motors," p 115; Thompson et al., "Magnetism and Its Relation to Electricity," p 124.

54. **(B)** If it is necessary to record images off of the image intensifier with either a cine or photospot camera, a device called a "beam splitter" is essential to divide the light stream into two different paths. The beam splitter is a semitransparent mirror in which some of the light is reflected up for recording and some is allowed to pass through for viewing on the television monitor (CRT).

Bushong, "Fluoroscopy," p 328; Carlton and McKenna-Adler, "Fluoroscopy," pp 542–543; Carroll, "Fluoroscopic Imaging," p 426.

55. **(C)** *Off-focus radiation* is any radiation that has been produced outside the target, or focal spot. This radiation is also emitted through the port window but appears outside of the collimated area; thus it is often mistaken for scatter radiation. *Scatter radiation* is produced when radiation strikes an object, typically the patient, and is scattered off in another direction from the primary beam. *Remnant*, or *exit, radiation* is any radiation that has not been absorbed by the patient and exits to expose the film; it is also referred to as the "exit beam." *Leakage radiation* is any radiation that is emitted through the x-ray tube other than through the port window. This radiation should be limited to 100 mR/h at a distance of 1 m from the tube.

Bushong, "The X-Ray Tube," p 108; Carlton and McKenna-Adler, "The X-Ray Tube," p 124; Curry et al., "Protection," p 385.

56. **(D)** In a modern x-ray tube, there are two electrodes: (1) the positive anode that serves as the target and (2) the negative cathode that serves as the source of electrons at the filament. Both the filament and the anode target are composed of tungsten for several reasons, including its high atomic number and its high melting point. At the cathode end, there is also a focusing cup that surrounds the filament and also contains a negative charge. The focusing cup serves to focus the electrons into a stream so that they will be narrowly aimed at the target, thus increasing resolution.

The material for the focusing cup is most often made up of nickel, but it may also consist of molybdenum.

Carlton and McKenna-Adler, "The X-Ray Tube," p 114; Curry et al., "Production of X-Rays," p 12; Thompson et al., "X-Ray Tube Components and Design," p 139; Wolbarst, "X-Ray Tubes," p 85.

57. **(C)** The brightness gain in a modern image intensifier is found by finding the product of the flux gain and the minification gain. The brightness in the output phosphor is increased from the input phosphor because of an increased emission of light in response to electron stimulation (flux gain) and because of the squared ratio of the size of the input phosphor to the size of the output phosphor, known as minification gain.

Bushong, "Fluoroscopy," p 325; Carlton and McKenna-Adler, "Fluoroscopy," p 539; Thompson et al., "Fluoroscopy: Viewing Motion with X-Ray," p 366.

58. **(D)** The waveform produced during the x-ray exposure in a battery-powered mobile unit most closely resembles that of a high-frequency generator. Because batteries operate on DC power and the high-voltage transformer necessary to produce x rays can operate only on AC power, it is necessary to incorporate a device in the battery-powered x-ray unit that causes a change in the direction of the current. This is accomplished with a "DC chopper." The current is then reverted back to pulsating DC through the use of rectifiers similar to those in an AC–powered x-ray unit; only the current has much higher frequency (1000 to 2000 Hz) when compared with the typical 60-Hz frequency seen in a fixed AC–powered generator. A high-frequency x-ray generator is supplied by 60 Hz AC power. However, the generator also contains a DC chopper that serves to greatly increase the frequency. Both of these generators are highly efficient, achieving a voltage ripple of less than 1 percent.

Carlton and McKenna-Adler, "X-Ray Equipment," p 103; Thompson et al., "X-Ray Machine Operation: The X-Ray Circuit," pp 190–193; Wolbarst, "The Nuts and Bolts of Generators," p 82.

59. **(B)** The emulsion in radiographic film is known as the "active" layer. It is composed of photosensitive silver halide crystals that form the basis of the image suspended in gelatin. Polyester forms the base of the radiographic film and serves as a support to hold the emulsion in place.

Bushong, "Radiographic Film," pp 166–167; Carlton and McKenna-Adler, "Radiographic Film," p 282; Thompson et al., "Radiographic Film," pp 238–239.

60. **(C)** When performing tube warm-up procedures, it is important to follow the guidelines suggested

by the manufacturer. If a large exposure is applied to a cold anode, the anode may crack. Most radiographic equipment manufacturers suggest a tube warm-up procedure that consists of very low milliamperes (no higher than 200), with a 1- to 2-second time setting and a medium setting of kilovolts (peak) (70 to 80 kVp). Although using a high-milliampere setting would be the most damaging to a cold anode, the use of a high-kilovolt (peak) setting is also not recommended. Of these four choices, C would be the best combination for a proper warm-up procedure.

Bushong, "The X-Ray Tube," p 120; Carlton and McKenna-Adler, "The X-Ray Tube," pp 128–129; Selman, "X-Ray Tubes and Rectifiers," p 223.

SECTION III: IMAGE PRODUCTION AND EVALUATION

61. **(B)** Careful collimation is extremely important when using an AEC device. If the radiographer overcollimates (collimates too tightly), the sensor may act as if the tissue of interest is very dense, thus prolonging the exposure time and overexposing the image. The opposite is also true. If the radiographer does not satisfactorily collimate, the scatter created may be excessive, causing the sensor to prematurely cut off, resulting in an underexposed image.

Carlton and McKenna-Adler, "Automatic Exposure Controls," pp 508–509; Carroll, "Automatic Exposure Controls," p 362.

62. **(A)** Processors must be carefully cleaned and monitored daily to avoid degradation of the image due to dirty rollers, misaligned parts, or inadequate chemistry. Crescent marks are caused from rough handling of the film in the darkroom, not from any mechanical error in the processor, and can appear anywhere on the image. Both wet-pressure sensitization and guide-shoe marks are lines that run across the film in the same direction that the film travels as it is fed through the processor. Pi lines are caused from dirty processor rollers and run opposite or perpendicular to the direction that the film travels as it is fed through the processor.

Bushong, "Film Artifacts," p 422; Papp, "Additional Quality Management Procedures," p 159.

63. **(C)** To differentiate between different screen speeds, most manufacturers use a numbering system, rather than depend on ambiguous terms such as "par" speed, "detail" speed, or "fast" speed. These numbers are based on relative speed (RS) of the screen and are designated as follows: RS = 100, RS = 200, RS = 400, RS = 800, and so

forth. Knowing these numbers for relative speed, the radiographer can then make proper adjustments in technical factors accordingly through the use of the milliamperage-second-screen formula:

$$\frac{\text{Original mAs}}{\text{New mAs}} = \frac{\text{New RS}}{\text{Original RS}}$$

Bushong, "Intensifying Screens," p 192; Carlton and McKenna-Adler, "Intensifying Screens," p 335; Papp, "Radiographic Ancillary Equipment," p 102; Wallace, "Intensifying Screens," p 165.

64. **(A)** When calibrating equipment, there are several quality assurance tests that must be performed to ensure that the equipment is working properly. One of these tests is called the test for reproducibility. This test ensures that the intensity of the beam will not vary by more than 5 percent for successive exposures when the same technical factors of kilovolts (peak), milliamperes, and time are used. Another test called reciprocity, or linearity, is done by adjusting the milliamperes and time between exposures with the equivalent in milliamperage-seconds and kilovolts (peak). For the reciprocity test, the intensity of the beam should not vary by more than 10 percent, or a 0.10 density point, on the radiograph.

Bushong, "Designing for Radiation Protection," p 511; Papp, "Radiographic Ancillary Equipment," pp 97–98.

65. **(D)** The density of the patient's tissue has a pronounced effect on the appearance of the radiographic image. The greater the density (mass per unit volume) of the tissue is, the more likely that the radiation will be absorbed because of the excess number of electrons that would be available for interaction. Differential absorption is the difference between how much radiation is absorbed by one tissue in comparison with an adjacent tissue. For instance, not taking into account the high atomic number of bony tissue will lead to more absorption. Bone also will absorb and scatter twice as many x rays as soft tissue because of its greater concentration of electrons. This will affect both the radiographic density and the radiographic contrast in the image.

Bushong, X-Ray Interaction with Matter," p 158; Carlton and McKenna-Adler, "Density," p 378, and "Contrast," p 398; Carroll, "Patient Status and Contrast Agents," pp 155–156.

66. **(B)** For this problem, the milliamperage-second screen formula should be used. First solve for mAs (800 × 0.25 = 200 mAs):

$$\frac{\text{Original mAs}}{\text{New mAs}} = \frac{\text{New RS}}{\text{Original RS}};$$

$$\frac{200}{x} = \frac{400}{100};$$

$$\frac{200}{4} = x; x = 50 \text{ mAs}$$

Carlton and McKenna-Adler, "Film/Screen Combinations," p 346; Dennis and Eisenberg, "Radiographic Calculations," p 94; Wallace, "Intensifying Screens," pp 165–167.

67. **(D)** The main purpose of a radiographic grid is to absorb radiation that is emitted from the patient (remnant or exit beam) so that the ultimate result is an improvement in image contrast. When a grid is used, it is important to make the appropriate technical adjustments because there will be a substantial loss of radiographic density. Although the grid greatly improves image quality, one disadvantage is an increased dose to the patient.

Bushong, "The Grid," p 216; Carlton and McKenna-Adler, "The Grid," p 265; Carroll, "Grids," p 181.

68. **(A)** Sodium sulfite is the preservative in both the developer and the fixer solutions. In the developer, it serves to prevent oxidation. In the fixer, it helps to dissolve the unexposed silver and improves the function of the clearing agent, ammonium thiosulfate. Glutaraldehyde is the hardener in the developing solution that serves to harden the emulsion, making transport through the automatic processor easier and also preventing scratches and abrasions in the emulsion. Hydroquinone is the reducing agent that serves to convert the latent image into the manifest image on the film.

Bushong, "Processing the Latent Image," pp 179–182; Carlton and McKenna-Adler, "Radiographic Processing," pp 296–300; Papp, "Film Processing," pp 26–32.

69. **(C)** For obvious financial benefits as well as environmental reasons, all imaging departments that use automatic processing systems should employ a system of active silver recovery. Unexposed silver is removed by the fixing solutions, but 50 percent of the silver remains on the film. Therefore, not only should each automatic processor be equipped with a silver recovery system attached to the fixer tank, but also the facility should have a place to store any rejected films. These rejected films should also be sent for reimbursement of silver recovery from the emulsion.

Carlton and McKenna-Adler, "Radiographic Processing," p 309; McKinney, "Silver Recovery," p 201; Papp, "Silver Recovery," p 65.

70. **(B)** When considering an alteration in technical factors because of a patient's pathology, there are usually two broad categories to consider: (1) additive pathology and (2) destructive pathology. Additive pathology increases the tissue density and sometimes the tissue thickness. requiring an increase in technical factors. Destructive pathology does the opposite; it decreases tissue density and thickness, requiring a decrease in technical factors. Aseptic necrosis, emphysema, and osteoporosis are examples of destructive pathology in their later stages. Initially, aseptic necrosis may actually increase tissue density but will eventually cause destruction in the later stages. Hemothorax is a type of pleural effusion and is an example of an additive pathology because blood is introduced into the lung cavity, requiring an increase in technique.

Carlton and McKenna-Adler, "The Pathology Problem," p 257; Carroll, "Pathology and Casts," pp 166–167; Eisenberg and Dennis, "Introduction to Pathology," p 3; Laudicina, "Respiratory System," p 27.

71. **(A)** An increase in the normal range of developer temperature will result in radiographs with increased radiographic density and decreased radiographic contrast due to chemical fog. Because of the profound effect of the automatic processor on image quality, it is essential to perform daily quality assurance on the automatic processor.

Carlton and McKenna-Adler, "Density," p 381, and "Contrast," p 399; Carroll, "Development Variables," pp 489–490; Wallace, "Radiographic Film and Development," p 144.

72. **(A)** When using an AEC device, if the radiographer wishes to decrease the exposure time, there are three choices to make. First, the SID may be decreased, thereby increasing the number of photons striking the film according to the inverse-square law. However, this may not be desirable because magnification would increase and recorded detail would also decrease. Another solution would be to increase the kilovolts (peak). Based on the 15 percent rule, an increase in kilovolts (peak) would require a decrease in milliamperage-seconds to maintain image density; therefore, the exposure time would also decrease. However, this also has its drawbacks in that changing the kilovolts (peak) alters the scale of contrast. A final solution would be to increase the milliampere setting, which would result in the same milliamperage-seconds but decreased exposure time. Changing the backup time would not decrease exposure time unless the radiographer decreased the backup time to a fraction of a second, which is not a wise practice. If a radiographer attempts to adjust the backup time to manipulate the exposure time, manually set technical factors would be best.

Cullinan, "The X-Ray Circuit," p 22; Wallace, "Automatic Exposure Control," p 217.

73. **(A)** To calculate the percentage of magnification, use the following formula:

$$\frac{SID}{(SID - OID)} - 1.0 \times 100 = \text{Percent magnification } or$$

$$\frac{SID}{SOD} - 1.0 \times 100 = \text{Percent magnification}$$

$$\frac{40}{40-8} = \frac{40}{32} - 1.0 \times 100 = 1.25 - 1.0 \times 100 = 25\%$$

Carlton and McKenna-Adler, "Distortion," pp 420–421; Carroll, "Distance Ratios," pp 271–272.

74. **(B)** The smallest amount of change in milliamperage-seconds necessary to produce a visible effect on the radiographic image is 30 percent. However, if a film needs to be repeated due to insufficient or excessive radiographic density, the milliamperage-seconds would probably need to be doubled or halved to produce a quality image.

Carlton and McKenna-Adler, "Density," p 370; Carroll, "Milliampere-Seconds," pp 83–85; Cullinan, "Technical Formulas and Related Data," p 293; Wallace, "mAs and Reciprocity," p 55.

75. **(B)** To calculate the new milliamperage-seconds, use the density maintenance formula, sometimes called the direct-square law, as follows:

$$\text{New mAs} = \frac{\text{Old mAs} \times \text{New distance}^2}{\text{Old distance}^2} ; x = 20\frac{(72 \text{ in.})^2}{(40 \text{ in.})^2} ;$$

$$x = 20(1.8)^2; x = 20 \times 3.24; x = 64.8 \text{ mAs}$$

Carlton and McKenna-Adler, "Exposure Conversion Problems," p 514; Carroll, "Source-Image Receptor Distance," p 257; Wallace, "The Inverse Square Law," p 68.

76. **(A)** Dirt or a chemical stain on a roller may cause scratches or tears in the emulsion at regular intervals as the film is transported through the automatic processor. If these artifacts specifically occur every time a sheet of film encircles a roller (3.1416 inches apart), they are referred to as pi lines. Wet-pressure sensitization and guide-shoe marks tend to cause scratches or marks all the way along the path the film travels, from one end to the other, and appear as lines. Improperly mixed chemicals will tend to cause artifacts throughout the entire image and may even cause the entire emulsion to smear in what is called the "curtain effect."

Bushong, "Film Artifacts," pp 421–422; McKinney, "Film Artifacts," p 179; Papp, "Additional Quality Management Procedures," pp 154–159.

77. **(C)** Panchromatic film is a type of film that is sensitive to all colors of the spectrum. A special type of film that is used in infrared (thermal) photography is especially sensitive to light in the red region of the spectrum. Orthochromatic film is sensitive to all colors of the light spectrum with the exception of red. Most rare earth film used in radiography is orthochromatic.

Bushong, "Radiographic Film," p 169; Carlton and McKenna-Adler, "Radiographic Film," p 285; Cullinan, "X-Ray Film," p 89; Papp, "Film Darkrooms," p 16.

78. **(B)** "Short-scale contrast" is another term used for an image exhibiting high contrast. Short scale is meant to give a visual representation of the contrast; "short" means that there are very few gray tones, with mostly black and white and great differences between adjacent densities. Conversely, "long-scale contrast," or low contrast, is an image that possesses many shades of gray, with very little difference in density between adjacent tissues.

Bushong, "Radiographic Technique," p 266; Carlton and McKenna-Adler, "Contrast," p 387; Wallace, "Radiographic Contrast," p 75.

79. **(A)** For this technique problem, it is important to know the grid conversion factor for each type of grid (e.g., 5:1, 6:1, 8:1, etc.), so that this number may be "plugged" into the formula. The following grid conversion factors are commonly accepted by most credentialing examinations:

Grid Ratio	Conversion Factor
No grid	1
5:1	2
6:1	3
8:1	4
10:1 & 12:1	5
16:1	6

Once the grid conversion factor is known, the following formula may be used:

$$\text{New mAs} = \frac{\text{Old mAs} \times \text{New grid conversion}}{\text{Old grid conversion}} ;$$

$$\text{New mAs} = 20 \times \frac{6}{4} ; = 20 \times \frac{3}{2} ;$$

$$\text{New mAs} = \frac{60}{2} = 30 \text{ mAs}$$

Cullinan, "Control of Scatter Radiation," p 77; Dennis and Eisenberg, "Radiographic Calculations," p 99; Wallace, "Grids and the Bucky," p 113.

80. **(D)** To figure out this problem, simply use the formula for geometric unsharpness (blur): GU = OID/SID − OID × FSS or OID/SOD × FSS.
A. 10/26 × 1 = 0.38
B. 8/32 × 2 = 0.5
C. 6/54 × 2 = 0.22
D. 4/68 × 1 = 0.058

The answer with the smallest blur would yield the greatest recorded detail. "Geometric unsharpness" is the term used for the blurred area around the perimeter of an image. Blur increases with a decrease in SID and an increase in OID and FSS.

Bushong, "Radiographic Quality," p 244; Cullinan, "Technical Formulas and Related Data," p 297; Dennis and Eisenberg, "Radiographic Calculations," p 103.

81. **(B)** The ability of an imaging system to differentiate between two small adjacent structures is the definition of resolution. The main QC tool that is used to test for resolution is the resolution grid, or resolution bar pattern (see Fig. 4–2). The grid is placed on an imaging system (i.e., a film-screen combination) and the ability of the system to image separate line-pairs is measured. The unit to measure resolution is line-pairs per millimeter. In other words, how many lines can one see when looking at the image.

Carroll, "Qualities of the Radiographic Image," pp 48–49; Papp, "Radiographic Ancillary Equipment," p 105; Wallace, "Geometric Factors Affecting Recorded Detail," pp 131–132.

82. **(C)** If any adjustment in radiographic density is to be made, usually the best technical factor to adjust is milliamperage-seconds. This is because the density of the film is directly proportional to the amount of milliamperage-seconds used. Kilovolts (peak) also has an effect on density, but to a much greater degree than the milliamperage-seconds. The radiographer should be aware that alterations in kilovolts (peak) will also change the scale of contrast, which is not always desirable. A change of 15 percent in the kVp is equivalent to either a 50 percent decrease (halving) or a 100 percent increase (doubling) in milliamperage-seconds. Therefore, milliamperage-seconds should be the primary controlling factor for radiographic density, and kilovolts (peak) should be the primary controlling factor for radiographic contrast in the image.

Carlton and Adler, "The Prime Factors," p 184; Carroll, "Kilovoltage-Peak," pp 107–110; Dennis and Eisenberg, "Radiographic Calculations," p 83; Wallace, "mAs and kVp Relationship," p 93.

83. **(A)** When performing a sensitometric strip, there are three important factors that the radiographer or QC technologist should check for using a densitometer. First, the radiographer should measure the clear area of the film, which gives an indication of the "base-plus-fog" inherent on the film. Second, a measurement should be taken of the optical step that measures closest to a density reading of 1.0 above base-plus-fog; this gives an indication of the "speed," or medium density, of

the test film. The last measurement is for the contrast or density difference on the test film. This is found by measuring the step closest to 2.0 above base-plus-fog and subtracting the step that measures closest to 0.25 above base-plus-fog. It is essential that all of these measurements be taken daily on each test strip, because all three factors may be affected by changes in processor temperature, replenishment rate, and/or chemical activity. If any measurements are found out of range of the normal limits, adjustments to the automatic processor or darkroom should be made.

Bushong, "Radiographic Quality," p 231; Carroll, "Sensitometry and Darkroom Quality Control," p 532; Papp, "Processor Quality Control," p 50.

84. **(B)** *Blur* is the area of unsharpness around the borders of an image. *Umbra* is the very sharp area of an image. There are mainly three factors in radiography that can have an effect on the size of the image blur: (1) FSS, (2) OID, and (3) SOD. They can be used in combination to calculate the geometric unsharpness mathematically as follows: $GU = FSS \times OID/SOD$.

The relationship between OID and the blur in the image is directly proportional. As the OID decreases, the blur decreases proportionately. A good visual example of this is when we see our shadows grow larger and less sharp as we increase our distance from a wall, whereas stepping closer to the wall will make our shadows smaller and very distinctly sharper.

Bushong, "Radiographic Quality," p 243; Carlton and McKenna-Adler, "Recorded Detail," pp 407–410; Carroll, "Distance Ratios," p 274.

85. **(C)** Using a small focal spot will produce images with greater recorded detail because the blur will decrease. Therefore, it would be desirable to use a smaller FSS when the blur is going to be large. There are only three instances when the geometric unsharpness (blur) would increase in radiography and those are when using (1) a large focal spot, (2) a large OID, or (3) a short SID. In only one of the choices, magnification procedures, would the blur increase substantially. That is because for magnification radiography both a large OID and a short SID are used, thus requiring the use of a small focal spot to compensate for the loss of recorded detail. If short exposure times are necessary, then a large focal spot allowing for greater milliampere settings would be more practical. If a large SID is used, it is not essential that a small focal spot be used because a large SID will decrease image blur. High-speed rotational anodes allow for greater heat dissipation when using a smaller FSS. Thus, most tubes that are to be used specifically for magnification radiography

come equipped with high-speed anodes, but a small focal spot would not be "useful" for a high-speed anode; in reality, the converse would be true.

Bushong, "Alternative Film Procedures," p 291; Carlton and McKenna-Adler, "Technical Aspects of Mammography," p 585; Carroll, "Distance Ratios," p 273–274.

86. **(A)** A film-screen combination with wide latitude will exhibit a long scale of contrast or low contrast. A film possessing wide latitude will give the radiographer more "room for error" when selecting technical factors. For example, if a radiographer inadvertently uses a high-speed screen to image a small extremity instead of using the slower-speed ("detail") screen, the milliampere-second setting is more critical and must be exact. Whereas when the same extremity is radiographed with the slower-speed screen (detail), there is a greater range of milliamperage-second settings that may be selected and still obtain a diagnostically useful radiograph.

Bushong, "The Radiographic Image," p 238; Carlton and McKenna-Adler, "Film/Screen Combinations," p 350; Carroll, "Image Receptor Systems," pp 227–228.

87. **(D)** The washing stage of automatic development is essential for the "archival quality of the film." *Archival quality* means that the radiograph will still be clear and readable several months or years after development because during the washing process, the chemicals from the fixer—mainly the clearing agent, ammonium thiosulfate—are removed from the film. If ammonium thiosulfate remains, the film will turn brown, yellow, or cloudy and will be difficult to interpret diagnostically. The developing solution is usually cleared off in the fixing tank and is not as much of a concern in the wash bath as the fixing solution.

Carlton and McKenna-Adler, "Radiographic Processing," p 300; McKinney, "Chemistry System," p 74; Papp, "Film Processing," p 31.

88. **(C)** Choice A describes the grid ratio and is usually represented as 5:1, 6:1, 8:1, and so forth. Choice B, the number of grid lines per inch or centimeter, is called the grid frequency. The "grid radius" is a term used only for focused grids that are restricted for use at specific distances because of the canting, or outward angling, of the grid lines. The grid radius is therefore the proper focusing distance that may be effectively used for a particular focused grid, Choice C.

Carroll, "Grids," p 190; Thompson, "Improving Image Quality," p 328.

89. **(D)** As screen speed in an imaging system increases, the latitude will decrease or become narrower, requiring a more specific selection of technical factors. A faster-speed screen will decrease resolution because faster screens employ larger crystals and/or thicker active layers. A faster-speed screen will produce higher contrast, or an image with more black and white shades and fewer shades of gray. The larger crystals and thicker active layers used in high-speed screens will produce a higher density with lower milliamperage-seconds than a slower-speed screen and therefore will decrease patient dose.

Bushong, "Intensifying Screens," pp 192–195; Carlton and McKenna-Adler, "Intensifying Screens," pp 333–337; Carroll, "Intensifying Screens," pp 209–217.

90. **(C)** There are three main portions of the characteristic curve as represented on a graph. The lowest end of the "S" curve is referred to as the "toe" portion represented by the letter A in Figure 4–3. It is usually the very lowest densities on the image or the base-plus-fog (clear part) and therefore does not represent the diagnostically useful portion. The highest end of the S curve represented by the letter C is referred to as the "shoulder" portion and represents the darkest areas on the image, also known as D-max. These areas are usually out of the diagnostically useful range of radiographic densities. The middle portion of the S curve represented by the letter B in Figure 4–3 is referred to as the straight-line portion, or "body," of the curve and does represent the diagnostically useful range, typically having a density measurement of between 0.25 and 2.5. How steep or shallow the slope of the straight-line portion is will be indicative of the contrast of the image.

Bushong, "Radiographic Quality," pp 231–238; Carlton and McKenna-Adler, "Sensitometry," pp 319–320; Carroll, "Sensitometry and Darkroom Quality Control," pp 530–531; Thompson et al., "Quality Control," p 400.

91. **(C)** The characteristic curve, or "D log E" curve as it is sometimes called, is a graphic representation of the relationship between the exposure and the optical density on the film. The x-axis represents the log-relative exposure (letter E in Figure 4–3), based on the milliamperage-second setting selected. The y-axis represents the optical density reading (letter D in Figure 4–3) on the film as measured by a densitometer. As expected, when the exposure increases along the x-axis, the optical density also increases along the y-axis in a sigmoidal fashion.

Bushong, "Radiographic Quality," pp 231–232; Carlton and McKenna-Adler, "Sensitometry," p 319; Carroll, "Sensitometry and Darkroom Quality Control," pp 530–531.

92. **(D)** The active chemicals in a developing solution work best in an alkaline-based solution having a pH level above 7.0. The activator in the developer that maintains its alkalinity is usually sodium carbonate. The chemicals in a fixing solution are acid-based, having a pH level below 7.0. The acidity of the fixer, mainly acetic acid, stops the action of the alkaline-based chemicals, thereby stopping development of the image.

    Bushong, "Processing the Latent Image," p 181; Carlton and McKenna-Adler, "Radiographic Processing," p 298; Papp, "Film Processing," p 27.

93. **(C)** The repeat rate is a very important consideration in any quality assurance program. A good repeat rate should be between 5 percent and 7 percent. In mammography, it should be much lower (about 2.5 percent or less). The repeat rate can be calculated by counting the number of films in the reject bin that needed to be repeated and dividing by the total number of films that were developed during that same time frame (usually a 1-week or 1-month period) times 100. In this example, the result would be as follows: $165/1240 \times 100$; $00.133 \times 100 = 13.3\%$.

    Bushong, "Mammography Quality Control," p 313; Carroll, "Quality Control," p 382; Papp, "Additional Quality Management Procedures," p 154.

94. **(A)** The ability of a substance such as a phosphor to emit light in response to radiation is termed *luminescence*. There are two types of luminescence: (1) *fluorescence*, which occurs only during stimulation such as during radiation exposure, and (2) *phosphorescence*, which refers to the continuous emission of light after the radiation has ceased and is undesirable in radiographic imaging systems. *Incandescence* is the emission of light by a substance when heated, such as what happens during thermionic emission when the filament is heated to the point that it glows. *Effervescence* refers to bubbling or sparkling, as in giving off gas bubbles in a carbonated drink.

    Bushong, "Intensifying Screens," p 192; Carlton and McKenna-Adler, "Intensifying Screens," p 332; Thompson et al., "Radiation: Its Atomic & Nuclear Origins," p 67.

95. **(A)** If the developer tank becomes heavily oxidized, which is often a problem in automatic processors, an ammonia-like smell will be noticeable in the darkroom. An oxidized developer may be avoided by using deep, narrow tanks rather than shallow, wide tanks. Also, a floating lid on top of the developing solution is very helpful in preventing oxidation because it minimizes contact with the outside air.

    Papp, "Film Processing," p 27.

96. **(A)** The milliamperage-seconds is the primary factor that determines the quantity of x-ray photons that are produced at the target. That is because there is a direct linear relationship to the amount of milliamperage-seconds used and the number of x-ray photons produced. The kilovolts (peak) also has a major influence on the quantity of x rays produced, because as the speed of the electrons hitting the target increases (as a result of an increase in kilovolts [peak]), the number of photons greatly increases. However, the relationship between kilovolts (peak) and x-ray quantity is not as predictable as the relationship between milliamperage-seconds and quantity and thus should not be used as the main variable for adjustments in quantity. The relationship between SID and quantity is inverse-square and also will affect other qualities in the image and should therefore not be of primary consideration when adjusting for x-ray quantity. The anode bevel does not have any affect on the quantity of x-ray photons produced, although the steeper the angle of the anode, the greater the resolution of the image.

    Bushong, "X-Ray Emission," pp 140–142; Carlton and McKenna-Adler, "X-Ray Production," p 138, and "The Prime Factors," p 182; Cullinan, "Glossary of Related Terminology," p 272; Wallace, "mAs and kVp Relationship," p 91.

97. **(A)** Excessive radiographic contrast is defined as an image that does not display enough shades of gray. All radiographs should be exposed using the optimum kilovolts (peak) required to produce sufficient radiographic contrast. In Figure 4–4, film B has been exposed using the optimum kilovolts (peak) of 70 and thus displays good contrast for diagnosis. Film A, on the other hand, was exposed using 55 kVp and was not sufficient to penetrate the part. Notice the lack of visibility of certain structures in the radiograph, such as the skull sutures, the sella turcica, and the mastoid air cells in film A, whereas film B demonstrates these structures more clearly.

    Carlton and McKenna-Adler, "Contrast," pp 392–394; Carroll, "Kilovoltage-Peak," pp 105–107; Wallace, "mAs and kVp Relationship," pp 87–90.

98. **(D)** A good quality assurance program should include routine annual QC tests on all radiographic equipment. Often, the term used for annual equipment inspection is "calibration." A technical engineer or a physicist usually performs equipment calibration. Some of the more common QC tests performed annually on radiographic equipment include tests for reciprocity, reproducibility, filtration, timer accuracy, beam alignment, and so forth.

Carroll, "Quality Control," pp 380, 388–402; Papp, "Quality Control of Radiographic Equipment," pp 73–74, 78–79; Thompson et al., "Quality Control," pp 403–408.

99. **(D)** This question requires knowledge of multiple technical factors and their effect on radiographic density and involves many steps. The first step involves noticing the change in three technical factors: (1) the SID, (2) the screen speed, and (3) the exposure time. So, the first step involves calculating the milliamperage-seconds: 100 mA × 0.25 = 25 mAs. The next step requires the use of the distance density maintenance formula for milliamperage-seconds:

$$\frac{mAs_1}{mAs_2} = \frac{(D_1)^2}{(D_2)^2}; \frac{25}{x} = \frac{40^2}{48^2}; \frac{25}{x} = \frac{1600}{2304};$$

$$\frac{25}{x} = 0.69; \frac{25}{0.69} = x; x = 36 \text{ mAs}$$

After finding the adjusted milliamperage-seconds for the new SID, next find the adjusted milliamperage-seconds for the new screen: Old relative screen speed/New relative screen speed × Old mAs = New mAs ; 400/100 × 36; 4 × 36 = 144 mAs. Finally, to find the new milliamperes, simply take the milliamperage-seconds and divide by the new time, 0.18 second: 144/0.18 = 800 mA.

Carlton and McKenna-Adler, "Exposure Conversion Problems," pp 514–516; Eisenberg and Dennis, "Radiographic Calculations," pp 59, 65, 94; Wallace, "Exposure Compensation," pp 186–190.

100. **(A)** If a radiograph appears with adequate radiographic density in the center, but with insufficient radiographic density on both sides, the most likely causes are peripheral grid cutoff. Peripheral grid cutoff can be caused by grids in three different situations: (1) an upside-down focused grid, (2) insufficient SID with a focused grid, and (3) excessive SID with a focused grid. If the central ray was not properly centered to the grid, the image would appear with insufficient radiographic density throughout the image, with more prominent grid cutoff to one side; it would not have sufficient radiographic density in the center.

Bushong, "The Grid," pp 224–225; Carlton and McKenna-Adler, "The Grid," pp 274–276; Carroll, "Grids," pp 190–193; Wallace, "Grids and the Bucky," pp 108–111.

101. **(B)** The base-plus-fog measurement as read by a densitometer is the "clear," or unexposed, area of the film. This reading is never at zero because there is some inherent optical density due to the blue base, and also, some fog that is attributed to manufacturing, storage, and development. Although some natural background radiation may contribute to the fog density on the film, x rays should not be responsible for fog in an effective quality assurance program. Most of the fog is due to development because the reducing agents in the developer will develop some of the unexposed silver halide crystals, causing a slight amount of fog density. The total base-plus-fog density should never exceed a reading of 0.20, or it may begin to affect the image quality.

Carlton and McKenna-Adler, "Sensitometry," p 319; Carroll, "Sensitometry & Darkroom Control," p 532; Papp, "Processor Quality Control," p 50.

102. **(C)** If the grid ratio is increased from one exposure to another, it will have no effect on blur or recorded detail if used properly. An increase in the grid ratio will, however, cause an increase in radiographic contrast and also a decrease in radiographic density due to the greater reduction of scatter.

Carlton and McKenna-Adler, "The Grid," p 271; Carroll, "Grids," pp 185–188; Wallace, "Grids and the Bucky," pp 112–113.

103. **(D)** The dryer temperature in most automatic processors ranges from 120° to 150°F. This is so that the film emulsion will shrink and seal dry in one pass through the dryer rollers, making the film immediately available to read. Most developer temperatures in an automatic processor range from 92° to 96°F. Most fixer temperatures are much cooler, ranging from about 65° to 75°F. Most wash tanks have water that is about 5°F cooler than the other solutions to control vast temperature differences from developer to fixer to wash. If the temperature difference is too great between solutions, the emulsion may crack, or reticulate.

Carlton and McKenna-Adler, "Radiographic Processing," p 300; Carroll, "Automatic Processors," p 503; McKinney, "Dryer System," p 113.

104. **(C)** If a radiographer changed screen speeds for the purpose of repeating an unsatisfactory radiograph, an AEC should not be used. Most AEC machines are calibrated for a specific type of screen and/or screen speed. If the screen speed is increased, the radiographic density will be too dark because the AEC will not be able to detect the difference in screen speed. If the screen speed is decreased as in this question—a change was made from a 400-RS screen to a 200-RS screen— the radiograph will have insufficient radiographic density.

Thompson et al., "Equipment and Accessory Malfunctions or Misapplications," pp 382–383.

105. **(B)** There are three types of shape distortion: (1) elongation, (2) foreshortening, and (3) spatial

distortion. Sometimes shape distortion is used intentionally to emphasize the appearance of a specific body structure, making it appear either longer or shorter. Shape distortion may occur when the alignment of the direction of the central ray, the position of the film, and/or the position of the part are different from the accepted method of positioning. This may often happen when uncooperative, immobile, or trauma patients are radiographed. A special challenge to the radiographer is taking an image with a portable unit in the patient's room when conditions are less than ideal. Often, because of patient's condition and the sheer size and structure of a patient's hospital room, the proper part-tube-film alignment may not be attainable.

Carlton and McKenna-Adler, "Distortion," p 422; Thompson et al., "Production of the Radiographic Image," p 271; Wallace, "Shape Distortion," pp 35–36.

106. **(D)** This answer would be found by using the following formula:

$$mAs = mA \times time; \text{ or } mAs/time = mA;$$

$$30/0.025 = 1200 \text{ mA}.$$

Bushong, "Radiographic Exposure," p 253; Carlton and McKenna-Adler, "Exposure Conversion Problems," p 514; Dennis and Eisenberg, "Radiographic Calculations," p 59; Wallace, "mAs and Reciprocity," p 53.

107. **(A)** Find the new technical factors by employing the 15 percent kilovolt (peak) rule. When kilovolts (peak) is increased by 15 percent, the milliamperage-seconds will need to be decreased by 50 percent, or ½ of the original setting. The original kilovolts (peak) is 61, and 61 ×0.15 = 9.15; 61 + 9 = 70. So, the radiographer should know that the kilovolts (peak) has increased by 15%. Therefore, the new milliamperage-seconds should be as follows: 6 × ½ = 3 mAs.

Carlton and McKenna-Adler, "The Prime Factors," p 184; Carroll, "Kilovoltage-Peak," pp 107–110; Dennis and Eisenberg, "Radiographic Calculations," p 83; Wallace, "mAs and kVp Relationship," p 93.

108. **(D)** The grid ratio can be found by dividing the height of the lead strips by the distance between the lead strips, most commonly represented as r = h/d. The thickness and grid frequency have very little impact on the grid ratio. For this example, if the height of the lead strips is 4 mm and the distance separating them is 0.25 mm, 4/0.25 = 16:1.

Bushong, "The Grid," p 216; Dennis and Eisenberg, "Radiographic Calculations," p 97; Wallace, "Grids and the Bucky," pp 105–106.

109. **(D)** Most conventional cassettes are manufactured with a lead-foil backing to absorb back-scatter radiation that will degrade the image quality. Light-absorbing dyes are sometimes added to improve resolution in detail screens. Reflective backing, which serves to reflect light back onto the film, serves to increase screen speed, and conversion efficiency can only increase by changing the type of light-emitting phosphor; rare earth phosphors such as gadolinium and lanthanum have the highest conversion efficiency.

Bushong, "Intensifying Screens," p 196; Carlton and McKenna-Adler, "Intensifying Screens," p 338; Wallace, "Methods to Control Scatter," p 125.

110. **(B)** Both elongation and foreshortening are types of shape distortion. Both types of distortion occur as a result of angling of the central ray, anatomic part, or the cassette. If the anatomic part is distorted in such a way that it appears longer than its actual size, it is called *elongation*, and if the part is distorted in such a way that it appears shorter than its actual size, it is called *foreshortening*. Size distortion occurs when the shape remains the same, but the size has been enlarged or magnified. Magnification, or size distortion, is caused by the use of a short SID or a long OID.

Carlton and McKenna-Adler, "Distortion," p 422; Thompson et al., "Production of the Radiographic Image," p 271; Wallace, "Shape Distortion," pp 35–36.

SECTION IV: RADIOGRAPHIC PROCEDURES AND RELATED ANATOMY

111. **(D)** It is important for radiographers to become familiar with all of the body planes to use precise positioning skills. There are four main planes in the body: (1) sagittal, (2) coronal, (3) horizontal, and (4) oblique. Both the sagittal and coronal planes run parallel with the longitudinal axis of the body, but at right planes to each other. The horizontal plane cuts through the body from side to side and is perpendicular to the longitudinal axis. The oblique plane cuts through the body at an angle, usually between the sagittal and coronal planes.

Ballinger, Vol 1, p 49; Bontrager, "Terminology," p 15; Cornuelle and Gronefeld, "Introduction to Radiography," p 10; Greathouse, "Introduction to Radiographic Positioning & Procedures," Vol 1, pp 7–8.

112. **(B)** The hypersthenic body habitus is the classification of body shape that is the largest in stature. Hypersthenic patients comprise about 5 percent of the population. They are characterized by broad lungs and a heart that is wider at the base and, in general, have organs that are more superior and lateral (away from the midline) com-

pared with those of other body types. It is essential to recognize the different body habitus of all patients, so that proper positioning techniques may be employed.

Ballinger, Vol 1, p 41; Bontrager, "Positioning Principles," p 53. Cornuelle and Gronefeld, "Introduction to Radiography" p 8; Greathouse, "Introduction to Radiographic Positioning and Procedures," Vol 1, pp 9–10.

113. **(D)** A general rule in radiographing any trauma patient, especially when the long bones are involved, is to "obtain a minimum of two radiographs for each body part at 90° angles to each other." These two projections may not be the typical AP/PA or lateral projections, but it is essential that they be 90° apart.

Ballinger, Vol 1, p 519; Bontrager, "Trauma & Mobile Radiography," p 551; Greathouse, "Trauma Head Positioning," Vol 1, p 570.

114. **(B)** To enhance filling of the renal pelves and calyces, a compression device is sometimes used. This device, if properly placed over the distal ureters at the level of the pelvic brim, will maintain contrast media in the kidneys and keep it from draining. This device should be used only for a short time following injection of the contrast media, and there are contraindications, such as suspected kidney stones, aneurysm, or an abdominal mass.

Ballinger, Vol 2, p 166; Bontrager, "The Urinary System," p 515; Cornuelle and Gronefeld, "Urinary System," p 425; Greathouse, Vol 1, "Urinary System," p 680.

115. **(A)** The anterior and posterior ethmoid and sphenoid sinuses lie toward the midline of the skull, whereas the maxillary sinuses lie lateral and inferior, and the frontal sinuses lie just superior to the ethmoids. In a PA projection, the maxillary sinuses will be projected most inferior and laterally, and on a lateral projection, they will be projected most inferior, as seen in Figure 4–5.

Ballinger, Vol 2, p 379; Bontrager, "Paranasal Sinuses," p 397.

116. **(D)** To ensure adequate visualization of the AC joints, it is essential that the patient be radiographed in the erect position and have weights secured to each wrist weighing at least 5 to 8 lb apiece. AC separations are best seen in this projection using the proper weight-bearing method.

Ballinger, Vol 2, p 152; Bontrager, "Acromioclavicular (AC) Joints," p 166; Cornuelle and Gronefeld, "Shoulder Girdle," p 166; Greathouse, "Upper Limb & Shoulder Girdle," Vol 1, p 186.

117 and 118. **(A)** and **(B)** Figure 4–6 is a lateral projection of the foot: the number 1 corresponds to

the talus, 2 to the navicular bone, 3 to the cuneiform bones, 4 to the calcaneus, 5 to the cuboid bone, 6 to the tibia, and 7 to the fibula.

Ballinger, Vol 1, pp 180, 207; Bontrager, "Lower Limb," p 177; McKinnis, pp 296–297.

119. **(C)** The duodenum takes a very sharp curve after leaving the stomach often called the "C-Loop" before attaching to the next section of the small intestine at the duodenojejunal flexure. This sharp flexure is held tightly in place by the ligament of Treitz. The falciform ligament is a very large band of tissue that separates the right and left lobes of the liver. In the large intestine, there is a thick muscular layer consisting of three fibrous bands called the taeniae coli. The taeniae coli serve to draw the lining of the colon into several puckers called haustra, which aids in the movement of waste products. The crypts of Lieberkühn are the microscopic cells found in the villi of the small intestine, which serve to absorb nutrients from digested food into the bloodstream.

Bontrager, p 447; Cornuelle and Gronefeld, "Digestive System," p 445.

120. **(B)** The best way to visualize the transthoracic lateral humerus is by using a breathing technique by which the patient is allowed to breathe normally for at least 2 to 5 seconds during the exposure. This allows the lung markings to be sufficiently blurred to demonstrate bony detail of the humerus. However, some equipment will not allow the radiographer to use this method. In that case, the patient should be instructed to suspend respiration on full inhalation. This will best demonstrate contrast between the lung and bone tissue.

Ballinger, Vol 1, p 130; Bontrager, "Shoulder: Trauma Routine," p 163; Cornuelle and Gronefeld, "Upper Limb (Extremity), p 144; Greathouse, "Upper Limb and Shoulder Girdle," Vol 1, p 180.

121. **(D)** The radial head in the elbow joint has two articulations. It articulates superiorly with the capitulum of the humerus, and it articulates medially with the radial notch of the ulna to form the proximal radioulnar joint.

Ballinger, Vol 1, pp 61, 63; Bontrager, "Forearm," p 106; Cornuelle and Gronefeld, "Upper Limb (Extremity)," p 104; Greathouse, "Upper Limb and Shoulder Girdle," Vol 1, p 94.

122. **(C)** The most superior aspect of the lung that extends above the clavicle is known as the apex. The hilum is the most medial portion where the main bronchus and pulmonary vessels enter and exit. The base is the most inferior aspect of the lung and comes to a point laterally at the costophrenic angle. The mediastinum is the mid-

section of the thorax where all of the most medial organs of the chest lie (i.e., esophagus, trachea, heart, and thymus gland).

Ballinger, Vol 1, p 438; Bontrager, "Chest," p 62; Cornuelle and Gronefeld, "Respiratory System," p 32.

123. **(C)** Long-bone measurement, also known as "orthoroentgenography," is a procedure done to measure discrepancies in bone length between two extremities. Although the difference in bone length may vary in the upper limbs, the most common developmental differences are found in the lower limbs. When long-bone measurement is performed on the lower limbs, three projections on one 14 × 17 size cassette are taken of each limb. The three projections consist of an AP hip, an AP knee, and an AP ankle as the patient lies on a radiopaque ruler. Each radiograph with the ruler is compared for discrepancies in bone length. This procedure can be done on adults for back pain or other symptoms, but it is most commonly ordered on children who may develop differences in their limb lengths.

Ballinger, Vol, 1, p 482; Bontrager, "Orthoroentgenography," p 612; Greathouse, "Long Bone Measurement," Vol 2, pp 116–117.

124. **(D)** When radiographing the mandible in either the AP or PA projection, the positioning is essential to best demonstrate the areas of primary interest, which are the lateral aspect of the body and the rami. In the PA projection with the central ray perpendicular, the cassette and central ray should be centered at the lips (Ballinger says at the acanthion). For the PA axial projection with the central ray angled 20° cephalad, Ballinger says to have the central ray exit at the tip of the nose; Bontrager says at the acanthion. The nasion would be too superior, and both the mental point and inferior alveolar processes would be too inferior.

Ballinger, Vol 2, p 342; Bontrager, "Mandible," p 374; Eisenberg et al, "Mandible," p 307; Greathouse, "Skull and Facial Bones," Vol 1, p 530.

125. **(D)** An accepted practice in radiography when positioning patients for GI studies is to vary the degree of obliquity according to the patient's body habitus. For a right anterior oblique (RAO) projection of the stomach, the degree of obliquity can vary from 40° to 70°. In general, those patients with thinner body habitus (asthenic and hyposthenic patients) have organs that are positioned more inferior and closer to the spine. Therefore, these patients will need to be rotated to a lesser degree than those with a larger body habitus (sthenic and hypersthenic patients) whose organs tend to lie in a more lateral position away from the spine.

Ballinger, Vol 2, p 105; Bontrager, "Upper GI Series," p 440; Cornuelle and Gronefeld, "Digestive System," p 455; Greathouse, "Upper Gastrointestinal Tract," Vol 1, p 600.

126. **(A)** The parietoacanthial projection (Waters method) is specifically done to demonstrate the maxillary sinuses. The patient's head should be adjusted so that the orbitomeatal line (OML) forms a 37° angle to the plane of the cassette, or so that the mentomeatal line is perpendicular to the cassette. With the OML properly adjusted and the central ray perpendicular to the cassette, the petrous ridges should be projected below the maxillary sinuses. The petrous ridges fill the orbits when the OML and central ray are perpendicular to the cassette. The petrous ridges will be projected to the lower one-third of the orbits when the OML is perpendicular and the central ray is angled 15° caudal (Caldwell method).

Ballinger, Vol 2, p 382; Bontrager, "Paranasal Sinuses," p 399; Cornuelle and Gronefeld, "Facial Bones and Paranasal Sinuses," p 373; Greathouse, "Skull and Facial Bones," Vol 1, p 542.

127. **(A)** To demonstrate the maximum joint space and to relax the muscles of the leg, the knee should be flexed at an angle of no more than 20° to 30° from full extension (Bontrager says 15° to 20°).

Ballinger, Vol 1, p 243; Bontrager, "Knee," p 208; Cornuelle and Gronefeld, "Lower Limb (Extremity)," p 202; Greathouse, "Lower Limb & Pelvis," Vol 1, p 260.

128. **(C)** Spina bifida is clearly demonstrated on an AP projection of the lumbar spine in Figure 4–7. Spina bifida is a congenital defect in which the posterior laminae fail to unite. With spina bifida occulta, the most common type, the patient is usually asymptomatic, so often a newborn will not be diagnosed with the disorder. Spondylolysis is also known as a "pars" defect and appears in an oblique projection of the lumbar spine as a collar on the "Scottie dog." Spondylolisthesis can be best diagnosed with a lateral projection of the spine; in this disorder, one vertebra slips forward on another vertebral body. Herniated nucleus pulposus can usually not be demonstrated on a routine radiograph, but only in specialized imaging procedures that demonstrate soft-tissue anatomy, such as myelography, computed tomography (CT), or magnetic resonance imaging (MRI).

Eisenberg and Dennis, "Skeletal System," p 67; Laudicina, "Central Nervous System," pp 217–218; McKinney, "Lumbosacral Spine and Sacroiliac Joints," p 205.

129. **(C)** When a person ingests food containing fat, a hormone called cholecystokinin is released in the

bloodstream, which stimulates the gallbladder to contract, releasing the bile contents. The bile is first excreted from the gallbladder to the cystic duct, where it descends and joins the hepatic duct to form the common bile duct. The common bile duct descends about 3 inches inferior, where it joins the pancreatic duct to form the ampulla of Vater, where the bile eventually drains into the duodenum through the sphincter of Oddi.

Ballinger, Vol 2, pp 33–34; Bontrager, "Gallbladder and Biliary Ducts," p 485; Cornuelle and Gronefeld, "Biliary System," pp 488–489; Greathouse, "Hepatobiliary System," Vol 1, pp 647–648.

130. **(D)** The best way to demonstrate pneumothorax, which is air in the thoracic cavity outside the lung, usually associated with a collapsed lung (atelectasis), is with a radiograph taken on full expiration. Most physicians request that the radiographer take two AP or PA projections, one on full inspiration and one on full expiration for comparison, and these should be taken with the patient erect if possible. A PA or AP projection with the patient in the lateral decubitus position may also be taken using a horizontal beam to demonstrate air-fluid levels with the affected side up. A lateral or AP projection with the patient in the recumbent position will be of little value in demonstrating a pneumothorax.

Bontrager, "Chest," p 66; Eisenberg and Dennis, "Respiratory System," p 53; Ballinger, Vol 1, pp 444, 476–477; Greathouse, "Chest and Upper Airway," Vol 1, p 59.

131. **(D)** When radiographing abdominal structures, involuntary motion from peristalsis and aortic circulation should always be a consideration. Therefore, it is best to radiograph abdominal structures with the shortest time possible. In this case, choice D has the shortest time at 0.02 second.

Ballinger, Vol 1, p 12; Bontrager, "Imaging Principles," p 33.

132. **(A)** A small-bowel series can take several hours to complete. This is because the patient usually ingests contrast media orally, and radiographs are taken every 15 to 20 minutes until the contrast has made its way through the entire small intestine. Typically, after about 2 to 4 hours, the radiologist will request a terminal ileum spot, or he or she will ask to "spot" the ileocecal junction using fluoroscopy. Thus, the examination is considered complete when the contrast has reached the cecum of the large intestine. However, some radiologists will continue to monitor the patient until the contrast reaches the ascending colon.

Bontrager, "Small Bowel Series," p 456; Cornuelle

and Gronefeld, "Digestive System," p 450; Ballinger, Vol 2, p 116.

133. **(B)** A narrowing or constriction of the aorta is referred to as *coarctation*. This pathology is often hard to demonstrate using routine chest radiography, and thus other methods such as a barium swallow, aortography, and CT or MRI scans are ordered in cases of suspected coarctation.

Eisenberg and Dennis, "Cardiovascular System," pp 227–229; Mace and Kowalczyk, "The Cardiovascular System," pp 204–205; Tortorici and Apfel, "Thoracic Aortography," pp 206, 210, 1995.

134. **(C)** Stress views are done specifically to demonstrate ligamentous injuries to the ankle. A ruptured ligament may best be demonstrated by widening of the joint space on the same side of the injury. This is usually performed by the orthopedic surgeon and may require a local anesthetic because it can be a painful procedure. With the ankle in inversion stress, the lateral ligament is best demonstrated, and with eversion stress, the medial ligament is best demonstrated.

Ballinger, Vol 1, p 233; Bontrager, "Ankle," p 203; Cornuelle and Gronefeld, "Lower Limb (Extremity)," p 178; Greathouse, "Lower Limb and Pelvis," Vol 1, pp 248–249.

135. **(B)** Whenever there is the presence of overlapping fragments in a skull fracture, this is usually indicative of a depression fracture caused by blunt trauma. Some depression fractures appear stellate (star-shaped) and may project outward from a centralized location. Blunt trauma is usually the result of trauma from a heavy, specifically shaped object such as a hammer, whereas a multilinear fracture is caused from the head hitting a large flat surface such as a windshield and usually does not cause a deep depression with overlapping fragments. A depression fracture is a very serious form of skull trauma because it usually results in massive injury to the brain. It may best be demonstrated using a tangential projection.

Eisenberg and Dennis, "Nervous System Disease," p 243; Laudicina, "Central Nervous System," p 215; Mace and Kowalczyk, "Traumatic Disease," p 261.

136. **(D)** The submentovertex projection is used specifically to demonstrate the sphenoid and ethmoid sinuses. The maxillary and frontal sinuses are not well demonstrated in this projection.

Ballinger, Vol 2, p 385; Cornuelle and Gronefeld, "Facial Bones and Paranasal Sinuses," p 375; Greathouse, "Skull and Facial Bones," Vol 1, p 546.

137. **(A)** The diaphragm is very important in chest radiography because it needs to expand and contract to reach its lowest position. This occurs on

full inspiration and is best for demonstrating the structures of the lung. When the patient exhales, the diaphragm relaxes and moves upward.

Cornuelle and Gronefeld, "Respiratory System," p 34; Greathouse, "Chest and Upper Airway," Vol 1, p 33; Tortora and Grabowski, "The Respiratory System," pp 737–739.

138. **(B)** With the patient in the supine position and the sacrum of primary interest, the central ray should be directed to enter at a level 2 inches superior to the symphysis pubis at a 10° caudal angle. When the patient is prone for a PA projection, the central ray should be directed 15° cephalad. This angulation will compensate for the natural curvature of the spine; it should appear more elongated than on an AP projection of the lumbar spine.

Ballinger, Vol 1, p 387; Bontrager, "Sacrum and Coccyx," p 300; Cornuelle and Gronefeld, "Vertebral Column," p 312; Greathouse, "Lumbar Spine, Sacrum and Coccyx," Vol 1, p 414.

139. **(D)** Myelography is the radiographic study of the central nervous system structures within the spinal canal. For this examination, the contrast material must be injected into the subarachnoid space. Usually the injection occurs at the level of the L2–3 or L3–4 disk interspace. This is because the spinal cord ends at approximately the level of L1, and it is safest to perform a spinal puncture below that level.

Ballinger, Vol 2, p 500; Bontrager, "Myelography," p 621; Cornuelle and Gronefeld, "Vertebral Column," p 284; Greathouse, Vol 2, p 376.

140. **(A)** A typical vertebra is classified as an irregular bone. It is very complex and has many intricate structures that serve to protect the spinal cord and the branching spinal nerves. The most anterior part of a typical vertebra is the vertebral body, which is the weight-bearing structure and is cushioned both on its superior and inferior surfaces by the intervertebral disks. The pedicles "jut" out posteriorly off of the vertebral body. The transverse processes project laterally from the pedicles, and the laminae project posteriorly and medially from the transverse processes to form the spinous process.

Ballinger, Vol 2, p 314; Bontrager, "Vertebral Column," p 250; Cornuelle and Gronefeld, "Vertebral Column," pp 269–270.

141. **(C)** The intracerebral circulation is very complex. At the area of the midbrain, the blood supply to the brain is fed by an intricate network of branching arteries which all meet together at the circulosis arteriosus (also known as the "circle of Willis"). The vertebral arteries arise superiorly

from the cervical foramina and through the foramen magnum, where they eventually unite to form the basilar artery in the brain. The basilar artery then branches into the posterior cerebral arteries that feed the cerebellum. The common carotid arteries arise superiorly from the aortic arch and right brachiocephalic artery. These eventually branch into the external and internal carotid arteries at the level of C4. The internal carotid artery enters the cranium through the temporal bone, where it then bifurcates into the anterior and middle cerebral arteries. The connection between the anterior and posterior communicating branches is made possible by the circle of Willis, which joins these arteries.

Ballinger, Vol 2, pp 544, 595; Bontrager, "Angiography," p 634; Spence, "Anatomy of the Vascular System," pp 313–314; Tortora and Grabowski, "The Cardiovascular System: Blood Vessels and Hemodynamics," pp 652, 654.

142. **(C)** There are three accepted methods of positioning for the intercondyloid fossa. In all three methods, the central ray should be perpendicular to the long axis of the lower leg. The AP axial projection, known as the "Beclere" method, is the only projection where the patient is supine. A curved cassette may be used with this method, and the central ray is angled 40° to 45° cephalad to the joint space. There are two variations of the PA axial projection. The first variation is better known as the "Camp-Coventry" method, in which the patient lies prone and raises the lower leg to a 40° to 50° angle from the cassette. The central ray should be perpendicular to the lower leg and thus should match the degree of flexion of the knee. The second method is called the "Holmblad" method in which the patient is radiographed while kneeling on the cassette. The patient should then lean forward so that the femur forms a 60° to 70° angle to the tabletop and the central ray is perpendicular to both the lower leg and cassette.

Ballinger, Vol 1, p 252; Bontrager, "Knee-Intercondyloid Fossa," p 210.

143. **(C)** To best demonstrate the zygapophyseal joints in the lumbar vertebra, the patient should be rotated 45° toward the side of interest in the posterior oblique position. If the joints of interest are in the lower lumbar and sacral region, the patient may only need to be rotated 30° to the side of interest.

Ballinger, Vol 2, p 374; Bontrager, "Lumbar Spine," p 290.

144. **(B)** There are many classifications of fractures. A more accepted term for compound fracture is an

"open fracture," in which a fragment of bony tissue protrudes through the skin. An impacted fracture is seen mostly in long bones where one end of the fracture is firmly imbedded into the other end. A torus fracture is a partial or incomplete fracture in which the cortex is not completely broken through and there is no displacement. A comminuted fracture is usually typical of blunt trauma in which the middle of the bone is broken into many fragmented pieces at the site of injury.

Bontrager, "Trauma and Fracture Terminology," p 548; Eisenberg and Dennis, "Skeletal System," p 98.

145. **(D)** The falciform ligament separates the right and left lobes of the liver. Radiographically, an important sign of pathology in children is when the falciform ligament can be demonstrated on a routine KUB. This may happen when the patient has pneumoperitoneum, or air in the peritoneum.

Ballinger, Vol 1, and Vol 2, p 32; Bontrager, "Gallbladder and Biliary Ducts," p 484; Cornuelle and Gronefeld, "Digestive System," p 447; Eisenberg and Dennis, "Gastrointestinal System," p 170; Tortora and Grabowski, "The Digestive System," p 789.

146. **(B)** The mediastinum is the cavity of the thorax that lies between both lungs. Only specific organs lie within this central cavity, such as the trachea, esophagus, the thymus gland, and the heart and great vessels, which include the superior vena cava. The lungs lie within the pleural cavity on either side of the mediastinum.

Ballinger, Vol 1, p 438; Bontrager, "Chest," p 62; Cornuelle and Gronefeld, "Respiratory System," p 32.

147. **(D)** The most proximal part of the stomach is the cardia. The cardia is the small area that surrounds the opening from the esophagus, the cardiac orifice, so named because of its proximity to the heart. The other three sections of the stomach in their proximal order are the (1) fundus, (2) body, and (3) pylorus.

Ballinger, Vol 2, p 85; Cornuelle and Gronefeld, "Digestive System," p 442; Tortora and Grabowski, "The Digestive System," pp 780–781.

148. **(B)** To best demonstrate the intervertebral disk spaces on an AP projection of the lumbar spine, the radiographer should have the patient flex both knees and hips. A cushioned support under the knees is usually helpful to overcome the natural lordosis of the lumbar area and is more comfortable for the patient.

Ballinger, Vol 1, p 366; Bontrager, "Lumbar Spine," p 289.

149. **(C)** Spondylolisthesis is a slipping forward of one vertebral body onto another. It is most commonly

seen at the L5–S1 disc space. Spondylolysis is also known as the pars defect, and a typical radiographic sign is a "collar on the Scottie dog" in the 45° oblique projection of the lumbar spine. Ankylosing spondylitis is also known as "bamboo spine" or Strümpell-Marie disease. This disorder is characterized by fusion (ankylosing) of the entire spine; thus the nickname bamboo spine. Spondylosis is a disorder of the spine that is usually associated with degenerative disease and osteoarthritis in which there is a breaking down of the vertebrae.

Eisenberg and Dennis, "Skeletal System," pp 114–115; Laudicina, "Osseous System and Joints," pp 156, 165–166; Mace and Kowalczyk, "The Skeletal System," p 34.

150. **(D)** The olecranon process is the most proximal part of the ulna. It is also most posterior and makes up part of the elbow joint. During extension of the forearm, the olecranon process of the ulna articulates with the olecranon fossa on the posterior aspect of the distal humerus.

Ballinger, Vol 1, p 61; Bontrager, "Forearm," p 106; Cornuelle and Gronefeld, "Upper Limb (Extremity)," p 104; Tortora and Grabowski, "The Skeletal System: The Appendicular Skeleton," p 203.

151. **(D)** Pneumoconiosis is a disorder of the respiratory system that is caused by inhalation of inorganic particles such as coal dust, asbestos, or silica. It is usually job-related, and many companies now go to great lengths to protect their workers who are exposed to these substances. There are many forms of pneumoconiosis depending on the type of particle to which the individual was exposed. The three most common are (1) asbestosis, (2) silicosis, and (3) anthracosis (coal miner's disease). Other forms may also be caused by exposure to dusts such as: tin, iron oxide, barium, and/or beryllium. Ewing's sarcoma is a rare type of malignancy found in the lower extremity that usually affects young males. *Pneumocystis carinii* pneumonia is a very rare type of pneumonia that is usually only seen in immunosuppressed patients, such as those with AIDS. Some other rare diseases prevalent in patients with AIDS include Kaposi's sarcoma (type of skin cancer), toxoplasmosis, cytomegalovirus, and herpes virus.

Eisenberg and Dennis, "Introduction to Pathology," pp 14–15, and "Respiratory System," pp 36–38; Laudicina, "Respiratory System," p 42; Mace and Kowalczyk, "The Respiratory System," pp 68–70, and "The Hemopoietic System," p 342.

152. **(D)** The coronoid process is often difficult to see on routine AP or lateral projections. Therefore, an AP projection in the medial oblique position is

often ordered to demonstrate this structure. The AP projection in the lateral oblique position is used to demonstrate the radial head free of superimposition.

Ballinger, Vol 1, p 104; Bontrager, "Elbow," p 138; Cornuelle and Gronefeld, "Upper Limb (Extremity)," p 136.

153. **(A)** The zygomatic arch, or cheekbone, is formed by part of two different bones. The anterior portion is formed by the malar, or zygomatic, bone, and the posterior portion is formed by the zygomatic process of the temporal bone.

Ballinger, Vol 2, p 231; Bontrager, "Facial Bones," p 334; Cornuelle and Gronefeld, "Facial Bones and Paranasal Sinuses," pp 359–360.

154. **(B)** Cephalopelvic disproportion (CPD) is sometimes seen in women who are in labor and are failing to progress, especially in primigravid (first-time pregnancy) female patients. CPD is often ruled out to determine if the fetal head is too large for the maternal pelvis, and this is why the labor is not progressing normally. This condition may be diagnosed with pelvic sonography or with pelvimetry using a Colcher-Sussman pelvimeter. Hysterosalpingography is a radiographic examination of the uterus and fallopian tubes and is not helpful in pregnant women, especially women in labor.

Ballinger, Vol 2, pp 200, 204, 206–208; Bontrager, "Proximal Femur and Pelvic Girdle," p 225; Cornuelle and Gronefeld, "Pelvic Girdle," p 226.

155. **(C)** When performing cystography, the AP oblique projection is done specifically to demonstrate the distal ureters and proximal urethra. To best see these structures, the patient must be rotated at least 40° to 60°. This position is often used to show possible reflux and/or prostate enlargement, and is thus a common position for a voiding cystourethrogram.

Ballinger, Vol 2, p 186; Bontrager, "Cystography," p 527; Cornuelle and Gronefeld, "Urinary System," p 434.

156. **(D)** If the central ray is centered to the first metacarpophalangeal joint, this will demonstrate the first digit, or thumb. When the hand is in a true lateral position and the fingers are extended, the image will demonstrate a PA projection of the thumb. This projection is used only when the patient cannot assume the position for an AP projection of the thumb. It is not advisable because of the increased OID and thus loss of recorded detail that is seen using this method.

Ballinger, Vol 1, p 72; Bontrager, "Upper Extremities," p 118.

157. **(A)** When the patient is positioned properly for an oblique projection of the spine, an appearance of a Scottie dog should be outlined on the radiograph for each vertebra. The ear of the Scottie dog is the superior articulating process of the vertebra. The front leg of the Scottie dog is the inferior articulating process. The eye of the Scottie dog is the pedicle. The neck of the Scottie dog is the pars interarticularis, and the body of the Scottie dog is the lamina.

Ballinger, Vol 1, p 373; Bontrager, "Lumbar Spine, Sacrum and Coccyx," p 284; Cornuelle and Gronefeld, "Vertebral Column," p 303.

158. **(B)** Arthrography is usually performed on diarthrodial, or freely movable, joints, such as the knee, shoulder, or temporomandibular joint. A distinguishing characteristic about diarthrodial joints is that they contain a synovial cavity with synovial fluid. The other two broad classifications of joints include (1) amphiarthrodial (slightly movable joints), which are typically cartilaginous and contain no joint cavity such as the intervertebral disk joint; and (2) synarthrodial (immovable joints), which are separated by fibrous tissue and include joints such as the sutures of the skull or the epiphyseal plate of a typical long bone.

Bontrager, "Arthrography," p 615; Tortora and Grabowski, "Articulations," p 217; Tortorici and Apfel, "Knee Arthrography," p 31, 1995.

159. **(D)** It is important to know all of the topographic landmarks of the body, especially when positioning the vertebral column. The third lumbar vertebra is located by finding the umbilicus as a topographic landmark. The inferior costal margin is located at about the level of L2–3. The iliac crest is located at about the level of the L4–5 disc interspace. The anterosuperior iliac spine indicates the level of approximately S1–2. Knowing the topographic landmark for the first sacral segment is useful when positioning the hips, pelvis, and sacrum.

Ballinger, Vol 1, p 40; Bontrager, "Positioning Principles," p 52.

160. **(B)** The maxillary sinuses can best be demonstrated in the parietoacanthial (Waters) projection. This method should project the petrous pyramids well below the maxillary sinuses, allowing complete demonstration. The PA (Caldwell) projection is done mainly for the frontal and anterior ethmoid sinuses. The SMV projection is done mainly for the sphenoid and ethmoid sinuses, and although the maxillary sinuses can be seen, they are not well demonstrated. The lateral projection demonstrates all sets of sinuses, but it is done mainly to demonstrate the sphenoid sinuses and is *not* the best method for demonstrating the maxillary sinuses.

Ballinger, Vol 2, pp 382–383; Bontrager, "Paranasal Sinuses," pp 397–399; Cornuelle and Gronefeld, "Facial Bones and Paranasal Sinuses," p 373; Greathouse, "Skull and Facial Bones," Vol 1, pp 542–543.

161. **(A)** Radiography is important for visualizing bony tissue as well as associated soft tissue. In some cases, minor changes in the appearance of the soft tissue, such as the fat pads, may be the only indicator of a pathology or disease process. This is mainly true in children whose soft bones may easily hide a greenstick fracture or a supracondylar fracture. The main soft-tissue areas of concern are those located around the joints of the upper limb, such as the elbow and wrist. To best demonstrate the fat pads of the elbow, the elbow must be in a true lateral position flexed at a 90° angle.

Ballinger, Vol 1, p 102; Bontrager, "Upper Limb," p 111.

162. **(D)** The flexures in the colon turn sharply from one section to another and are often hard to see on a routine AP or PA projection. Thus, the patient must be rotated to open up the flexures. The right hepatic flexure is best demonstrated with the left posterior oblique or the RAO projection, and the left splenic flexure is best demonstrated using the right posterior oblique or the left anterior oblique projection.

Ballinger, Vol 2, pp 135 & 140; Bontrager, "Lower Gastrointestinal Tract," pp 473 & 475; Cornuelle and Gronefeld, "Digestive System," pp 474–475.

163. **(B)** The proximal row of carpal bones in the wrist from lateral to medial are (1) the scaphoid (navicular) bone, (2) lunate (semilunar) bone, (3) triquetrum (triangular or cuneiform bone), and (4) pisiform bone. Of these four, the scaphoid, or navicular, bone is the largest carpal bone. The distal row from lateral to medial consists of (1) the trapezium (greater multangular), (2) trapezoid (lesser multangular) bone, (3) capitate bone (os magnum), and (4) hamate (unciform) bone. Of all of the carpal bones, the capitate bone, or os magnum, is the largest.

Ballinger, Vol 1, p 60; Bontrager, "Hand and Wrist," p 104; Cornuelle and Gronefeld, "Upper Limb (Extremity)," p 103.

164. **(C)** There are four main chambers of the heart. The upper chambers called the atria receive blood from veins. The lower chambers called ventricles pump blood out through arteries. The right atrium receives blood from the systemic circulation from both the superior and inferior venae cavae. It next travels to the *right ventricle, which pumps the deoxygenated blood out through the pulmonary trunk; the pulmonary trunk splits into right and left pulmonary arteries,* which send blood to the lungs for oxygen. After receiving oxygen from the lungs, the blood then returns through the pulmonary veins and dumps the oxygenated blood into the left atrium. It then travels to the left ventricle, where the oxygenated blood is then pumped out through the aortic arch and sent to the rest of the body.

Ballinger, Vol 2, p 516; Tortora and Grabowski, "The Cardiovascular System: The Heart," p 597; Tortorici and Apfel, "Pulmonary Angiography," p 226.

165. **(B)** The transthoracic lateral projection of the upper humerus is used to demonstrate fractures and/or dislocations when the patient is unable to move his or her upper arm. To best demonstrate pathology in this area, the humerus should be radiographed with the epicondyles perpendicular to the plane of the cassette. However, this may be contraindicated in the case of suspected fractures or dislocations. In that case, the patient's arms should not be moved, but the patient's body should be rotated to place the arm midway between the vertebral column and sternum, ensuring that the epicondyles are placed perpendicular to the plane of the cassette.

Ballinger, Vol 2, p 118; Bontrager, "Shoulder: Trauma Routine," p 163; Cornuelle and Gronefeld, "Upper Limb (Extremity)," pp 144–145; Eisenberg et al., "Humerus," p 77.

166. **(A)** The movement of a body part toward the midline is termed *adduction.* Movement away from the midline is termed *abduction. Eversion* is rotation of a part outward, as in moving the toes laterally. *Supination* refers to rotating a part into the supine position (on one's back); it is the opposite of pronation.

Ballinger, Vol 1, p 56; Bontrager, "Terminology," pp 24–27; Cornuelle and Gronefeld, "Introduction to Radiography," pp 11–13.

167. **(D)** The hilum of an organ is a depression usually located on the medial aspect of that organ where the blood vessels, nerves, and other structures enter or exit. On the kidney, the hilum allows the entrance of the renal artery and the exit of the renal vein as well as the ureter.

Ballinger, Vol 2, pp 137–139; Bontrager, "Urinary System," p 507; Tortora and Grabowski, "Urinary System," p 865.

168. **(C)** With the patient's head properly positioned using the Rhese method, the optic foramen should be demonstrated in the lower outer quadrant of the orbit. For this position, the patient's head should be rotated from the true PA so that the midsagittal plane forms an angle of 53° to the plane of the cassette. Also, the acanthiomeatal

line should be aligned so that it is perpendicular to the cassette.

Ballinger, Vol 2, pp 258–259; Bontrager, "Optic Foramen," p 374.

169. **(B)** Normally, diverticula and ulcers (often seen in Crohn's disease) are easily filled with barium or water-soluble contrast medium. Polyps, on the other hand, do not easily fill with barium and will cause a void in the filling of the colon. Therefore, if the colon is not properly prepared and traces of fecal material are still in the large intestine, these will not fill with barium and may easily be mistaken for polyposis.

Ballinger, Vol 2, p 211; Bontrager, "Lower Gastrointestinal Tract," p 460.

170. **(B)** The routine projections for a sternum usually include an RAO and a lateral projection. The oblique requires a breathing technique with a long exposure. However, for the lateral projection, the sternum is best demonstrated when the patient is instructed to suspend respiration on full inhalation.

Ballinger, Vol 1, p 372; Bontrager, "Sternum," p 315.

SECTION V: PATIENT CARE

171. **(B)** A specific type of shock that is associated with the pooling of blood in the peripheral vessels is *neurogenic shock,* also called *vasogenic shock.* It is most often seen in cases of severe trauma, such as head injuries or injuries to the spinal cord. Damage to the central nervous system results in decreased arterial resistance and pooling of blood in the peripheral vessels of the upper and lower limbs. A similar type of shock is called *cardiogenic shock,* caused by insufficient cardiac output usually due to a myocardial infarction, pulmonary embolus, or cardiac tamponade. *Hypovolemic shock* is caused by a decrease in blood volume due to a massive hemorrhage from severe trauma. *Septic shock* occurs when the bloodstream has been exposed to a toxin such as bacteria.

Adler and Carlton, "Medical Emergencies," p 260; Kowalczyk, "Patient Care in Critical Situations," pp 211–213; Torres, "Medical Emergencies in Diagnostic Imaging," p 154.

172. **(D)** If a patient is suffering from respiratory arrest and still has a pulse, the rescuer should breathe for the adult victim once every 5 seconds (12 times per minute). For infants and children up to 8 years old, the rescue breaths should be given at a rate of one breath every 3 seconds (20 times per minute).

AHA, "Adult Basic Life Support," pp 4–7.

173. **(A)** When the body temperature in an adult consistently falls below 95°F during oral temperature monitoring, the patient is labeled as hypothermic. Hypothermia may be medically induced, such as in cases of heart surgery, or it may be as a result of a disease process.

Adler and Carlton, "Vital Signs and Oxygen," p 181; Mosby's Medical, Nursing and Allied Health Dictionary, p 803.

174. **(C)** One of the most important vital signs is a patient's arterial blood pressure. The blood pressure is measured for both phases of the heart rhythm and is measured in units of millimeters of mercury (mm Hg). Systole is the phase in which blood pressure is the highest because it is the contraction phase when the ventricles contract to force blood into the arterial system. Diastole is the phase of relaxation in which blood is allowed to drain back into the top chambers (atria) of the heart. The blood pressure is designated by how much force is exerted on the walls of the arteries during both phases. The systolic pressure is mentioned first and is the top number. The diastolic pressure is the bottom number. Thus, in this example, the systolic pressure is 120 mm Hg.

Adler and Carlton, "Vital Signs and Oxygen," pp 185–186; Kowalczyk, "Patient Assessment & Assistance," p 113.

175. **(A)** Whenever there is suspicion of an obstructed airway, the first step should be to perform the Heimlich maneuver so that air may be forced through the trachea to dislodge the foreign body. Inserting an ET tube after emergency tracheostomy should be a last resort after all efforts of dislodging the foreign body have failed.

Adler and Carlton, "Medical Emergencies," pp 262–263; AHA, "Adult Basic Life Support," pp 416–417; Kowalczyk, "Patient Care in Critical Situations," pp 202–203.

176. **(D)** The proper medical term for a nosebleed is *epistaxis.*

Adler and Carlton, "Medical Emergencies," p 258; Mosby's Medical, Nursing and Allied Health Dictionary, p 578.

177. **(A)** A patient's head injury can vary in severity based on level of consciousness. The patient with the least serious head injury is said to be alert and responsive. The worst-case scenario would be a patient in a comatose state who does not respond to any stimuli. If a radiographer is examining a patient with a head injury, it is imperative that the level of consciousness be noted so any changes may alert the radiographer to ask for medical assistance. The first priority of the radiographer when caring for the patient with a head

injury should be to maintain an open airway. A head injury may cause airway obstruction as a result of a loss of the gag reflex, relaxation of the tongue, or the presence of fluid drainage (e.g., blood, cerebrospinal fluid, etc.) into the throat.

Adler and Carlton, "Medical Emergencies," p 260; Torres, "Care of Patients with Special Problems," p 186.

178. **(B)** The normal respiration rate for an adult at rest can range from 12 to 20 breaths per minute. If the respiration rate falls below 10 breaths per minute, the person may suffer from cyanosis, apprehension, restlessness, or loss of consciousness. If the rate exceeds 20 breaths per minute, the patient may suffer from hyperventilation and may also lose consciousness. The respiration rate for a child under the age of 10 is much faster and may range from 20 to 30 breaths per minute.

Adler and Carlton, "Vital Signs and Oxygen," p 162; Kowalczyk, "Patient Assessment and Assistance," p 112; Torres, "Vital Signs and Oxygen Administration," pp 136–137.

179. **(C)** Barium sulfate is categorized as a suspension, not a solution, meaning that it cannot dissolve in water. Barium will temporarily be suspended in a solution, but eventually it will settle to the bottom of a cup or enema bag. Barium sulfate cannot be absorbed by the body, and if it is introduced to the pelvic or peritoneal cavity, it must be surgically removed. This is why it cannot be used as a contrast material for any type of IV or intrathecal injections, or when there may be a possibility of a bowel perforation.

Adler and Carlton, "Contrast Media," pp 303–308; Kowalczyk, "Medication Administration," p 190; Torres, "Patient Care during Imaging Examinations of the Gastrointestinal System," p 200.

180. **(C)** The most common method of assessing the body temperature is orally. Therefore, the radiographer should be familiar with the normal oral body temperature, which is 98.6°F or 37°C.

Kowalczyk, "Patient Assessment and Assistance," pp 129–130; Torres, "Vital Signs and Oxygen Administration," pp 73–74.

181. **(C)** Universal precautions, as set forth by the Centers for Disease Control and Prevention, advise all health-care workers to assume that all patients may be infectious. Certain guidelines should be considered mandatory practice, such as frequent hand washing and the wearing of proper protective gear such as gloves, gowns, masks, and/or eye shields as necessary. Needles should *never* be recapped, but rather discarded in a proper "sharps guard" container. Recapping

needles is one of the leading causes of infection among health-care workers and is considered a very dangerous practice because so many serious infectious diseases can be transmitted by contact with blood and body fluids. Latex gloves should be worn routinely whenever cleaning up any type of spill, especially those that contain blood or body fluids. Latex gloves are very effective barriers to microorganisms. Unfortunately, they are not effective protection against sharp objects such as needles or razors, which should be handled extremely carefully. When dealing with a surgical or trauma case, or even a barium enema on an uncooperative patient, a protective eye shield and mask should be worn to protect against any body fluids that may splash onto the face.

Centers for Disease Control Infection Control Guidelines, 1997; Kowalczyk, "Infection Control and Aseptic Technique," p 86; Torres, "Infection Control," p 52.

182. **(D)** Freely discussing a patient's medical information with any individual who is not directly responsible for that patient's care is not only morally and ethically wrong, but also may expose a health-care worker to a lawsuit. All patients have the right to confidential medical care. The legal grounds may be based on a patient's right to privacy, and the patient may sue based on breech of patient confidentiality. Another form of invasion of privacy may be improper covering of a patient, negating a person's right to privacy.

Kowalczyk, "Medical Ethics and Legalities," pp 69–70; Obergfell, "Standard of Care, Patient Rights, and Informed Consent," p 85; Wilson, "Basic Concepts of Medical Law," p 147.

183. **(B)** When a radiographer is involved in venipuncture during the administration of a contrast medium, infiltration or extravasation of fluids may occur. Some signs and symptoms of extravasation include redness, swelling, and a painful burning sensation around the injection site. If the radiographer sees signs of extravasation, the first thing to do is to remove the needle and to apply pressure. A warm compress is also helpful in aiding the surrounding tissues to absorb some of the excess fluid. However, leaving the needle in and continuing contrast administration is never good practice because this will only worsen the condition.

Kowalczyk, "Medication Administration," p 188.

184. **(C)** A radiographer who performs the wrong examination on a patient may be charged with battery. *Battery* is defined as the unlawful laying of hands on a patient. *Assault* is the threat of touching a patient without actually ever touching the

patient. *Negligence* is failing to provide proper care or safety to a patient, such as not strapping an elderly patient to a table who then falls and fractures a hip. *Breech of patient confidentiality* is usually charged as an invasion of privacy in which confidential records are discussed with persons not directly involved with that patient's care.

Adler and Carlton, "Medical Law," p 348; Kowalczyk, "Medical Ethics & Law," pp 68–69; Obergfell, "Civil Liability," pp 44–45; Wilson, "Basic Concepts of Medical Law," p 145.

185. **(A)** Whenever a patient is under respiratory distress, oxygen administration is usually recommended. Not all respiratory diseases require a high rate of flow. For instance, chronic respiratory diseases, such as pulmonary emphysema, usually require oxygen therapy through a nasal cannula at a flow rate of about 2 to 3 L/min. This lower flow rate is required because the long-term prescription of oxygen can dry out the nasal mucosa.

Ehrlich and McCloskey, "Dealing with Acute Situations," pp 220–221; Torres, "Vital Signs and Oxygen Administration," p 142.

186. **(D)** It is essential that a patient have no stomach contents prior to receiving a UGI examination to ensure proper diagnosis. Most patients are told to withhold food and water for a period of at least 8 hours prior to the procedure. Also, smoking and/or chewing gum may stimulate the stomach to release gastric enzymes that may dilute some of the barium suspension, thus interfering with its coating ability. Therefore, the patient should be instructed to refrain from food, smoking, and gum chewing after midnight prior to the UGI examination.

Ballinger, Vol 2, p 98; Bontrager, "Upper GI Series," p 432.

187. **(B)** *Postural hypotension*, also called *orthostatic hypotension*, is a condition in which the blood pressure will suddenly fall when a patient rises quickly from the recumbent position, causing dizziness and sometimes syncope. This is a very common problem in elderly patients, as well as those who have suffered hemorrhage due to trauma or who are under the influence of certain drugs. Thus, a radiographer should be very gentle and carefully observe patients as they are sitting a patient up from the recumbent position.

Ehrlich and McCloskey, "Safety, Transfer & Positioning," p 98; Kowalczyk, "Patient Assessment and Assistance," p 116.

188. **(B)** The pulse rate is usually measured in units of beats per minute. The normal resting pulse rate for an adult ranges anywhere from 80 to 100 beats per minute. The blood pressure is measured in millimeters of mercury (mm Hg) and is taken twice, once at systole and once at diastole. In the United States, the body temperature is usually measured in °F.

Adler and Carlton, "Vital Signs & Oxygen," p 183; Kowalczyk, "Patient Assessment and Assistance," p 112.

189. **(B)** The most common means of spreading a respiratory disease is by airborne or droplet infection. This occurs when an infectious person coughs or sneezes and microscopic droplets are dispersed into the air. A host will then inhale these droplets and become infected. Respiratory diseases can also be spread by direct contact and by touching contaminated objects, but these are far less common modes of transmission. The best protection against droplet infection is a mask worn by both the patient and the health-care workers involved in that patient's care.

Ehrlich and McCloskey, "Infection Control," p 147; Kowalczyk, "Infection Control and Aseptic Technique," p 82.

190. **(C)** Whenever preparing for an invasive procedure, it is always important to thoroughly clean the injection site of the patient. This is done with some form of topical antiseptic that is meant to kill most of the germs of the surrounding area. The two most commonly used agents for this purpose are povidone-iodine and isopropyl alcohol. Surgical asepsis is required for all medical personnel performing certain invasive procedures and for all of the invasive equipment, such as needles, catheters, guide wires, contrast media, and so forth. However, the patient cannot be completely sterilized without damaging the skin. Alcohol and povidone-iodine are highly effective and are also safe topical treatments.

Ehrlich and McCloskey, "Infection Control," p 172; Mosby's Medical, Nursing and Allied Health Dictionary, pp 56, 1304; Torres, "Surgical Asepsis," pp 120.

191. **(B)** An infusion port is sometimes inserted into a large vein in the chest and fed through to the right atrium of the heart. The port is usually placed into the patient surgically under a local anesthetic. This is for the purpose of continuous infusion of fluids such as blood products, medications, chemotherapy treatment, and parenteral nutrition. A common type of infusion port is called a *Hickman catheter*, which is used for very ill chemotherapy patients who cannot receive treatment by any other means.

Kowalczyk, "Tubes, Catheters and Vascular Access Lines," p 144; Taber's Cyclopedic Medical Dictionary, p 900.

192. **(B)** An *emetic* is an agent that is sometimes used to induce vomiting. A common "over-the-counter" example would be ipecac. It is most often used in emergency situations when a patient has swallowed a toxic chemical or substance.

Gylys and Wedding, "Gastrointestinal System," p 106; Taber's Cyclopedic Medical Dictionary, p 626.

193. **(A)** Nonionic contrast agents have gained great popularity within the last decade because of their low incidence of patient reactions. There are two reasons for this. One is that because the iodine is nonionic, it is much less likely to cross the cellular membrane through osmosis to interact with tissues in the body; this is termed *low osmolality*. The second is that it is much less toxic because it is less likely to interact chemically through ionic bonding. One drawback of nonionic contrast agents, however, is their high cost. In general, they usually cost three times as much as their ionic counterparts. So, the benefits to the patient have to be weighed against the added cost of the procedure.

Bontrager, "Urinary System," p 511; Kowalczyk, "Medication Administration," p 192; Torres, "Assisting with Drug Administration," p 211.

194. **(D)** A *host*, or *reservoir*, is any environment that promotes the growth of microbes, such as a warm, moist atmosphere with an appropriate pH and sufficient light. The most common reservoir is the human body. An inanimate object, such as a table or door handle, may also become a carrier of an infectious microorganism. If a person becomes infected through contact with inanimate objects, this mode of transmission is known as *fomes* transmission. If an individual becomes infected through contact with an animal or insect, this mode of transmission is called a *vector*. If an individual becomes infected through contaminated food or water, this is known as a *vehicle* transmission.

Ehrlich and McCloskey, "Infection Control," p 146–147; Kowalczyk, "Infection Control and Aseptic Technique," pp 80–82; Torres, "Infection Control," p 46.

195. **(B)** Some types of IV contrast agents are categorized according to their viscosity (density or thickness). Some contrast agents are so viscous that they may be difficult to inject without the use of a power injector. If a power injector is not available, most manufacturers recommend warming the contrast to body temperature to make it less viscous and easier to inject. This is usually done in a contrast warmer, but may also be done by placing the bottle into a tub of tepid water.

Ehrlich and McCloskey, "Contrast Media and Spe-

cial Imaging Techniques," p 268; Tortorici, "Contrast Media," p 20.

196. **(B)** Emphysema is a chronic disease of the lungs in which the patient has great difficulty in breathing due to increased dilation of the alveoli. A patient with emphysema has difficulty breathing especially when lying down. The most comfortable position for them is the upright position. This condition is called *orthopnea*, which literally means "straight breathing." *Bradycardia* is a slow heart rate, which is usually not indicative of emphysema. *Epistaxis* means nosebleed, and *dysphagia* is difficulty in swallowing.

Gylys and Wedding, "Respiratory System," p 126.

197. **(C)** There are two major blood tests that should be done prior to administering IV contrast. These are the BUN and the creatinine laboratory tests that are meant to check for urinary function. If either of these two results are found "out-of-range," the physician should be informed immediately because they could be indicative of renal failure. The normal BUN range should fall between 8 and 23 mg/100 mL. The normal creatinine range should fall between 0.6 and 1.5 mg/100 mL.

Cornuelle and Gronefeld, "The Urinary System," p 421; Laudicina, "Genitourinary System," p 110; Mosby's Medical, Nursing and Allied Health Dictionary, pp 1837, 1838; Taber's Cyclopedic Medical Dictionary, pp 2199, 2201; Tortora and Grabowski, "The Urinary System," p 888.

198. **(C)** The gauge indicates the diameter of the needle. The diameter is one of the most important factors in choosing a needle for injection because this will determine the flow rate of the IV fluids. Usually larger gauges, such as 15- or 18-gauge, are selected for withdrawing blood, and smaller gauges (21, 23, or 25) are used for injections of medications.

Ehrlich and McCloskey, "Medications and Their Administration," p 193; Garza and Becan-McBride, "Collection Reagents, Supplies, and Interfering Chemical Substances," p 78; Torres, "Drug Administration," p 278.

199. **(C)** When a patient is brought into the emergency room with a cardiac arrest, sometimes it is because the heart has gone into spasms and cannot assume its normal cardiac rhythm. This is called *ventricular fibrillation*, or *V-fib*. This can often be corrected by the use of an electrical stimulation device called a *defibrillator*. Also, a patient can "code" in the radiology department for the same reason, so all crash carts in the department should have a defibrillator located on the top

of the cart. A sphygmomanometer and pulse oximeter are both monitoring devices and should not affect the normal sinus rhythm of the heart.

Kowalczyk, "Patient Care in Critical Situations," p 205; Taber's Cyclopedic Medical Dictionary, p 498.

200. **(D)** An intrathecal injection is an injection into the spinal canal; it can be epidural, subdural, or subarachnoid. This type of injection requires the patient to be either in a prone position, a lateral position, or seated and bent forward. If the patient is supine, the spinal canal is much harder to access.

Ballinger, Vol 2, p 501; Bontrager, "Myelography," p 621; Tortorici and Apfel, "Myelography," pp 78–79.

BIBLIOGRAPHY

Adler, AM, and Carlton RR: Introduction to Radiography and Patient Care. WB Saunders, Philadelphia, 1993.

American Heart Association (AHA): Basic Life Support for Healthcare Providers. Author, Dallas, TX, 1997.

Ballinger, PW: Merrill's Atlas of Radiographic Positions and Radiologic Procedures, ed 8. Mosby-Year Book, St. Louis, 1995.

Bontrager, KL: Textbook of Radiographic Positioning and Related Anatomy, ed 4. Mosby-Year Book, St. Louis, 1997.

Burns, EF: Radiographic Imaging: A Guide to Producing Quality Radiographs. WB Saunders, Philadelphia, 1992.

Bushong, S: Radiologic Science for Technologists: Physics, Biology and Protection, ed. 6. Mosby-Year Book, St. Louis, 1997.

Carlton, RR, and McKenna-Adler, A: Principles of Radiographic Imaging: An Art and A Science. ed 2. Delmar, Albany, 1996.

Carroll, QB: Fuchs's Radiographic Exposure, Processing and Quality Control, ed 6. Charles C Thomas, Springfield, IL, 1998.

Centers for Disease Control and Prevention: Infection Control Standards & Guidelines for Healthcare Workers. Author, Atlanta, 1997.

Cornuelle, AG, and Gronefeld, DH: Radiographic Anatomy & Positioning: An Integrated Approach, Appleton & Lange, Stamford, CT, 1998.

Cullinan, AM: Producing Quality Radiographs, ed 2. Lippincott, Philadelphia, 1994.

Curry, TS, et al: Christensen's Physics of Diagnostic Radiology, ed 4. Lea & Febiger, Philadelphia, 1990.

Dennis, CA, and Eisenberg, RL: Applied Radiographic Calculations, WB Saunders, Philadelphia, 1993.

Dowd, SB, and Tilson, ER: Practical Radiation Protection and Applied Radiobiology. WB Saunders, Philadelphia, 1999.

Ehrlich, RA, and McCloskey, ED: Patient Care in Radiography, ed 5. Mosby, St. Louis, 1999.

Eisenberg, RL, and Dennis, CA: Comprehensive Radiographic Pathology, ed 2. Mosby, St. Louis, 1995.

Eisenberg, RL, et al: Radiographic Positioning. Little Brown and Co., Boston, 1989.

Garza, D, and Becan-McBride K: Phlebotomy Handbook, ed 3. Appleton & Lange, Norwalk, CT, 1993.

Gould, BE: Pathophysiology for the Health Related Professions. WB Saunders, Philadelphia, 1997.

Gray, JE, et al: Quality Control in Diagnostic Imaging. University Park Press, Baltimore, 1983.

Greathouse, JS: Radiographic Positioning & Procedures, 3 vols. Delmar, Albany, NY, 1998.

Gurley, LT, and Callaway, WJ: Introduction to Radiologic Technology, ed 4. Mosby, St. Louis, 1996.

Gylys, BA, and Wedding, ME: Medical Terminology: A Systems Approach, ed 3. FA Davis, Philadelphia, 1995.

Hendee, WR: Medical Radiation Physics: Roentgenology, Nuclear Medicine and Ultrasound, ed 2. Year Book Medical Publishers, Chicago, 1979.

Hiss, SS: Understanding Radiography, ed 3. Charles C Thomas, Springfield, IL, 1993.

Ireland, SJ: Integrated Mathematics of Radiographic Exposure. Mosby, St. Louis, 1994.

Kowalczyk, N: Integrated Patient Care for the Imaging Professional. Mosby, St. Louis, 1996.

Laudicina, P: Applied Pathology for Radiographers. WB Saunders, Philadelphia, 1989.

Linn-Watson, TA: Radiographic Pathology. WB Saunders, Philadelphia, 1996.

Mace, JD, and Kowalczyk, N: Radiographic Pathology, ed 2. Mosby-Year Book, St. Louis, 1994.

Mallett, M: Anatomy and Physiology for Students of Medical Radiation Technology. Burnell, Mankato, MN, 1981.

Malott, JC, and Fodor, J: The Art and Science of Medical Radiography, ed 7. Mosby, St. Louis, 1993.

McKinney, WEJ: Radiographic Processing and Quality Control. Lippincott, Philadelphia, 1988.

McKinnis, LN: Fundamentals of Orthopedic Radiology. FA Davis, Philadelphia, 1997.

Memmler, RL, and Wood, DL: The Human Body in Health & Disease, ed 5. JB Lippincott, Philadelphia, 1983.

Mosby's Medical, Nursing and Allied Health Dictionary, ed 3. Mosby, St. Louis, 1993.

National Council on Radiation Protection and Measurements (NCRP): Limitation of Exposure to Ionizing Radiation. Report No. 116. National Council on Radiation Protection and Measurement, Bethesda, MD, 1993.

NCRP: Medical X-ray Electron Beam and Gamma-Ray Protection for Energies up to 50 MeV (Equipment Design, Performance and Use.) Report No. 102. National Council on Radiation Protection and Measurements, Bethesda, MD, 1989.

NCRP: Quality Assurance for Diagnostic Imaging. Report No. 99. National Council on Radiation Protection and Measurements, Bethesda, MD, 1988.

NCRP: Radiation Protection for Medical and Allied Health Personnel. Report No. 105. National Council on Radiation Protection and Measurements, Bethesda, MD, 1989.

Obergfell, AM: Law and Ethics in Diagnostic Imaging and Therapeutic Radiology. WB Saunders, Philadelphia, 1995.

Papp, J: Quality Management in the Radiologic Sciences. Mosby, St. Louis, 1998.

Scanlon, VC, and Sanders, T: Essentials of Anatomy and Physiology, ed 2. FA Davis, Philadelphia, 1991.

Selman, J: The Fundamentals of X-ray and Radium Physics, ed 8. Charles C Thomas, Springfield, IL, 1994.

Sheldon, H. Boyd's Introduction to the Study of Disease, ed 10. Lea & Febiger, Philadelphia, 1988.

Snopek, AM: Fundamentals of Special Radiographic Procedures, ed 3. WB Saunders, Philadelphia, 1992.

Spence, AP: Basic Human Anatomy, ed 3. Benjamin/Cummings, Redwood City, CA, 1990.

Springhouse Medication Administration & I.V. Therapy Manual: Process & Procedures. Springhouse Corporation, Springhouse, PA, 1988.

Statkiewicz-Sherer, MA, et al: Radiation Protection in Medical Radiography, ed 3. Mosby, St. Louis, 1998.

Sweeney, RJ: Radiographic Artifacts: Their Cause and Control. Lippincott, Philadelphia, 1983.

Taber's Cyclopedic Medical Dictionary, ed 18. FA Davis, Philadelphia, 1996.

Tamparo, CD, and Lewis, MA: Diseases of the Human Body, ed 2. FA Davis, Philadelphia, 1995.

Thompson, MA, et al: Principles of Imaging Science and Protection. WB Saunders, Philadelphia, 1994.

Torres, LS: Basic Medical Techniques and Patient Care in Imaging Technology, ed 5. Lippincott, Philadelphia, 1997.

Tortora, GJ, and Grabowski, SR: Principles of Anatomy and Physiology, ed 7. Harper-Collins, New York, 1993.

Tortorici, MR, Concepts in Medical Radiographic Imaging: Circuitry, Exposure and Quality Control. WB Saunders, Philadelphia, 1992.

Tortorici, MR, and Apfel, PJ: Advanced Radiographic and Angiographic Procedures. FA Davis, Philadelphia, 1995.

Travis, EL: Primer of Medical Radiobiology, ed 2. Year Book, Chicago, 1989.

Wallace, JE: Radiographic Exposure: Principles & Practice. FA Davis, Philadelphia, 1995.

Wilson, BG: Ethics and Basic Law for Medical Imaging Professionals. FA Davis, Philadelphia, 1997.

Wolbarst, AB: Physics of Radiology. Appleton & Lange, Norwalk, CT, 1993.

SIMULATION TEST #4

NAME_____

Last   First   Middle

ADDRESS _____

Street

_____

City   State   Zip

· ·

MAKE
ERASURES
COMPLETE

PLEASE USE NO. 2 PENCIL ONLY.

↓ BEGIN HERE

**Radiation Protection
and Radiobiology**

01 Ⓐ Ⓑ Ⓒ Ⓓ	21 Ⓐ Ⓑ Ⓒ Ⓓ	41 Ⓐ Ⓑ Ⓒ Ⓓ	**Image Production and Evaluation** 61 Ⓐ Ⓑ Ⓒ Ⓓ
02 Ⓐ Ⓑ Ⓒ Ⓓ	22 Ⓐ Ⓑ Ⓒ Ⓓ	42 Ⓐ Ⓑ Ⓒ Ⓓ	62 Ⓐ Ⓑ Ⓒ Ⓓ
03 Ⓐ Ⓑ Ⓒ Ⓓ	23 Ⓐ Ⓑ Ⓒ Ⓓ	43 Ⓐ Ⓑ Ⓒ Ⓓ	63 Ⓐ Ⓑ Ⓒ Ⓓ
04 Ⓐ Ⓑ Ⓒ Ⓓ	24 Ⓐ Ⓑ Ⓒ Ⓓ	44 Ⓐ Ⓑ Ⓒ Ⓓ	64 Ⓐ Ⓑ Ⓒ Ⓓ
05 Ⓐ Ⓑ Ⓒ Ⓓ	25 Ⓐ Ⓑ Ⓒ Ⓓ	45 Ⓐ Ⓑ Ⓒ Ⓓ	65 Ⓐ Ⓑ Ⓒ Ⓓ
06 Ⓐ Ⓑ Ⓒ Ⓓ	26 Ⓐ Ⓑ Ⓒ Ⓓ	46 Ⓐ Ⓑ Ⓒ Ⓓ	66 Ⓐ Ⓑ Ⓒ Ⓓ
07 Ⓐ Ⓑ Ⓒ Ⓓ	27 Ⓐ Ⓑ Ⓒ Ⓓ	47 Ⓐ Ⓑ Ⓒ Ⓓ	67 Ⓐ Ⓑ Ⓒ Ⓓ
08 Ⓐ Ⓑ Ⓒ Ⓓ	28 Ⓐ Ⓑ Ⓒ Ⓓ	48 Ⓐ Ⓑ Ⓒ Ⓓ	68 Ⓐ Ⓑ Ⓒ Ⓓ
09 Ⓐ Ⓑ Ⓒ Ⓓ	29 Ⓐ Ⓑ Ⓒ Ⓓ	49 Ⓐ Ⓑ Ⓒ Ⓓ	69 Ⓐ Ⓑ Ⓒ Ⓓ
10 Ⓐ Ⓑ Ⓒ Ⓓ	30 Ⓐ Ⓑ Ⓒ Ⓓ	50 Ⓐ Ⓑ Ⓒ Ⓓ	70 Ⓐ Ⓑ Ⓒ Ⓓ
11 Ⓐ Ⓑ Ⓒ Ⓓ	**Equipment Operation and Maintenance** 31 Ⓐ Ⓑ Ⓒ Ⓓ	51 Ⓐ Ⓑ Ⓒ Ⓓ	71 Ⓐ Ⓑ Ⓒ Ⓓ
12 Ⓐ Ⓑ Ⓒ Ⓓ	32 Ⓐ Ⓑ Ⓒ Ⓓ	52 Ⓐ Ⓑ Ⓒ Ⓓ	72 Ⓐ Ⓑ Ⓒ Ⓓ
13 Ⓐ Ⓑ Ⓒ Ⓓ	33 Ⓐ Ⓑ Ⓒ Ⓓ	53 Ⓐ Ⓑ Ⓒ Ⓓ	73 Ⓐ Ⓑ Ⓒ Ⓓ
14 Ⓐ Ⓑ Ⓒ Ⓓ	34 Ⓐ Ⓑ Ⓒ Ⓓ	54 Ⓐ Ⓑ Ⓒ Ⓓ	74 Ⓐ Ⓑ Ⓒ Ⓓ
15 Ⓐ Ⓑ Ⓒ Ⓓ	35 Ⓐ Ⓑ Ⓒ Ⓓ	55 Ⓐ Ⓑ Ⓒ Ⓓ	75 Ⓐ Ⓑ Ⓒ Ⓓ
16 Ⓐ Ⓑ Ⓒ Ⓓ	36 Ⓐ Ⓑ Ⓒ Ⓓ	56 Ⓐ Ⓑ Ⓒ Ⓓ	76 Ⓐ Ⓑ Ⓒ Ⓓ
17 Ⓐ Ⓑ Ⓒ Ⓓ	37 Ⓐ Ⓑ Ⓒ Ⓓ	57 Ⓐ Ⓑ Ⓒ Ⓓ	77 Ⓐ Ⓑ Ⓒ Ⓓ
18 Ⓐ Ⓑ Ⓒ Ⓓ	38 Ⓐ Ⓑ Ⓒ Ⓓ	58 Ⓐ Ⓑ Ⓒ Ⓓ	78 Ⓐ Ⓑ Ⓒ Ⓓ
19 Ⓐ Ⓑ Ⓒ Ⓓ	39 Ⓐ Ⓑ Ⓒ Ⓓ	59 Ⓐ Ⓑ Ⓒ Ⓓ	79 Ⓐ Ⓑ Ⓒ Ⓓ
20 Ⓐ Ⓑ Ⓒ Ⓓ	40 Ⓐ Ⓑ Ⓒ Ⓓ	60 Ⓐ Ⓑ Ⓒ Ⓓ	80 Ⓐ Ⓑ Ⓒ Ⓓ

081 Ⓐ Ⓑ Ⓒ Ⓓ

Radiographic Procedures and Related Anatomy

082 Ⓐ Ⓑ Ⓒ Ⓓ
083 Ⓐ Ⓑ Ⓒ Ⓓ
084 Ⓐ Ⓑ Ⓒ Ⓓ
085 Ⓐ Ⓑ Ⓒ Ⓓ
086 Ⓐ Ⓑ Ⓒ Ⓓ
087 Ⓐ Ⓑ Ⓒ Ⓓ
088 Ⓐ Ⓑ Ⓒ Ⓓ
089 Ⓐ Ⓑ Ⓒ Ⓓ
090 Ⓐ Ⓑ Ⓒ Ⓓ
091 Ⓐ Ⓑ Ⓒ Ⓓ
092 Ⓐ Ⓑ Ⓒ Ⓓ
093 Ⓐ Ⓑ Ⓒ Ⓓ
094 Ⓐ Ⓑ Ⓒ Ⓓ
095 Ⓐ Ⓑ Ⓒ Ⓓ
096 Ⓐ Ⓑ Ⓒ Ⓓ
097 Ⓐ Ⓑ Ⓒ Ⓓ
098 Ⓐ Ⓑ Ⓒ Ⓓ
099 Ⓐ Ⓑ Ⓒ Ⓓ
100 Ⓐ Ⓑ Ⓒ Ⓓ
101 Ⓐ Ⓑ Ⓒ Ⓓ
102 Ⓐ Ⓑ Ⓒ Ⓓ
103 Ⓐ Ⓑ Ⓒ Ⓓ
104 Ⓐ Ⓑ Ⓒ Ⓓ
105 Ⓐ Ⓑ Ⓒ Ⓓ
106 Ⓐ Ⓑ Ⓒ Ⓓ
107 Ⓐ Ⓑ Ⓒ Ⓓ
108 Ⓐ Ⓑ Ⓒ Ⓓ
109 Ⓐ Ⓑ Ⓒ Ⓓ
110 Ⓐ Ⓑ Ⓒ Ⓓ

111 Ⓐ Ⓑ Ⓒ Ⓓ
112 Ⓐ Ⓑ Ⓒ Ⓓ
113 Ⓐ Ⓑ Ⓒ Ⓓ
114 Ⓐ Ⓑ Ⓒ Ⓓ
115 Ⓐ Ⓑ Ⓒ Ⓓ
116 Ⓐ Ⓑ Ⓒ Ⓓ
117 Ⓐ Ⓑ Ⓒ Ⓓ
118 Ⓐ Ⓑ Ⓒ Ⓓ
119 Ⓐ Ⓑ Ⓒ Ⓓ
120 Ⓐ Ⓑ Ⓒ Ⓓ
121 Ⓐ Ⓑ Ⓒ Ⓓ
122 Ⓐ Ⓑ Ⓒ Ⓓ
123 Ⓐ Ⓑ Ⓒ Ⓓ
124 Ⓐ Ⓑ Ⓒ Ⓓ
125 Ⓐ Ⓑ Ⓒ Ⓓ
126 Ⓐ Ⓑ Ⓒ Ⓓ
127 Ⓐ Ⓑ Ⓒ Ⓓ
128 Ⓐ Ⓑ Ⓒ Ⓓ
129 Ⓐ Ⓑ Ⓒ Ⓓ
130 Ⓐ Ⓑ Ⓒ Ⓓ
131 Ⓐ Ⓑ Ⓒ Ⓓ
132 Ⓐ Ⓑ Ⓒ Ⓓ
133 Ⓐ Ⓑ Ⓒ Ⓓ
134 Ⓐ Ⓑ Ⓒ Ⓓ
135 Ⓐ Ⓑ Ⓒ Ⓓ
136 Ⓐ Ⓑ Ⓒ Ⓓ
137 Ⓐ Ⓑ Ⓒ Ⓓ
138 Ⓐ Ⓑ Ⓒ Ⓓ
139 Ⓐ Ⓑ Ⓒ Ⓓ
140 Ⓐ Ⓑ Ⓒ Ⓓ

141 Ⓐ Ⓑ Ⓒ Ⓓ
142 Ⓐ Ⓑ Ⓒ Ⓓ
143 Ⓐ Ⓑ Ⓒ Ⓓ
144 Ⓐ Ⓑ Ⓒ Ⓓ
145 Ⓐ Ⓑ Ⓒ Ⓓ
146 Ⓐ Ⓑ Ⓒ Ⓓ
147 Ⓐ Ⓑ Ⓒ Ⓓ
148 Ⓐ Ⓑ Ⓒ Ⓓ
149 Ⓐ Ⓑ Ⓒ Ⓓ
150 Ⓐ Ⓑ Ⓒ Ⓓ
151 Ⓐ Ⓑ Ⓒ Ⓓ
152 Ⓐ Ⓑ Ⓒ Ⓓ
153 Ⓐ Ⓑ Ⓒ Ⓓ
154 Ⓐ Ⓑ Ⓒ Ⓓ
155 Ⓐ Ⓑ Ⓒ Ⓓ
156 Ⓐ Ⓑ Ⓒ Ⓓ
157 Ⓐ Ⓑ Ⓒ Ⓓ
158 Ⓐ Ⓑ Ⓒ Ⓓ
159 Ⓐ Ⓑ Ⓒ Ⓓ
160 Ⓐ Ⓑ Ⓒ Ⓓ
161 Ⓐ Ⓑ Ⓒ Ⓓ
162 Ⓐ Ⓑ Ⓒ Ⓓ
163 Ⓐ Ⓑ Ⓒ Ⓓ
164 Ⓐ Ⓑ Ⓒ Ⓓ
165 Ⓐ Ⓑ Ⓒ Ⓓ
166 Ⓐ Ⓑ Ⓒ Ⓓ
167 Ⓐ Ⓑ Ⓒ Ⓓ
168 Ⓐ Ⓑ Ⓒ Ⓓ
169 Ⓐ Ⓑ Ⓒ Ⓓ
170 Ⓐ Ⓑ Ⓒ Ⓓ

Patient Care

171 Ⓐ Ⓑ Ⓒ Ⓓ
172 Ⓐ Ⓑ Ⓒ Ⓓ
173 Ⓐ Ⓑ Ⓒ Ⓓ
174 Ⓐ Ⓑ Ⓒ Ⓓ
175 Ⓐ Ⓑ Ⓒ Ⓓ
176 Ⓐ Ⓑ Ⓒ Ⓓ
177 Ⓐ Ⓑ Ⓒ Ⓓ
178 Ⓐ Ⓑ Ⓒ Ⓓ
179 Ⓐ Ⓑ Ⓒ Ⓓ
180 Ⓐ Ⓑ Ⓒ Ⓓ
181 Ⓐ Ⓑ Ⓒ Ⓓ
182 Ⓐ Ⓑ Ⓒ Ⓓ
183 Ⓐ Ⓑ Ⓒ Ⓓ
184 Ⓐ Ⓑ Ⓒ Ⓓ
185 Ⓐ Ⓑ Ⓒ Ⓓ
186 Ⓐ Ⓑ Ⓒ Ⓓ
187 Ⓐ Ⓑ Ⓒ Ⓓ
188 Ⓐ Ⓑ Ⓒ Ⓓ
189 Ⓐ Ⓑ Ⓒ Ⓓ
190 Ⓐ Ⓑ Ⓒ Ⓓ
191 Ⓐ Ⓑ Ⓒ Ⓓ
192 Ⓐ Ⓑ Ⓒ Ⓓ
193 Ⓐ Ⓑ Ⓒ Ⓓ
194 Ⓐ Ⓑ Ⓒ Ⓓ
195 Ⓐ Ⓑ Ⓒ Ⓓ
196 Ⓐ Ⓑ Ⓒ Ⓓ
197 Ⓐ Ⓑ Ⓒ Ⓓ
198 Ⓐ Ⓑ Ⓒ Ⓓ
199 Ⓐ Ⓑ Ⓒ Ⓓ
200 Ⓐ Ⓑ Ⓒ Ⓓ

SIMULATION EXAM 5

Questions

Directions: (Questions 1 to 200) For each of the following items, select the best answer among the four possible choices (A, B, C, or D). For ease of scoring, it is suggested that you use the bubble sheet provided in the back of this examination. Make sure to answer all questions. You should allow yourself a maximum of 3 hours to take this examination.

Refer to the scale in the back of the book to determine a passing score in each section. It is not necessary that you pass each section, but you must receive a total "scaled" score of 75 to pass the examination.

SECTION I: RADIATION PROTECTION AND RADIOBIOLOGY

1. If a person's office is situated adjacent to the wall of a radiographic room, this person's annual dose-equivalent limit as recommended by the National Council on Radiation Protection and Measurement (NCRP) should not exceed:
   A. 50 mSv (5 rem)
   B. 10 mSv (1 rem)
   C. 5 mSv (0.5 rem)
   D. 1 mSv (0.1 rem)

2. Which statement is true concerning the properties of x-radiation?
   A. X rays can be focused by a lens.
   B. X rays are affected by a magnetic field.
   C. X rays are heterogeneous.
   D. X rays travel at one-third the speed of light.

3. When would it not be appropriate to use lead as a shielding material?
   A. When radiographing a patient who has been injected with a gamma-emitting source
   B. When radiographing a patient who has been injected with a beta-emitting source
   C. When radiographing a patient who has been injected with an alpha-emitting source
   D. When radiographing a patient who has received a 10–megaelectron-volts (MeV) treatment of x rays

4. What is the minimum amount of total filtration required when the tube is operating at 100 kilovolts (peak) (kVp)?
   A. 0.5 mm aluminum (Al)
   B. 1.5 mm Al
   C. 2.5 mm Al
   D. 3 mm Al

5. In the United States, the annual genetic significant dose (GSD) per person is estimated to be approximately:
   A. 5 mrad
   B. 10 mrad
   C. 20 mrad
   D. 40 mrad

6. Which of the following responses to radiation would be considered a deterministic effect?
   A. Thyroid cancer
   B. Leukemia
   C. Genetic defects
   D. Cataracts

7. During which gestational stage will high doses of radiation to the embryo or fetus most likely result in congenital defects?
   A. During the first 2 weeks
   B. Between weeks 3 to 10
   C. During the second trimester
   D. During the third trimester

8. A unit of measure that is used to specify radiation "exposure" is one that is actually measuring:
   A. Energy deposited in tissue
   B. Occupational exposure
   C. Ionization in air
   D. Radioactivity

9. What is the annual dose limit as recommended by the NCRP for the lower extremities of occupational personnel?
   A. 10 mSv (1000 mrem)
   B. 50 mSv (5000 mrem)
   C. 150 mSv (15,000 mrem)
   D. 500 mSv (50,000 mrem)

10. When water molecules are irradiated, the principal molecular byproducts are:
    A. Triphosphates
    B. Nucleic acids
    C. Free radicals
    D. Proteins

11. Which of the following types of electrons are most tightly bound in their shells?
    A. The ones inside the nucleus
    B. The ones closest to the nucleus
    C. The ones in the outermost shell
    D. The free radical types

12. Which of the following x-ray procedures has one of the lowest entrance skin exposures (ESE)?
    A. Chest
    B. Abdomen
    C. Skull
    D. Breast

13. Which set of technical factors would produce the lowest patient dose?
    A. Low kilovolts (peak), high milliamperage-seconds
    B. High kilovolts (peak), low milliamperage-seconds
    C. High milliamperes, short exposure time
    D. Low milliamperes, long exposure time

14. The nucleolus of a typical cell contains which of the following?
    A. Ribosomes
    B. DNA
    C. RNA
    D. Lysosomes

15. Ionizing radiation has been documented as a well-known teratogen, which means that it causes:
    A. Genetic effects from damage done to the ova or sperm cell before conception
    B. Congenital abnormalities induced by exposure of the embryo or fetus after conception
    C. Cancer or other long-term late effects from natural background exposure
    D. Somatic effects, such as cataractogenesis, from occupational exposure

16. Which of the following is the radiation unit that is used for calibration measurements of diagnostic radiographic equipment?
    A. coulomb per kilogram (roentgen)
    B. Gray (rad)
    C. Sievert (rem)
    D. Curie (becquerel)

17. What type of filter is located in the film badge when it is used as a personnel monitor?
    A. Cadmium or lead
    B. Lead or zinc
    C. Aluminum or copper
    D. Aluminum or lead

18. The principal piece of test equipment that is used to measure the radiation output of an x-ray unit is the
    A. Scintillation-type meter
    B. Pinhole camera
    C. Milliroentgen per milliamperage-seconds ionization-type meter
    D. Line-pair test pattern

19. During fluoroscopy, a protective curtain or sliding panel having a minimal lead thickness of 0.25 mm is used for the purpose of absorbing:
    A. Primary radiation
    B. Scatter radiation
    C. Remnant radiation
    D. Leakage radiation

20. During which stage of the cell cycle is radiation-induced chromosome damage most evident?
    A. Prophase
    B. Metaphase
    C. Interphase
    D. Telophase

21. A dose of 30 rem is equal to:
    A. 3 mSv
    B. 30 mSv
    C. 300 mSv
    D. 3000 mSv

22. The probability of the photoelectric interaction _____ as the atomic number of the irradiated tissue _____ .
    A. Increases, decreases
    B. Decreases, increases
    C. Increases, increases
    D. Stays consistent, changes

mR/mAs at a 100 cm SID

KVp	60	70	80	90	100
mR/mAs	1.4	2.5	3.2	4.0	5.2

FIGURE 5–1. mR/mAs chart.

23. In the early part of the twentieth century, which radiation unit of measure was used to designate occupational exposure?
    A. Roentgen
    B. Skin erythema dose (SED)
    C. rem
    D. rad

For questions 24 and 25, refer to Figure 5–1:

24. What is the approximate skin dose to the patient using technical factors of 400 mA, 100 ms, and 80 kVp at a 100-cm source-image receptor-distance (SID)?
    A. 8 mR
    B. 12.5 mR
    C. 128 mR
    D. 256 mR

    mR/mAs 3.2mR
    400 mA / 100ms (.01) = 40 × 3.2 = 128

25. What would the estimated entrance skin exposure (ESE) be if the technical factors were changed to 600 mA, 50 ms, and 90 kVp?
    A. 7.5 mR
    B. 13 mR
    C. 120 mR
    D. 150 mR

    50ms = .05s × 600mA = 30mAs
    4.0 × 30 = 120mR

For questions 26 and 27, refer to Figure 5–2:

26. According to the graph, the linear, threshold-type relationship is illustrated by:
    1. Curve A
    2. Curve B
    3. Curve C

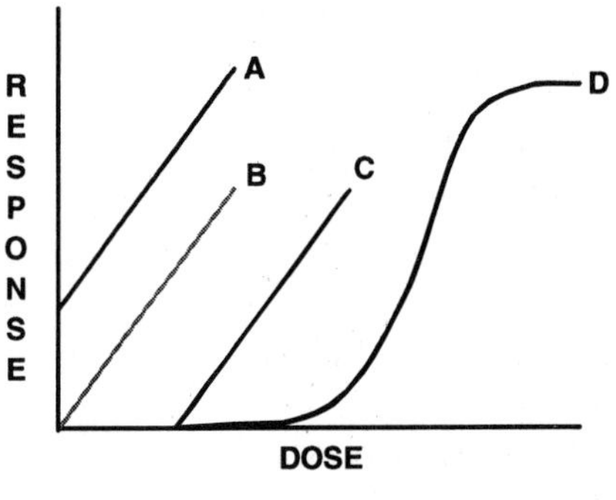

FIGURE 5–2. Dose-response curves.

A. 1 only
B. 2 only
C. 3 only
D. 1, 2, and 3

27. Which curve is the basis for NCRP dose-equivalent limits for stochastic effects?
    A. Curve A
    B. Curve B
    C. Curve C
    D. Curve D

28. A radiographer is helping to stabilize a patient during a fluoroscopic procedure at the same position where the radiation intensity measured 250 mR/h. What would the radiographer's total exposure be if the entire procedure had a fluoroscopic "ON time" of 5 minutes?
    A. 21 mR
    B. 25 mR
    C. 50 mR
    D. 1250 mR

29. What is the radiation protection philosophy that is meant to reduce the amount of radiation used in medical imaging procedures?
    A. NCRP
    B. LET
    C. GSD
    D. ALARA

30. Which of the following is a type of particulate radiation?
    A. Alpha rays
    B. X rays
    C. Gamma rays
    D. Ultraviolet radiation

SECTION II: EQUIPMENT OPERATION AND MAINTENANCE

31. Which device may be used to maintain the x-ray intensity incident on the input phosphor of an image intensifier?
    A. Photocathode
    B. Electrostatic lenses

C. Plumbicon
D. Automatic brightness control (ABC)

32. Which device may be used to determine accuracy of multiple technical factors for quality control (QC) of x-ray equipment?
A. Sensitometer
B. Pinhole camera
C. Digital dosimeter
D. Synchronous spinning top

33. Which of the following generators would not be capable of providing long exposure times for procedures such as tomography or breathing techniques?
A. High-frequency generator
B. Battery-powered generator
C. Capacitor discharge generator
D. Falling-load generator

34. The minimum exposure time most modern generators are capable of producing is:
A. 0.0001 millisecond
B. 0.01 millisecond
C. 1 millisecond
D. 10 milliseconds

35. If the x-ray intensity at 70 kVp is 100 mR, what is the intensity if the kilovolts (peak) is increased to 81 and all other factors remain constant?
A. 50 mR
B. 67 mR
C. 134 mR
D. 200 mR

36. Which of the following will result in an increase in speed of an intensifying screen?
1. Increased kilovolts (peak)
2. Thicker phosphor layer
3. Larger focal spot
A. 1 and 2 only
B. 1 and 3 only
C. 2 and 3 only
D. 1, 2, and 3

37. The smallest effective focal spot will always be projected:
A. Equally on both sides of the radiograph
B. In the center of the radiograph
C. On the anode side of the radiograph
D. On the cathode side of the radiograph

38. Which of the following will result if a 9-inch image intensification field is used instead of a 6-inch field during fluoroscopy?
A. Less dose to the patient
B. Greater resolution
C. Less quantum mottle
D. Greater magnification

39. Federal regulations state that when using an automatic exposure control system with technical factors above 50 kVp, the x-ray exposure must terminate at:
A. 100 mAs or less
B. 300 mAs or less
C. 600 mAs or less
D. 2000 mAs or less

40. What is the primary function of the positive beam limitation (PBL) mechanism?
A. Ensures the accuracy of the centering light
B. Automatically limits the primary beam field size
C. Opens the collimator to maximum primary beam field size
D. Restricts access to the Bucky tray

41. What is the secondary voltage if the primary voltage is 220 in a transformer with a turns ratio of 500:1?
A. 0.44 V
B. 110 V
C. 110 kV
D. 220 kV

42. The thickness of the focal plane during tomography is primarily dependent on the
A. SID
B. Exposure time
C. Amplitude of tube travel
D. Height of the fulcrum above the tabletop

43. An acceptance test on newly installed radiographic equipment should include a test for focal spot size (FSS) using the pinhole camera. When this device is used, it should be placed:
A. As close to the image receptor as possible
B. As close to the source as possible
C. Halfway between the source and image receptor
D. At the upper right corner of the image receptor

44. What type of current is usually found between the secondary side of the high-tension transformer and the rectification system?
A. High-voltage DC
B. High-voltage AC
C. Low-voltage DC
D. Low-voltage AC

45. Which type of radiographic equipment produces the lowest radiation output?
A. Full-wave rectified, single-phase
B. Full-wave rectified, 3-phase
C. Capacitor discharge mobile unit
D. High-frequency generator

46. With which of the following technical factors is the radiographer able to control the potential difference across the x-ray tube?

1. Milliamperage setting
2. Density control
3. Kilovolt (peak) setting

A. 1 only
B. 2 only
C. 3 only
D. 1, 2, and 3

47. Assuming the same exposure arc for each type, which of the following tomographic motions will produce the greatest length of tube travel?
A. Hypocycloidal
B. Trispiral
C. Figure-eight
D. Elliptical

For questions 48 and 49, refer to Figure 5–3:

48. Figure 5–3 represents a spectral distribution of x rays produced at a tungsten target for various kiloelectron-volt (keV) levels. What type of radiation production does the sharp vertical line appearing on the graph represent?
A. Characteristic
B. Photoelectric
C. *Bremsstrahlung*
D. Compton's

49. What is the average energy of the x-ray beam produced according to the graph?
A. 30 keV
B. 45 keV
C. 65 keV
D. 80 keV

50. How many half-value layers (HVLs) would be equivalent to one tenth-value layer (TVL)?
A. 2
B. 3.3

C. 5.5
D. 10

51. Various forms of electromagnetic (EM) radiation, such as x rays or gamma rays, are usually identified by their
A. Mass
B. Velocity
C. Energy
D. Origin

52. What is the electrical charge of the filament in an x-ray tube?
A. Positive
B. Negative
C. Neutral
D. It depends on the material it is made of

53. Which of the following technical factors controls the number of projectile electrons passing from cathode to anode during the exposure?
A. The milliamperage setting
B. The kilovolt (peak) setting
C. The HVL
D. The density control

54. If x rays cannot easily pass through a material, the material is said to be:
A. Radiolucent
B. Translucent
C. Transparent
D. Radiopaque

55. Which x-ray component uses a photomultiplier tube?
A. Anode induction motor
B. Automatic exposure control (AEC)
C. Rectification system
D. Filament rheostat

56. Which of the following interactions of x rays with matter is the least likely to occur in the diagnostic range?
A. Photoelectric interaction
B. Compton scattering
C. Classical scattering
D. Pair production

57. In a modern televised fluoroscopic system, the terms *vidicon* and *plumbicon* refer to the types of:
A. Television monitors
B. Television camera tubes
C. X-ray tubes
D. Fluoroscopic screen phosphors

58. The photocathode of an image intensification system is located:
A. On the input side
B. On the output side
C. In the television camera tube
D. In the x-ray tube

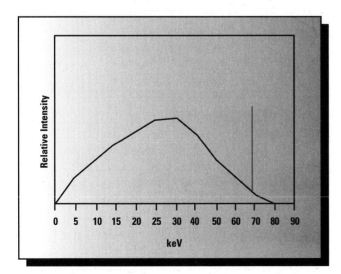

FIGURE 5–3. Spectral distribution of x rays produced at a tungsten target for various keV levels.

59. If a 3-phase, 12-pulse radiographic x-ray tube has an anode storage capacity of 350,000 heat units (HU), how many rapid exposures can be safely made on a cool anode using technical factors of 300 mA, 1 second, and 72 kVp?
   A. 6
   B. 11
   C. 12
   D. 16

60. X-ray tubes that possess very small FSSs (0.3 mm or less) are specifically designed for:
   A. The radiography of very large anatomic parts
   B. Use with low-milliampere and high-kilovolt (peak) exposure factors
   C. Procedures that generate consistently high heat loading on the x-ray tube
   D. Direct magnification radiography

SECTION III: IMAGE PRODUCTION AND EVALUATION

61. A radiograph taken with a film-screen combination having a wide latitude will likely exhibit:
   A. Low contrast
   B. High contrast
   C. Low recorded detail
   D. High density

62. If 76 kVp, 400 mA, and 50 milliseconds were used for a particular exposure with single-phase equipment, what milliamperage-seconds would be required using 3-phase, 12-pulse equipment to produce a similar radiograph?
   A. 10 mAs
   B. 40 mAs
   C. 100 mAs
   D. 400 mAs

63. Why is a cardboard cassette used when measuring FSS?
   A. To eliminate all sources of blur except that caused by the focal spot
   B. To permit use of higher milliamperage-seconds and to reduce quantum mottle
   C. To allow higher magnification with minimum focal spot blur
   D. Screens will result in focal spot images that are too dark

64. There are a total of 20 radiographs collected in the "discard" box. Five of the radiographs are clear, and five were retaken because of positioning errors. What percentage of the retakes is due to positioning errors?
   A. 3.3 percent
   B. 25 percent
   C. 33 percent
   D. More data needed to determine percentage

65. Which of the following is most efficient in absorbing scatter radiation?
   A. Compensating filter
   B. Grid
   C. Collimator
   D. Intensifying screen

66. A grid used with the SID set at the wrong focal distance will produce:
   A. Increased density along the periphery of the image
   B. Decreased density in the center of the image
   C. Decreased density along the periphery of the image
   D. Increased density across the entire image

67. What causes a black, crescent, half-moon artifact on a radiograph?
   A. Static discharge
   B. Handling the film with damp hands
   C. Bending the film
   D. Improper alignment of guide-shoe deflectors

68. What is the approximate fixer immersion time for a sheet of radiographic film in a 90-second processor?
   A. 1 to 5 seconds
   B. 20 to 25 seconds
   C. 45 to 60 seconds
   D. 65 seconds

69. Which of the following will minimize size distortion?
   A. Decrease the SID
   B. Decrease the grid ratio
   C. Decrease the object-image receptor-distance (OID)
   D. Decrease the FSS

70. Which of the following is within the range of resolving ability for a general diagnostic film-screen combination?
   A. 0.1 to 1 line-pair per millimeter
   B. 1 to 10 line-pairs per millimeter
   C. 10 to 20 line-pairs per millimeter
   D. 50 to 100 line-pairs per millimeter

71. For the Hurter and Driffield (H & D) curve, an increase of _____ on the log relative exposure axis is equal to a doubling of the exposure.
   A. 0.3
   B. 0.6
   C. 1
   D. 2

72. What percentage of light will be transmitted by radiographic film with a measured optical density of 2?
   A. 0.1 percent
   B. 1 percent

C. 10 percent

D. 100 percent

73. Which of the following will cause areas of decreased density on a radiograph?
    A. Dirt in the cassette
    B. Handling film with damp hands
    C. Abrasion on the film surface during handling
    D. Insufficient relative humidity in the darkroom

74. What is the appropriate relative humidity for proper film storage?
    A. 0 to 10 percent
    B. 40 to 60 percent
    C. 70 to 80 percent
    D. 90 to 100 percent

75. What is the most common type of filter used in most modern darkroom safelights?
    A. Wratten 2-B
    B. Wratten 4-B
    C. Wratten 6-B
    D. GBX

76. What is the cause of a "pi line" artifact on a radiograph?
    A. Static discharge
    B. Dirt on the processor transport roller
    C. Bending of the film
    D. Improper alignment of guide shoes

77. Which of the following will cause a loss of recorded detail?
    A. Milliamperage-second changes
    B. Kilovolt (peak) changes
    C. High grid ratios
    D. Patient motion

78. The advantages of using high kilovolts (peak) with a subsequent reduction in milliamperage-seconds include less
    1. Heat units generated
    2. Patient exposure
    3. Quantum mottle

    A. 1 and 2 only
    B. 1 and 3 only
    C. 2 and 3 only
    D. 1, 2, and 3

79. Exposed silver halide crystals are changed to black metallic silver by the
    A. Preservative
    B. Reducers
    C. Activators
    D. Clearing agent

80. What body part should be placed on the anode side of the beam to take advantage of the anode heel effect inherent in most x-ray tubes?

A. Homogeneous body tissue

B. Heterogeneous body tissue

C. Thinner body part

D. Thicker body part

For questions 81 to 84, use the following information:
A satisfactory lateral radiograph of the skull has been produced using the technical factors that follow. In each of the questions, one factor has been changed. Indicate the result that will be seen on the radiograph as a result of each factor change.

200 mA	100 relative film-screen speed
0.25 second	1.0-mm focal spot
65 kVp	10 × 12 in. field size
40-in. SID	2-in. OID
8:1 grid ratio	

81. Changing the OID to 4 inches would result in:
    A. Reduced magnification
    B. Greater magnification
    C. Better recorded detail
    D. Lower contrast

82. The use of a 400 relative film-screen speed combination would result in:
    A. Increased magnification
    B. Decreased magnification
    C. Increased density
    D. Decreased density

83. Collimating to a 4 × 4 in. primary beam field would result in:
    A. Increased density
    B. Decreased density
    C. Grid cutoff
    D. Focal spot blooming

84. Changing the grid ratio to 12:1 would result in:
    A. Decreased density and higher contrast
    B. Decreased density and lower contrast
    C. Increased density and higher contrast
    D. Increased density and lower contrast

85. A linear tomogram of the ankle requires a 120-cm amplitude and a 20 cm/s travel time. Which of the following technical factors could be set to make a satisfactory image?
    A. 50 mA, 2 seconds, at 75 kVp
    B. 50 mA, 3 seconds, at 70 kVp
    C. 25 mA, 4 seconds, at 75 kVp
    D. 25 mA, 6 seconds, at 70 kVp

86. A patient is to be radiographed using an AEC unit at 500 mA and 75 kVp. If the unit has a minimum response time of 20 milliseconds and a backup time set at 200 milliseconds, which of the following exposures are possible?
    1. 5 mAs
    2. 10 mAs
    3. 100 mAs

A. 1 and 2 only
B. 1 and 3 only
C. 2 and 3 only
D. 1, 2, and 3

87. What performance characteristic of the generator is tested by making four successive exposures using identical technical factors (milliamperes, time, and kilovolts [peak]) and then measuring and averaging the radiation output?
    A. Linearity
    B. Reproducibility
    C. Reciprocity
    D. HVL

88. Blurring of the radiographic image is often the result of:
    A. Insufficient kilovolts (peak)
    B. Poor film-screen contact
    C. Excessive drying temperature
    D. Conversion efficiency

89. The acceptable tolerance level for focal spot blooming when measuring a 1.0-mm focal spot is a variance of no more than:
    A. 10 percent
    B. 30 percent
    C. 40 percent
    D. 60 percent

For questions 90 and 91, refer to Figure 5–4:

90. Which QC test instrument was used to produce the image in Figure 5–4?
    A. Penetrometer
    B. Wisconsin test cassette
    C. Wire mesh
    D. Pinhole camera

91. The QC test instrument in Figure 5–4 is used to evaluate:
    A. Uniformity of screen fluorescence
    B. Uniformity of film-screen contact
    C. Central ray axis alignment
    D. Pi lines and guide-shoe marks

92. Which of the following will produce a change in contrast without changing density?
    A. Increasing kilovolts (peak) by 15 percent and decreasing milliamperage-seconds by 50 percent
    B. Increasing kilovolts (peak) by 15 percent and increasing milliamperage-seconds by 50 percent
    C. Decreasing milliamperage-seconds by 50 percent with no change in kilovolts (peak)
    D. Decreasing kilovolts (peak) by 15 percent with no change in milliamperage-seconds

93. What is the magnification factor (MF) for a kidney stone that casts an image 0.4 cm wide on an

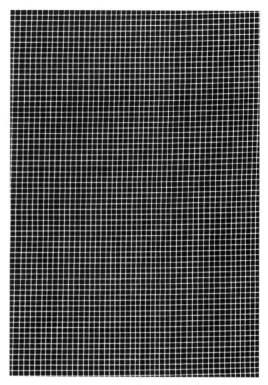

FIGURE 5–4. (Courtesy of JRMC Engineering Department.)

AP projection radiograph of the abdomen produced at a 100 cm when the stone is located 7.2 cm from the film?
    A. 0.37
    B. 1.08
    C. 2.32
    D. 2.70

For questions 94 and 95, refer to Figure 5–5:

94. Calculate the grid ratio for the grid illustrated in Figure 5–5.
    A. 6:1
    B. 8:1
    C. 12:1
    D. 16:1

95. This grid would be useful for which of the following types of equipment?
    A. Dedicated chest unit operating routinely above 110 kVp
    B. Dedicated Bucky unit used strictly for intravenous urography (IVU) examinations between 70 to 80 kVp
    C. Portable grid cassette used mainly for extremity and skull radiography
    D. Portable grid cassette used mainly for abdominal radiography

96. Which of the following QC tests would be performed to document several inaccurate milliamperage settings?

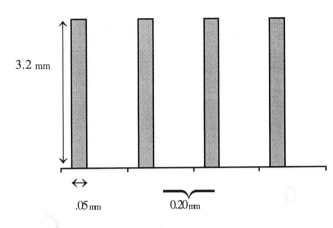

3.2 mm

↔

.05 mm   0.20 mm

FIGURE 5–5. Grid ratio graph.

A. Rectification failure test
B. Milliamperage HVL test
C. Milliamperage linearity test
D. Modulation transfer function

97. What is the primary reason intensifying screens must be cleaned on a regular basis?
    A. To reactivate the phosphors
    B. To remove film emulsion residue
    C. To remove dust and dirt particles
    D. To reactivate the light-absorbing dyes in the screen

98. Which of the following sets of technical factors would achieve the same radiographic density?
    1. 64 kVp, 400 mA, 0.008 second
    2. 64 kVp, 200 mA, 0.32 second
    3. 75 kVp, 400 mA, 0.16 second
    4. 86 kVp, 400 mA, 0.08 second

    A. 1 and 2
    B. 1 and 3
    C. 2 and 3
    D. 3 and 4

99. What does increased collimation of the primary beam do to the primary radiographic exposure factors of image contrast and density?
    A. Contrast increases and density increases
    B. Contrast decreases and density decreases
    C. Contrast increases and density decreases
    D. Contrasts decreases and density increases

100. Which of the following anatomic tissues has the lowest tissue density?
    A. Fat
    B. Muscle
    C. Water
    D. Bone

101. The Pyrex glass of the x-ray tube, the beryllium window, and the insulating oil through which the x rays pass all constitute part of the

A. Compensating filtration
B. Anode heel effect
C. Off-focus radiation
D. Inherent filtration

102. What alteration of technical factors is required for an extremity in a fiberglass cast as compared with one with no cast?
    A. A 40 percent increase in milliamperage-seconds
    B. Increase of 10 kVp
    C. Doubling of the mAs
    D. No increase necessary

103. Which of the following types of screens would be used in a 36-inch cassette to radiograph the entire vertebral column with an anteroposterior (AP) projection?
    A. Rare earth screen
    B. Gradient screen
    C. Ultra-detail screen
    D. Dual-sided screen

104. What type of material is now used as a base in modern x-ray film?
    A. Polyester
    B. Glass
    C. Cellulose nitrate
    D. Cellulose acetate

105. Technical factors of 75 kVp, 800 mA, and 1/16 second were required to produce a diagnostic radiograph using a single-phase radiographic machine. What single adjustment in technical factors—all other factors remaining constant—would be sufficient to produce a similar radiographic density using a 3-phase, 12-pulse unit?
    A. 0.0625 second
    B. 0.125 second
    C. 400 mA
    D. 1000 mA

106. Five rapid exposures set at technical factors of 200 mA, 50 milliseconds, and 70 kVp result in an average beam intensity of 77 mR. Which of the following individual values meets the prescribed limit for a test on reproducibility?
    1. 74 mR
    2. 80 mR
    3. 85 mR

    A. 1 and 2 only
    B. 1 and 3 only
    C. 2 and 3 only
    D. 1, 2, and 3

107. The artifact seen in Figure 5–6 was most likely caused by:
    A. Dirt on the processor rollers
    B. Dirt or dust on the intensifying screens
    C. Low humidity in the darkroom
    D. Mishandling of the film in the darkroom

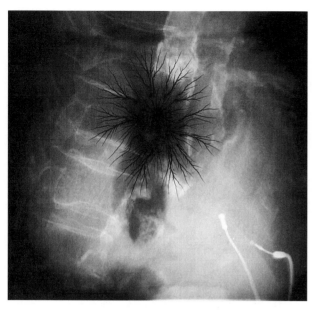

FIGURE 5–6. (Courtesy of JRMC Radiology Department.)

108. Which of the following sets of technical factors will produce a radiographic image displaying the greatest degree of magnification?

	mAs	kVp	SID	OID	FSS
A.	25	72	100	25	1.2 mm
B.	32	76	150	30	0.6 mm
C.	40	80	120	20	0.6 mm
D.	30	78	200	40	1.2 mm

109. Which type of grid has the greatest amount of centering and distance latitude?
   A. 5:1 ratio focused grid
   B. 6:1 ratio linear grid
   C. 8:1 ratio rhombic grid
   D. 12:1 ratio cross-hatched grid

110. What type of technical adjustment is required for the pathological condition demonstrated in Figure 5–7?
   A. A 15 percent decrease in kilovolts (peak)
   B. A 30 percent decrease in milliamperage-seconds

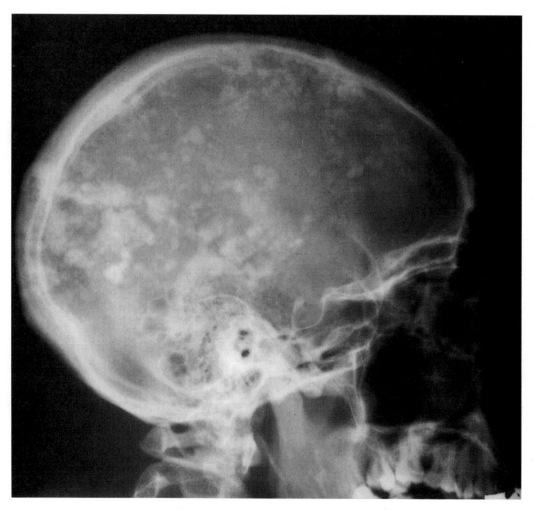

FIGURE 5–7.

C. A 50 percent decrease in milliamperage-seconds

D. A 15 percent increase in kilovolts (peak)

SECTION IV: RADIOGRAPHIC PROCEDURES AND RELATED ANATOMY

111. A specialized arterial structure in the brain that helps to prevent irreparable damage in cases of arterial blockage is called the
     A. Circle of Willis
     B. Corpus callosum
     C. Choroid plexus
     D. Cerebral peduncle

112. The right axillary ribs are best demonstrated by placing the patient in the _____ position.
     A. Prone
     B. Supine
     C. Left anterior oblique (LAO)
     D. Right anterior oblique (RAO)

113. Obstruction or infection may be indicated if air is seen in the _____ on a radiograph of the abdomen.
     A. Small intestine
     B. Fundus of the stomach
     C. Colon
     D. Rectum

114. Which of the following erect projections will demonstrate a fluid level in the sphenoid sinus?
     1. Parietoacanthial (Waters method)
     2. Parietoacanthial (open-mouth Waters method)
     3. Submentovertical (SMV)
     A. 1 only
     B. 1 and 2 only
     C. 2 and 3 only
     D. 1, 2, and 3

115. To place the right kidney parallel to the image receptor surface during renal tomography, the patient should be placed in the _____ position.
     A. 30° left posterior oblique (LPO)
     B. 30° right posterior oblique (RPO)
     C. 45° RPO
     D. Prone

116. Which of the following is adjusted perpendicular to the image-receptor surface to perform a lateral projection of the skull?
     A. Orbitomeatal line
     B. Infraorbitomeatal line (IOML)
     C. Interpupillary line
     D. Midsagittal plane (MSP)

117. Most carcinomas of the breasts are found in the _____ of the breast.

A. Upper outer quadrant (UOQ)
B. Lower outer quadrant (LOQ)
C. Upper inner quadrant (UIQ)
D. Lower inner quadrant (LIQ)

118. A frontal projection of the elbow with the patient in acute flexion would most likely be used to demonstrate:
     A. Fractures of the proximal humerus
     B. Fractures of the distal ulna
     C. Fractures of the coronoid process
     D. Fractures of the olecranon process

119. The anterior oblique projection of the shoulder (scapular "Y") is primarily useful in the demonstration of:
     A. The glenoid fossa
     B. Acromioclavicular (AC) joint separation
     C. Shoulder dislocation
     D. Fractures of the humeral head

120. Which of the following positions will best demonstrate the hepatic flexure of the colon without self-superimposition during a contrast procedure?
     A. RPO and LAO
     B. LPO and RAO
     C. RPO and LPO
     D. RAO and LAO

121. To direct the central ray through the joint space of the knee for the AP projection, the central ray should enter approximately ½ inch distal to the _____ of the patella.
     A. Lateral border
     B. Medial border
     C. Base
     D. Apex

122. With which of the following bones does the clavicle articulate?
     1. Humerus
     2. Scapula *acromion*
     3. Sternum
     A. 1 only
     B. 1 and 2 only
     C. 1 and 3 only
     D. 2 and 3 only

123. Which of the following may be diagnosed by operative cholangiography?
     1. Biliary tract calculi
     2. Patency of the biliary ducts
     3. Function of the sphincter of Oddi
     A. 1 only
     B. 2 only
     C. 2 and 3 only
     D. 1, 2, and 3

124. One unique characteristic of all cervical vertebrae is that each has:

A. Bifid-tipped spinous processes
B. Three foramina
C. Transverse processes arising from the body and pedicle
D. Facets for the articulations of ribs

125. The medical suffix -*plasia* refers to:
A. Downward displacement
B. Formation or development
C. State or condition of
D. Excessive flow

126. Which of the following bones help to form the hard palate?
A. Palatines and maxillae
B. Vomer and maxillae
C. Vomer and palatines
D. Mandible and maxillae

127. Which organs of the abdominopelvic cavity are most affected by variations in the patient's body habitus?
A. Kidneys and liver
B. Stomach and gallbladder
C. Kidneys and stomach
D. Liver and gallbladder

128. The bone that provides attachment for the muscles of the tongue and mouth is the _____ bone.
A. Cricoid
B. Thyroid
C. Hyoid
D. Sesamoid

129. Concerning the joints, the periosteum is continuous with which of the following?
A. Tendons
B. Ligaments
C. Bursa
D. Hyaline cartilage

130. Which of the following conditions correctly describes an infection in the peritoneal space?
A. Ascites
B. Gastroenteritis
C. Jaundice
D. Peritonitis

131. Which two carpal bones can normally be palpated on the anteromedial surface of the wrist?
A. Pisiform and hamate
B. Lunate and capitate
C. Scaphoid and trapezoid
D. Triquetrum and trapezium

132. Which of the following bones form all or part of the knee joint?
1. Fibula
2. Patella
3. Tibia

A. 1 and 2 only
B. 1 and 3 only

C. 2 and 3 only
D. 1, 2, and 3

133. Discrepancy in the length of the lower limbs would best be evaluated by:
A. Nuclear medicine bone scan
B. Scanogram
C. Bone densitometry scan
D. Magnetic resonance imaging (MRI) scan

134. When free air is suspected, it is most important that the left lateral decubitus projection of the abdomen should be centered to include the
A. Symphysis pubis
B. Diaphragm
C. Left side
D. Xyphoid tip

135. When radiographs are required during a hysterosalpingogram, where is the correct centering point?
A. Level of the lower rib margin
B. 2 inches above the symphysis
C. Level of the anterosuperior iliac spine
D. Level of the iliac crests

136. The most prominent aspect of the greater trochanter lies at approximately _____ the symphysis pubis.
A. 1 inch below
B. 1 inch above
C. The same level of
D. 2 inches lateral to

137. A suture may be classified as what type of joint?
A. Amphiarthrodial
B. Diarthrodial
C. Synarthrodial
D. Gompharthrodial

138. A properly positioned lateral projection of the humerus will demonstrate:
1. Lesser tubercle in profile
2. Glenoid fossa in profile
3. Humeral epicondyles nearly superimposed

A. 1 and 2 only
B. 1 and 3 only
C. 2 and 3 only
D. 1, 2, and 3

139. Which of the following projections or positions will best demonstrate the cuboid bone and its articulations?
A. AP
B. AP medial oblique
C. Lateral oblique
D. Tangential

140. When radiographing the lateral thoracic spine with the patient in the recumbent position, how should the central ray be directed if the lower vertebral column is not elevated to the horizontal position?

A. Perpendicular to the image receptor
B. 5°–8° caudad
C. 15°–20° caudad
D. 10°–15° cephalad

141. Which projection of the wrist will demonstrate the pisiform and triquetrum separated from one another?
 A. Posteroanterior (PA)
 B. PA oblique
 C. AP oblique
 D. Lateral

142. What type of joint classification is the pubic symphysis?
 A. Synarthrodial
 B. Diarthrodial
 C. Amphiarthrodial
 D. Fibrous connective

For questions 143 and 144, refer to Figure 5–8:

143. What is the best description of the radiograph shown in Figure 5–8?
 A. AP projection of the knee
 B. Tangential projection of the knee
 C. Axial projection of the knee
 D. "Sunrise" projection of the knee

144. How was the central ray angled for the radiograph obtained in Figure 5–8?
 A. Perpendicular to the long axis of the femur
 B. Parallel to the long axis of the femur
 C. Perpendicular to the long axis of the tibia
 D. Parallel to the long axis of the tibia

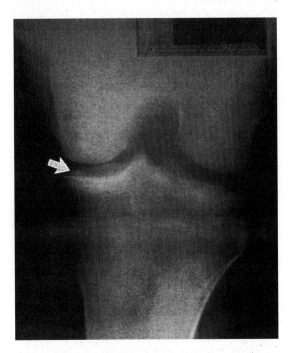

FIGURE 5–8. (Adapted from McKinnis, LN: Fundamentals of Orthopedic Radiology. FA Davis, Philadelphia, 1997, p 283.)

145. One of the main functions of the respiratory system is to make _____ available to the body.
 A. Carbon dioxide
 B. Erythrocytes
 C. Hemoglobin
 D. Oxygen

146. The spinal cord is protected along the vertebral column as it extends inferiorly from the brainstem by the
 A. Obturator foramina
 B. Intervertebral foramina
 C. Transverse foramina
 D. Vertebral foramen

147. Radiologists prefer that their AP projection radiographs be properly placed on the viewbox in such a way that the patient position appears to:
 A. Be facing the direction of the viewer
 B. Be looking at himself or herself in a mirror
 C. Have his or her anterior surface in contact with the view box
 D. Vary depending on the part that was radiographed

148. Which of the following positions best enhances peristaltic motion of barium through the stomach?
 A. RAO
 B. Trendelenburg
 C. Left lateral
 D. Lateral erect

149. Which organ is most responsible for maintaining the proper levels of glucose in the circulating blood and for the metabolism or breakdown of sugars in the body?
 A. Liver
 B. Kidney
 C. Pancreas
 D. Gallbladder

150. Where is the centering point for a lateral projection of the nasal bones?
 A. At the glabella
 B. At the zygoma
 C. ¾ inch superior to the acanthion
 D. ¾ inch inferior to the nasion

151. With which of the following bones does the vomer articulate?
 1. Ethmoid
 2. Maxilla
 3. Sphenoid

 A. 1 and 2 only
 B. 1 and 3 only
 C. 2 and 3 only
 D. 1, 2. and 3

152. When attempting to demonstrate any abnormal lordotic or kyphotic curvatures of the spine, which position or projection would be best?

A. AP
B. Weight-bearing PA
C. Lateral
D. Oblique

153. Which bones help to form the shoulder girdle?

    1. Humerus
    2. Clavicle
    3. Scapula

    A. 1 and 2 only
    B. 1 and 3 only
    C. 2 and 3 only
    D. 1, 2, and 3

For questions 154 to 156, refer to Figure 5–9:

154. The patient radiographed in Figure 5–9 was placed in the _____ position.
    A. Supine
    B. Internal oblique
    C. External oblique
    D. Prone

155. The number 1 in Figure 5–9 refers to what anatomic part?
    A. Lateral epicondyle
    B. Medial epicondyle

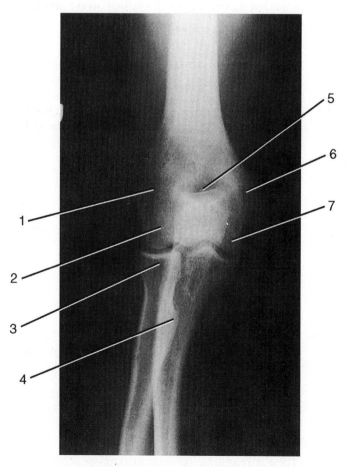

FIGURE 5–9. (Adapted from McKinnis, LN: Fundamentals of Orthopedic Radiology. FA Davis, Philadelphia, 1997, p 369.)

C. Trochlea
D. Capitulum

156. The number 5 in Figure 5–9 refers to the
    A. Coronoid process
    B. Trochlear notch
    C. Olecranon fossa
    D. Radial tuberosity

157. Which of the following is not one of the bones found in the middle ear?
    A. Malleus
    B. Cochlea
    C. Incus
    D. Stapes

158. When a patient has a sixth lumbar vertebra that articulates with the sacrum, it is sometimes referred to as:
    A. Spondylolysis
    B. Spondylolisthesis
    C. Lumbarization
    D. Sacralization

159. When attempting an AP projection of the atlas, the radiograph appears with the patient's teeth obscuring the odontoid process. How should this be corrected on the repeat examination?
    A. Angle the central ray 5° caudal
    B. Increase the kilovolts (peak) by 15 percent
    C. Extend the patient's neck
    D. Depress the patient's chin

160. Failure to dorsiflex the patient's ankle during an AP medial oblique projection of the ankle will result in:
    A. Inaccurate demonstration of the distal tibiofibular articulation
    B. Inaccurate demonstration of the lateral malleolus
    C. Superimposition of the malleoli
    D. Superimposition of the phalanges and the tarsal bones

161. Which anatomic structure is usually critiqued for unacceptable rotation of a PA projection of the lungs?
    A. AC joints
    B. Heart size
    C. SC joints
    D. Number of ribs

162. A lateral "shoot-through" projection of the cervical vertebrae on a trauma patient fails to demonstrate the body of the seventh cervical vertebra. What should be done to image this bone?
    A. Increase the kilovolts (peak) by 30 percent
    B. Increase the milliamperage-seconds by 50 percent
    C. Depress the patient's shoulders more
    D. Use a faster-speed screen

163. Failure to properly invert the lower extremities for an AP projection of the pelvis would be most noticeable in evaluating which anatomic structure?
    A. Femoral necks
    B. SI joints
    C. Acetabulum
    D. Symphysis pubis

164. An AP projection of the knee fails to demonstrate the patella. What are possible causes?
    1. Kilovolts (peak) is insufficient.
    2. Milliamperage-seconds is insufficient.
    3. SID is insufficient.
    A. 1 and 2 only
    B. 1 and 3 only
    C. 2 and 3 only
    D. 1, 2, and 3

165. A radiographer positions a patient for a lateral projection of the elbow and does not adjust the elbow and axilla in the same plane. The resultant radiograph will demonstrate:
    A. Superimposition of the humeral condyles
    B. An unobstructed projection of the radial head
    C. A distorted projection of the elbow joint
    D. A profile projection of the coronoid process

166. To prevent the medial femoral condyle from obscuring the femorotibial joint space on a lateral projection of the knee, the
    A. SID should be increased to 72 inches
    B. Screen speed should be 200 relative speed (RS) or greater
    C. Knee should be flexed 90°
    D. Central ray should be directed 5° cephalad

167. For a PA projection of the stomach on a hypersthenic patient following ingestion of a barium sulfate suspension, the central ray should be centered _____ the second lumbar vertebra:
    A. 1 to 2 inches inferior to
    B. 2 inches to the right of
    C. 2 inches to the left of
    D. 1 to 2 inches superior to

168. During an IVU examination, the radiographer notices that the patient is suffering from hydronephrosis. To ensure adequate filling of the ureters with contrast medium, which of the following positions should be used?
    A. Prone
    B. RPO
    C. LPO
    D. Supine

169. An AP projection of the chest is performed in the nursery. Seven pairs of ribs are visualized in the right lung field on inspection of the radiograph. What is the probable explanation for this image?

A. Kilovolts (peak) was excessive for this tiny patient.
B. The exposure time was too short.
C. The neonate was imaged while in the incubator.
D. The exposure was made on expiration.

170. Radiographs with the patient in the decubitus position are produced following an air-contrast barium enema examination. The radiographer fails to properly label the radiographs. To identify the right lateral decubitus image, the radiographer should see:
    A. Air in the lateral descending colon and medial ascending colon
    B. Barium in the lateral descending colon and medial descending colon
    C. Air in the descending colon and barium in the stomach
    D. Air in the stomach and barium in the lateral descending colon

SECTION V: PATIENT CARE

171. If a radiographer shares a patient's medical records with an individual not directly involved with that patient's care, the radiographer may be found guilty of:
    A. Slander
    B. Assault
    C. Defamation of character
    D. Breach of confidentiality

172. When performing cardiopulmonary resuscitation (CPR) on an infant, the pulse should be assessed using the
    A. Carotid artery
    B. Brachial artery
    C. Femoral artery
    D. Radial artery

173. A reduction in the normal number of erythrocytes circulating in the blood is called:
    A. Leukemia
    B. Anemia
    C. Hypoglycemia
    D. Hyperglycemia

174. Which of the following would be classified as a moderate reaction to an injection of an iodinated contrast medium?
    1. Difficulty breathing
    2. Reddening of the face
    3. Nausea and vomiting
    A. 1 only
    B. 2 only
    C. 3 only
    D. 1, 2, and 3

175. When the radiographer puts on sterile apparel for a surgical procedure, which of the following should be put on last?
    A. Gloves
    B. Face mask
    C. Shoe covers
    D. Gown

176. A barium sulfate suspension should not be used for a colon examination in a patient with suspected
    A. Rectal bleeding
    B. Intestinal tract perforation
    C. Vomiting
    D. Polyps

177. An enema tip should be inserted into the rectum _____ inches for a barium enema examination.
    A. 1 to 2
    B. 3 to 4
    C. 5 to 6
    D. 7 to 8

178. Which of the following are most resistant to aseptic techniques?
    A. Yeasts
    B. Molds
    C. Streptococci bacteria
    D. Bacillic spore bacteria

179. Which of the following practices is most helpful in communicating with very small children?
    A. Talking very loudly
    B. Placing your arms or hands around the child immediately
    C. Getting down to eye level with the child and maintaining distance
    D. Not smiling to avoid showing your teeth

180. What is the proper method of preparing the skin surface with an antiseptic prior to a surgical procedure?
    A. Beginning outside the area and moving in a circular motion toward the center
    B. Beginning at the center of the area and moving in a circular motion toward the outside
    C. Beginning in one corner and moving in a linear pattern
    D. Beginning in one corner in a linear pattern, followed by a second linear pattern in the opposite direction

181. Which of the following is the primary concern during enteric isolation precautions?
    A. Blood
    B. Airborne droplets
    C. Fecal material
    D. Vectors

182. Which of the following is classified as a sterile technique procedure?
    A. Insertion of a urinary catheter
    B. Insertion of a nasogastric tube
    C. Insertion of a barium enema tip
    D. Insertion of a thermometer

183. What is the proper treatment for a conscious patient experiencing hypoglycemia?
    A. Administering insulin
    B. Administering sugar
    C. Administering CPR
    D. Administering water

184. Diuretics are used for:
    A. Restricting urine production
    B. Promoting urine production
    C. Patients who are constipated
    D. Preventing vomiting

185. "Log rolling" is a method of moving patients with suspected
    A. Head injury
    B. Vertebral column injury
    C. Bowel obstruction
    D. Extremity fracture

186. The best communication method for dealing with preschool-age children having radiographic procedures that may be painful is to:
    A. Describe the sensation they may experience
    B. Reassure them that it will not hurt
    C. Let them know you will only need to take one film
    D. Tell them they will receive a treat if they behave

187. When radiographing elderly patients, special attention should be given to the patients'
    A. Allergies
    B. Radiosensitivity
    C. Skin
    D. Medications

188. Reactions to contrast media will most likely occur following what type of administration?
    A. Intrathecal
    B. Rectal
    C. Intradermal
    D. Intravenous

189. The most common side effect of the use of barium sulfate contrast medium is:
    A. Nausea
    B. Constipation
    C. Dyspnea
    D. Urticaria

190. The legal term that best describes failure to provide reasonable care or caution to the patient is:
    A. *Res ipsa loquitur*
    B. *Respondeat superior*
    C. Assault
    D. Unintentional tort

191. Which of the following patient care items is used to administer oxygen through the nose?
    A. Nasogastric (NG) tube
    B. Nasal cannula
    C. Hickman catheter
    D. Central line

192. Which of the following medical abbreviations is used to designate a heart attack?
    A. CVA
    B. HA
    C. MI
    D. TIA

193. A physician will often order a radiographic examination on a neonate with suspected atelectasis. Which part of the body would the radiographer be examining?
    A. Chest
    B. Colon
    C. Stomach
    D. Neck soft tissue

194. Prior to an invasive procedure on a 40-year-old male patient, a radiographer checks the vital signs of this anxious patient and notes that the patient's pulse rate is 115. This patient is said to have:
    A. Coronary artery disease (CAD)
    B. Bradycardia
    C. Hypertension
     D. Tachycardia

195. When a patient with a colostomy comes to the radiology department for a barium enema (BE) examination, the radiographer is usually required to place the enema tip into the
    A. Rectum
    B. Stoma
    C. Fistula
    D. Orifice

196. Which of the following guidelines are accepted means of controlling infection in the radiology department?
    1. Washing hands between patients
    2. Wearing gloves when emptying soiled linen
    3. Recapping any dirty needles

    A. 1 and 2 only
    B. 1 and 3 only
    C. 2 and 3 only
    D. 1, 2, and 3

197. A patient on a clear-liquid diet is restricted from ingesting which of the following?
    A. Gelatin
    B. Tea
    C. Bouillon
    D. Dry toast

198. When performing CPR on an adult victim, the chest compressions are considered effective when the sternum is depressed about:
    A. ½ to 1 inch
    B. 1 to 1½ inches
    C. 1½ to 2 inches
    D. 2 to 3 inches

199. Normal adult diastolic pressure usually ranges from:
    A. 30–50 mm of mercury
    B. 60–90 mm of mercury
    C. 100–120 mm of mercury
    D. 130–150 mm of mercury

200. Which of the following types of drugs would be the best to administer to a patient following an allergic reaction to contrast medium?
    A. Analgesic
    B. Cathartic
    C. Diuretic
    D. Antihistamine

Answers and Explanations

Each rationale is followed by a reference to a text listed in the bibliography at the end of this chapter.

SECTION I: RADIATION PROTECTION

1. **(D)** A person whose office is situated adjacent to a radiographic room would be considered part of the public frequently exposed to radiation because it can be assumed that this person would be in the office the majority of the 40-hour workweek. Therefore, the lead lining should be sufficient in the walls to limit exposure to this area to less than 1 mSv (0.1 rem) annually. An area outside the radiographic room that would provide *infrequent* exposure to the public would be a back hallway, stairwell, or waiting room where the same individual would not be exposed continuously during a 40-hour workweek.
    Bushong, "Health Physics," p 502; NCRP Report No. 116, pp 55–56; Statkiewicz-Sherer et al., "Limits for Exposure to Ionizing Radiation," p 64.

2. **(C)** X rays are a part of the EM spectrum and thus travel at the "speed of light." However, they also have their own unique properties due to their comparatively high energy. Some of these properties include the ability to ionize matter and the ability to cause certain materials to fluoresce. In addition, they are highly penetrating and invisible; they cannot be focused by a lens as light waves can; they are not affected by an electrical

or a magnetic field; and they are heterogeneous, meaning that they are produced with many different energies.

Carlton and McKenna-Adler, "Radiation Concepts," pp 35–36; Cullinan, "Energy, Atomic Structure and Electromagnetic Radiation," p 8; Selman, "X-Rays (Roentgen Rays)," p 160.

3. **(B)** Shielding materials made out of lead are best when used to protect from highly penetrating sources of EM radiation such as x rays or gamma rays. Any type of shielding material will protect from alpha radiation because it is not capable of penetrating even a sheet of paper. Lead shielding should not be the material of choice when the exposure is from beta radiation. Although beta particles are not very penetrating compared with x rays and gamma rays, beta particles are high-speed electrons and when coming into contact with material of high atomic number, such as lead, more radiation will be produced. This is similar to how x rays are produced at the anode when tungsten atoms, which have a high atomic number, decelerate high-speed electrons. Better shielding materials to use when exposed to a beta-emitting patient or other source are elements with low atomic number, such as glass or plastic.

Dowd and Tilson, "Radiation Protection in Nuclear Medicine," pp 266; Selman, "Protection in Radiology: Health Physics," pp 538–539.

4. **(C)** Whenever the energy of the x-ray tube exceeds 70 kVp, the minimum amount of total filtration should be equivalent to at least 2.5 mm Al. The NCRP also recommends that when the tube operates above an energy level of 50 kVp, but does not exceed 70 kVp, the minimum amount of total filtration should be equivalent to at least 1.5 mm Al. Special x-ray tubes, such as those used for mammography, operating routinely below 50 kVp should have a minimum of 0.5-mm Al equivalent.

Bushong, "Designing for Radiation Protection," p 510; Selman, "Protection in Radiology: Health Physics," pp 528–529.

5. **(C)** The *GSD* is defined as the average gonadal dose dispersed among the population based on those individuals in that population who were actually exposed to man-made ionizing radiation. Currently the GSD in the United States is estimated to average 20 millirad per individual, which is over and above the genetic load on the population of background radiation, which is approximately 40 millirad. However, many experts believe that despite efforts by the NCRP to limit the GSD to as low as reasonably achievable, it is steadily rising each year. This is due to many factors, including (1) de-

fensive medicine, (2) increased diagnostic efficacy of higher-dose procedures such as cardiac catheterization, and (3) an aging population.

Bushong, "Radiation Protection Procedures," p 529; Dowd and Tilson, "The Basis for Radiation Protection," p 9; Statkiewicz-Sherer et al., "Protection of the Patient During Diagnostic Radiologic Procedures," p 172.

6. **(D)** The NCRP categorizes dose limits to anatomic parts based on two types of effects: (1) stochastic and (2) deterministic. *Stochastic effects* are nonthreshold effects that may occur at any dose and are usually long-term late effects, such as cancer and genetic mutations. *Deterministic effects* usually occur above a certain threshold and may be either short term or long term depending on the dose. Examples of deterministic effects include skin erythema, alopecia, drop in the white blood cell count, and cataracts. The NCRP limits many of the very sensitive tissues of the body (bone marrow, thyroid, gonads, etc.) to low doses based on stochastic effects, which may occur at any dose (nonthreshold effects). The limits for more resistant tissues (skin, hands, and feet and lens of the eye) are slightly higher based on deterministic effects. Of the effects listed, only cataracts would be considered a deterministic effect because cataractogenesis produced by radiation will occur only above a threshold dose of 2 Gy (200 rads).

Bushong, "Late Effects of Radiation," pp 478–479; Dowd and Tilson, "Further Concepts of Radiobiology," pp 111–113; NCRP Report No. 116, p 36; Carlton and McKenna-Adler, "Radiation Protection Procedures for Patients and Personnel," p 156.

7. **(B)** The gestational stage when the fetus is *most* susceptible to congenital defects is during the period called major *organogenesis,* which occurs between the 2nd and the 10th week. The first stage, called the *preimplantation stage,* is probably the safest time to radiate a fetus because radiation effects will be all-or-nothing; either the damage will be so severe that the result is spontaneous abortion, or the fetus will be carried to term with no ill effects. During the final stage of development, the *fetal stage,* from the 10th week to full term, the developing baby is more likely to suffer long-term effects such as leukemia or other forms of malignancy rather than congenital effects, which are obvious at birth.

Bushong, "Late Effects of Radiation," pp 490–491; Dowd and Tilson, "Late Effects of Radiation," pp 158–162; Travis, "Total Body Radiation Response," pp 152–161.

8. **(C)** The units that are used to specify radiation "exposure" are the roentgen, or coulomb per

kilogram in the International System of Units, and are used to measure the number of ionizing events produced in air by either x- or gamma radiation. The units that are used to specify energy absorbed by tissue are the gray or the rad. The units that specify occupational exposure are either the sievert or the rem. Radioactivity can be measured by either the curie or the becquerel.

Bushong, "Radiographic Definitions and Mathematics Review," pp 13–14; Carlton and McKenna-Adler, "Radiation Concepts and Equipment," pp 146–148; Dowd and Tilson, "Ionizing Radiation," pp 43–45.

9. **(D)** Occupational workers who are exposed daily to man-made ionizing radiation should be carefully monitored to ensure that their exposure is kept well below the recommended limits. The NCRP recommends that the annual total body dose be kept below a maximum of 50 mSv (5 rem or 5000 mrem). For more resistant tissues, such as the skin, hands, and feet, the NCRP recommends that doses should be kept well below the maximum of 500 mSv (50 rem or 50,000 mrem).

Bushong, "Health Physics," p 500, Table 38–4; Carlton and McKenna-Adler, "Radiation Protection Procedures for Patients and Personnel," p 157, Table 9–1; NCRP Report No. 116, Table 19.1.

10. **(C)** In general, the first stage of a biologic response to radiation damage is ionization. Because water (H_2O) is the most abundant chemical in the cell (approximately 65 to 70 percent), it is the most likely molecule to be struck by radiation. When ionization occurs in H_2O molecules due to radiation exposure, the molecules may break down further to form free radicals. Free radicals cause biologic damage to other molecules because they are chemically unstable by themselves and will thus look for other chemicals to combine with. *Free radicals* may be defined as an uncharged atom or molecule possessing only one free electron in its outer shell. Some atoms are naturally occurring free radicals, such as hydrogen. One hydrogen atom will normally combine with other atoms in a covalent bond, such as with two additional oxygen atoms to form H_2O. When water splits apart following irradiation, the free radicals that are produced may combine to make volatile or toxic chemicals in the cell, such as hydrogen peroxide (H_2O_2).

Bushong, "Molecular and Cellular Radiobiology," pp 452–453; Dowd and Tilson, "Principles of Radiobiology," p 106; Statkiewicz-Sherer et al., "Radiation Biology," pp 97–98; Travis, "Basic Biologic Interactions of Radiation," p 27.

11. **(B)** There are no electrons that exist inside the nucleus although beta particles, which are identical to electrons, may be emitted from an unstable atom when a neutron splits apart. There are also no electrons that may be categorized as free radicals of themselves; an entire atom or molecule may be classified as such. Thus, the electrons that are most tightly bound in their orbit around the nucleus are the ones closest to the nucleus. The K-shell electrons have the highest "binding" energy and are most difficult to eject from the atom.

Bushong, "The Atom," p 36; Carlton and McKenna-Adler, "Radiation Concepts," p 26; Dowd and Tilson, "Interactions of Radiation with Matter," p 66.

12. **(A)** The entrance skin exposure is a commonly used measure of patient exposure because the skin is always the tissue that receives the highest dose. ESE will increase with lower-energy x rays (low-kilovolts [peak]) and higher–milliamperage-second values. In general, those tissues with low inherent subject contrast, such as the breast, abdomen, and skull, require lower-kilovolt (peak) and higher–milliamperage-second technical factors to ensure satisfactory radiographic contrast. Thus, the ESE in these areas of the body would be greater than in the chest, which comparatively has very high subject contrast requiring a higher-kilovolt (peak) and lower–milliamperage-second selection. Thus, the lowest ESE of all of the radiographic examinations listed would be that of the chest, which has an ESE of about 10 to 20 millirad.

Bushong, "Radiation Protection Procedures," pp 526–530; Carlton and McKenna-Adler, "Minimizing Patient Dose," p 208, Table 13–2, and "Technical Aspects of Mammography," p 568; Dowd and Tilson, "Protecting the Patient in Radiography," p 196, Table 11–3.

13. **(B)** In most cases, when the kilovolts (peak) is increased and the milliamperage-seconds is decrease comparably to produce satisfactory radiographic density, the patient's radiation dose will also decrease. Only when the kilovolts (peak) is increased without a comparable decrease in milliamperage-seconds will the patient's dose increase. It is the milliamperage-seconds (Milliamperage × Time) that will have a direct effect on the patient's dose. In other words, if the milliamperage-seconds is doubled, without any other changes, the patient's dose will also double. Decreasing the milliamperes with a comparable increase in time that results in equal milliamperage-seconds should have no effect on patient dose as long as the equipment is functioning properly.

Bushong, "Radiation Protection Procedures," pp 537–538; Carlton and McKenna-Adler, "Minimizing Patient Dose," p 210, Table 13–4; Dowd and Tilson, "Protecting the Patient in Radiography," pp 219–221.

14. **(C)** There are two main parts of the cell: the nucleus and the cytoplasm. The cytoplasm contain most of the water and the functional organelles such as the lysosomes, ribosomes, mitochondria, and so forth. The nucleus contains the DNA in addition to one organelle—the nucleolus. The nucleolus contains most of the RNA but does not contain any DNA. The nucleolus is usually situated very close to the nuclear membrane to allow the passage of RNA from the nucleus to the cytoplasm.

Bushong, "Human Biology," p 435; Dowd and Tilson, "Cellular Biology," p 92; Statkiewicz-Sherer et al., "Overview of Cell Biology"; Travis, "Review of Cell Biology," pp 10–11.

15. **(B)** Ionizing radiation has long been known to induce *teratogenesis*, which means that it is capable of causing severe congenital anomalies to a developing embryo or fetus. Other well-known teratogens include alcohol, certain types of drugs, rubella (german measles), malnutrition, and so forth. This is why a radiographer should always ask women of childbearing age if there is any possibility of pregnancy, especially when performing abdominal radiographs.

Dowd and Tilson, "Late Effects of Radiation," p 159.

16. **(A)** Radiographic equipment is usually calibrated by using the units of exposure, which designate radiation intensity. The units that are used to specify radiation exposure are the roentgen, or coulomb/kg in the SI system, and are used by a radiation detector to measure the number of ionizing events produced in air by either x- or gamma radiation. The roentgen, or coulomb per kilogram, is not appropriate for other types of radiation because particulate radiation, such as alpha, beta, or other particles, ionizes differently than EM radiation.

Papp, "Quality Control of Radiographic Equipment," p 73; Selman, "X-Rays (Roentgen Rays)," pp 161–164; Statkiewicz-Sherer et al., "Radiation Monitoring," p 228; Thompson et al., "Radiological Health Physics," p 456.

17. **(C)** The film badge is the most commonly employed type of personnel monitor because of its low cost and because it can be kept as a permanent record. Filters are usually placed in front of the film's emulsion to estimate the average energies of radiation that exposed the film. The filters act much like a step wedge, casting an image on the exposed film underneath. The filters are typically made of aluminum, copper, and sometimes plastic or cadmium. Lead foil may be used as a backing to absorb any backscatter but is not used as a filter.

Bushong, "Radiation Protection Procedures," p 532; Selman, "Protection in Radiology: Health Physics," p 512; Statkiewicz-Sherer et al., "Radiation Monitoring," p 218.

18. **(C)** The principal piece of test equipment used to measure most radiation output is an ionization-type meter. The most common type of ionization chamber used for radiographic equipment is what is called the "cutie pie." The cutie pie is usually calibrated to measure radiation output in milliroentgens and can be coupled with a computer to automatically measure the milliroentgen per unit milliamperage-seconds.

Papp, "Quality Control of Radiographic Equipment," pp 71–73; Selman, "X-Rays (Roentgen Rays)," pp 161–164, and "Protection in Radiology," p 539; Statkiewicz-Sherer et al., "Radiation Monitoring," pp 226–228; Thompson et al., "Radiological Health Physics," p 456.

19. **(B)** The protective curtain or sliding panel, which is attached to the image intensifier above the examining table, is usually used during fluoroscopy to protect the radiographer and other personnel from scatter radiation exiting the patient. The radiographer should never be exposed to the primary beam, and this includes the exit beam, which is coming directly out of the patient to expose the image receptor. This is especially important to remember when assisting with fluoroscopic procedures because the dose is so much higher than it is for routine diagnostic procedures. Leakage radiation is that which exits the x-ray tube in directions other than through the port window. The lead housing is used to protect personnel from this type of radiation.

Dowd and Tilson, "Protecting the Radiographer and Other Workers," p 212; Selman, "Protection in Radiology: Health Physics," p 521; Statkiewicz-Sherer et al., "Protecting Occupationally Exposed Personnel during Diagnostic Radiologic Procedures," p 195.

20. **(B)** The four phases of *mitosis*, when the cell is undergoing division, are (1) prophase, (2) metaphase, (3) anaphase, and (4) telophase. *Prophase* is the first stage in which the nuclear membrane dissolves and the chromatin threads begin to migrate to the equator. During the second stage, *metaphase*, the chromosomes take on their definitive shape and line up along the equator of the cell. This is the best stage to study chromosomes for signs of radiation damage. *Anaphase* is the third stage in which the chromosomes split and divide and head toward the poles. Finally, *telophase* is when the two new nuclear membranes form at each pole and the chromosomes once again dissolve into chromatin threads and the

cytoplasm divides (cytokinesis) into two new cells. *Interphase* is often called the "resting" stage because it separates one mitotic stage from another; it is also the longest stage of the cell cycle, but chromosomes are not clearly visible until metaphase.

Bushong, "Human Biology," p 436; Travis, "Basic Biologic Interactions of Radiation," p 36.

21. **(C)** In 1989, the NCRP began using SI units to designate its dose-equivalent limits for occupational personnel. Thus, it is important for radiographers to become familiar with these new units. When converting from rem to millisievert, simply multiply by 10. Therefore, 3 rem would convert to 30 mSv, and 30 rem would convert to 300 mSv.

Dowd and Tilson, "Radiation Safety/Protection and Health Physics," pp 182–184; Carlton and McKenna-Adler, "Radiation Protection Concepts and Equipment," p 148; Statkiewicz-Sherer et al., "Radiation Quantities and Units," p 47.

22. **(C)** The photoelectric effect is more likely when x rays of lower photon energy are used and when interaction occurs with tissues of higher atomic number. Compton scattering, the other common interaction in the diagnostic range, is more likely to occur with x rays of higher photon energy and with tissues of lower atomic number. This is why a grid is necessary when technical factors above 80 kVp are used or when body parts with a higher fat content, such as the abdomen, are radiographed.

Bushong, "X-Ray Interaction with Matter," pp 151–154; Carlton and McKenna-Adler, "X-Ray Interactions," pp 199–201; Dowd and Tilson, "Interactions of Radiation with Matter," pp 67–70.

23. **(B)** Shortly after the discovery of x rays in 1895, it was found that exposure to x-radiation would cause changes in biologic tissues. The reason for these changes was unclear until the 1920s, when radiation physicists concluded that the biologic damage was due to ionization. Thus, the roentgen became the unit for radiation intensity, or ionization, in air in 1929. The units of rad and rem were implemented soon after. However, prior to the 1920s, the radiological community used the SED_{50} to set limits for radiation exposure. The *SED* was the dose that it would take to turn an occupational worker's skin red (approximately 600 rad). Early occupational workers were allowed only ⅒ of the SED annually (approximately 60 rad). This is totally unacceptable by today's standards. Our current limits are set at 50 mSv (5 rem) annually.

Bushong, "Early Effects of Radiation," p 468; Dowd and Tilson, "Early Effects of Radiation," p 131;

Statkiewicz-Sherer et al., "Radiation Quantities and Units," p 38.

24. **(C)** For questions 24 and 25, three steps are required. First, calculate the milliamperage-seconds. Second, look on the chart to determine what the exposure rate would be at the particular kilovolts (peak) in the question; in this case, 80 kVp is found to have a rate of 3.2 mR/mAs. The third step requires setting up a ratio and proportion equation. If there are 3.2 mR for every 1 mAs, how many milliroentgens are there in 40 mAs (400 mA × 0.1 second)?

$$\frac{mR}{mAs} = \frac{x}{40\ mAs}; \quad \frac{3.2\ mR \times 40\ mAs}{1\ mAs} = x;$$

$$x = 128\ mR$$

Bushong, "Radiation Protection Procedures," p 528.

25. **(C)** Follow these steps to solve the problem: (1) find the milliamperage-seconds, which is 30; (2) Find the exposure rate at 90 kVp, which is 4.0 mR/mAs; (3) set up a ratio and proportion as shown:

$$\frac{4\ mR}{1\ mAs} = \frac{x}{30\ mAs}; \quad \frac{4\ mR \times 30\ mAs}{1\ mAs} = x;$$

$$x = 120\ mR$$

Bushong, "Radiation Protection Procedures," p 528.

26. **(C)** When reading dose-response curves on a graph, the horizontal axis represents the dose received, whereas the vertical axis represents the effects that may be observed. There are two broad categories of curves: (1) threshold and (2) nonthreshold. There are also three distinct shapes that these curves can take: (1) linear, (2) linear quadratic, and (3) sigmoidal. A *linear curve* is one represented by a straight line. Curves A, B, and C are all linear curves because they are all straight lines. Curves A and B are both nonthreshold because the radiation effects are immediately noticeable above a dose level of zero on the graph. Curve A starts out higher on the vertical axis because some effects may occur naturally in a population prior to any radiation exposure (e.g., sterility, cancer, etc.). Curve C will begin to show an effect above a specific threshold. An example of a threshold effect would be cataracts because this effect is induced only by radiation doses exceeding 200 rads.

Dowd and Tilson, "Principles of Radiobiology," pp 109–111; Statkiewicz-Sherer et al., "Radiation Biology," pp 113–115.

27. **(B)** The NCRP determines its dose-equivalent limits based on the linear, nonthreshold dose curve

(curve B), meaning that even a very small dose can cause certain types of biologic damage. However, in reality, most experts believe that the effects seen at lower doses and with low–linear energy transfer (LET) radiation are negligible and thus follow more of a linear, quadratic shape. The NCRP prefers to take the more conservative approach by using the linear model for all nonthreshold effects to ensure minimum exposure to the public.

Dowd and Tilson, "Principles of Radiobiology," pp 109; Statkiewicz-Sherer et al., "Radiation Biology," pp 113–115.

28. **(A)** The total exposure can be determined by finding the product of Exposure rate × Time. The exposure rate is usually expressed in units of milliroentgen per hours or roentgen per minute. In this example, the rate is expressed as milliroentgen per hour, and assuming that the radiographer maintained the same distance throughout the procedure, the answer would be found by multiplying:

$$\frac{250 \text{ mR}}{h} \times \frac{5 \text{ min}}{60 \text{ min/h}} = \frac{1250}{60} = 21 \text{ mR}$$

Bushong, "Radiation Protection Procedures," p 524.

29. **(D)** The NCRP is the government entity established by the Food and Drug Administration (FDA) to protect the public from man-made ionizing radiation. LET is the measure of the rate of energy deposited by radiation as it travels through matter. The GSD is a representative number of the genetic load on the population based on the average gonadal dose. The ALARA philosophy states that all occupational personnel should strive to keep radiation exposures to patients, personnel, and the public to as low as reasonably achievable.

Bushong, "Basic Concepts of Radiation Science," p 8; Dowd and Tilson, "The Basis for Radiation Protection," p 2; Statkiewicz-Sherer et al., "Limits for Exposure to Ionizing Radiation," p 59.

30. **(A)** Ultraviolet radiation and x rays and gamma rays are all classified as EM radiation although only x rays and gamma rays are capable of ionization. All three are forms of energy and are not considered matter because they have no mass, no charge, and so forth. Other types of ionizing radiation may be categorized as particulate radiation because they are actually particles of matter. Typically, they have mass and most have some type of charge, either positive or negative. The only type of ionizing radiation among the possible choices that is categorized as particulate radiation is alpha. An alpha particle has a mass of 4 atomic mass units and a charge of +2.

Bushong, "The Atom," pp 40–41; Carlton and McKenna-Adler, "Radiation Protection Concepts and Equipment," p 144; Dowd and Tilson, "Ionizing Radiation," p 40.

SECTION II: EQUIPMENT OPERATION AND MAINTENANCE

31. **(D)** Without the use of the ABC, the brightness of the image on the fluoroscopic screen would vary greatly as the image intensifier was moved across the patient. The ABC automatically adjusts the technical factors of kilovolts (peak) and milliamperes as the patient thickness and/or tissue density increases or decreases. This is accomplished by the use of a photocell placed between the image intensifier and the television camera. The brightness may also be automatically adjusted on the TV monitor itself, and this is called the *automatic gain control*. The automatic gain control, unlike the automatic brightness control, does not have an effect on the technical factors of kilovolts (peak) and milliamperage-seconds, and thus does not affect patient dose. The photocathode is found on the input side of the image intensifier and serves to convert the light from the input phosphor into electrons. The electrostatic lenses are found within the image intensifier and help to focus the electron stream from the photocathode toward the output phosphor.

Bushong, "Fluoroscopy," pp 324–327; Curry et al., "Viewing and Recording the Fluoroscopic Image," p 185; Carlton and McKenna-Adler, "Fluoroscopy," pp 536–540.

32. **(C)** The synchronous spinning top is a QC test tool used for calibrating the accuracy of the timer in a 3-phase x-ray generator. It has little application for any other QC test. The pinhole camera is a tool used to measure the size of the effective focal spot, but it cannot be used to monitor the function of other parts of the radiographic tube or generator. The sensitometer is a device that projects an optical step wedge onto a QC test film to assess the function of the automatic processor. It also has little application anywhere else in radiography. Only the digital dosimeter may be used for multiple quality assurance purposes. It is usually coupled with a computerized system by which the dosimetric readings taken from the intensity of the x-ray tube may be automatically calculated. The calculations may be used to check the accuracy of multiple devices of the x-ray generator at the same time: (1) milliamperage accuracy, (2) timer accuracy, (3) kilovolt (peak) accuracy, (4) leakage radiation, (5) maximum flu-

oroscopic output, (6) minimum filtration (HVL), and (7) rectification system.

Carlton and McKenna-Adler, "Quality Control," p 444; Papp, "Quality Control of Radiographic Equipment," pp 71–72; Thompson et al., "Quality Control," pp 403–407.

33. **(D)** The falling-load generator is designed specifically to produce exposures using the highest possible milliamperes with the shortest possible time settings. The radiographer is limited to the selection of milliamperage-seconds, and the machine determines the milliamperage and time combination that would be safest to use to avoid heat damage to the tube. Therefore, it would not be useful when long exposure times are required, such as in breathing techniques for lateral thoracic spines. Of the four types of x-ray generators mentioned, the high-frequency generator has the highest constant potential and the widest variety of options available for the selection of technical factors (milliamperes, kilovolts [peak], and time). The battery-powered mobile unit also offers a wide selection of technical factors, including long exposure times; its main disadvantage is its need to be fully charged prior to use. The capacitor discharge unit offers a good selection of milliamperage and time variables, but the kilovolts (peak) varies during the exposure, somewhat limiting its use to certain body parts and thickness.

Bushong, "Radiographic Exposure," p 254; Carlton and McKenna-Adler, "X-Ray Equipment," pp 103–105; Curry et al., "X-Ray Generators," pp 56–57; Thompson et al., "X-Ray Machine Operation: The X-Ray Circuit," p 194.

34. **(C)** Most modern x-ray units are either 3-phase or high-frequency generators that use a device called an electronic timer. The electronic timer is the most complex and most accurate of all of the available timers and also is capable of producing the shortest exposure times, as small as 1 millisecond (0.001 second).

Bushong, "The X-Ray Unit," p 98; Carlton and McKenna-Adler, "X-Ray Equipment," p 98; Selman, "X-Ray Circuits," p 241.

35. **(C)** There is an exponential relationship between the kilovolt (peak) setting and the intensity of the x-ray beam. In other words, if the kilovolts (peak) is doubled, the intensity will increase by a factor of 4. To figure out this problem, use the kilovolt (peak) intensity formula:

$$\frac{kVp_1^2}{kVp_2^2} = \frac{I_1}{I_2};$$

$$\frac{70^2}{81^2} = \frac{100 \text{ mR}}{X};$$

$$X = \frac{100 \text{ mR} \times (81 \times 81)}{70 \times 70}; \frac{100 \text{ mR} \times 6561}{4900};$$

$$X = 133.8 \text{ mR or } 134 \text{ mR}$$

Bushong, "X-Ray Emission," pp 140–141; Curry et al., "Production of X-Rays," p 35.

36. **(A)** An increase in kilovolts (peak) and an increase in phosphor thickness will have a direct effect on the speed of an intensifying screen. The screen will emit more light at higher-kilovolt (peak) settings and also with thicker phosphor layers. The FSS should have no effect on the speed of the intensifying screen. Another factor that may affect screen speed is that extremely high temperatures may decrease the light emission and therefore the screen speed.

Carlton and McKenna-Adler, "Intensifying Screens," pp 334–335; Curry et al., "Luminescent Screens," pp 124–131.

37. **(C)** Because of the anode heel effect that is inevitable with an angled anode, the intensity not only varies from cathode to anode but also varies the effective FSS. The effective focal spot would be smaller on the anode side, and the x-ray intensity would be less toward the anode side than toward the cathode side. This is why the thinner anatomy should be placed under the anode and the thicker anatomy toward the cathode side. For example, when PA projection of the chest is performed, the cathode should be placed so that it faces the patient's feet, whereas the anode end of the tube should be placed so that it faces the patient's head, because the upper thorax is much thinner and requires less radiation.

Bushong, "The X-Ray Tube," p 118; Carlton and McKenna-Adler, "The X-Ray Tube," p 120; Selman, "Devices for Improving Radiographic Quality," pp 394–396.

38. **(A)** Reducing the field of view in an image intensifier serves to magnify the image. This image is magnified because of the change in the focal point, which ultimately changes the minification gain. Because minification gain affects the brightness, a decrease in brightness will cause the ABC to automatically increase the technical factors of milliamperes and kilovolts (peak) to compensate. The result is an increase in patient dose when smaller field sizes are used. Therefore, a 9-inch field size will cause a decrease in patient dose as compared with a 6-inch field size.

Bushong, "Fluoroscopy," pp 325–326; Carlton and McKenna-Adler, "Fluoroscopy," pp 538–539; Curry et al., "Fluoroscopic Imaging," p 173.

39. **(C)** The AEC unit should be calibrated so that the backup timer terminates the exposure within 6

seconds or 600 mAs, whichever comes first. This is a guideline as set forth by the Code of Federal Regulations (21 CFR) for x-ray tubes operating above 50 kVp. For x-ray tubes operating below 50 kVp, the maximum allowable exposure is 2000 mAs.

Carlton and McKenna-Adler, "X-Ray Equipment," p 108; Papp, "Radiographic Ancillary Equipment," p 96; Selman, "X-Ray Circuits," pp 243–244.

40. **(B)** The built-in mechanism of PBL was mandated in the 1970s by the federal government for the manufacture of all new radiographic equipment. This was to ensure that the x-ray field size would be limited to the size of the cassette in the Bucky tray. Most PBL systems have an override mechanism that allows the radiographer to collimate to a greater degree. This federal mandate is no longer enforced because the FDA believed that this would actually decrease the effectiveness of the ALARA (as low as reasonably achievable) principle. The agency cited that the PBL mechanism was "no substitute for properly trained and supervised operators."

Bushong, "Designing for Radiation Protection," p 510; Carlton and McKenna-Adler, "Beam Restriction," p 242; Carroll, "Field Size Limitation," p 137; Dowd and Tilson, "Protecting the Patient in Radiography," p 231.

41. **(C)** The turns ratio in a transformer is always the ratio of the number of turns in the secondary coil over the number of turns in the primary coil. Because the turns ratio in this transformer is greater than 1:1, it can be assumed that this must be a step-up transformer. In a step-up transformer, the voltage on the secondary side is always larger than the voltage on the primary side based on the following formula:

$$\frac{V_2}{V_1} = \frac{\text{No. of turns}_2}{\text{No. of turns}_1}$$

$$\frac{x}{220\,V} = \frac{500}{1}; x = 220 \times 500;$$

x = 110,000 V or 110 kilovolts (kV)

Bushong, "Electromagnetism," p 83; Carlton and McKenna-Adler, "Electromagnetism," p 74; Selman, "Production and Control of High Voltage," p 125.

42. **(C)** The amplitude of tube travel, or the degree of angulation, is the number one determinant of slice thickness in a tomographic image. The SID may affect the thickness, but only if it causes a change in the degree of angulation. The height of the fulcrum above the x-ray table will only change the pivot point, which serves to adjust the anatomy of interest demonstrated on the image.

The exposure time has nothing to do with the slice thickness.

Bushong, "Alternative Film Procedures," pp 282–284; Carlton and McKenna-Adler, "Tomography," pp 558–559; Curry et al., "Body Section Radiography," p 246.

43. **(C)** When a pinhole camera is used to test for the FSS, it should be placed halfway between the actual focal spot and the image receptor. In other words, if the SID is 40 inches, then the pinhole camera should be placed at a 20-inch OID or at a 20-inch source-object receptor-distance (SOD). Position of the camera is critical to obtain an accurate measurement of the focal spot.

Carroll, "Quality Control," p 401; Curry et al., "Geometry of the Radiographic Image," p 230; Papp, "Quality Control of Radiographic Equipment," p 80; Selman, "Radiographic Quality," p 324.

44. **(B)** On the secondary side of the high-tension transformer, the voltage has been "stepped up," usually to thousands of volts or kilovolts. However, it is still AC until it is rectified. Rectification is essential for radiographic equipment because the x-ray tube will not function properly and may in fact sustain irreparable damage if supplied by AC. The current is thus high-voltage AC between the high-tension transformer and the rectification system and high-voltage DC between the rectification system and the x-ray tube.

Carlton and McKenna-Adler, "Electromagnetism," pp 77–84; Curry et al., "X-Ray Generators," pp 42–43; Selman, "Rectification," pp 139–148.

45. **(C)** A capacitor discharge unit starts an exposure at the kilovolt (peak) setting but then drops off continuously throughout the entire exposure. Sometimes this drop in kilovolts (peak) as the capacitor loses its charge can be substantial, depending on the milliamperage-seconds selected for the exposure; typically, about 1 kVp is discharged for each milliamperage-second selected. This puts its efficiency at the lowest of all types of x-ray generators. Fully rectified single-phase generators also fluctuate throughout the exposure but are usually able to maintain a level of about 70 percent of the kilovolt (peak) setting. Fully rectified 3-phase generators fluctuate even less, achieving an efficiency of approximately 95 percent. High-frequency generators have the highest efficiency with almost no fluctuation, somewhere around 99 percent.

Curry et al., "X-Ray Generators," pp 51–54; Thompson et al., "Magnetism and Its Relation to Electricity," p 122.

46. **(C)** The potential difference is a measurement of the potential energy that exists between one side

of an electric circuit and the other. This potential difference is typically the difference in charge between two points in an electric circuit. The greater this difference, the higher the potential energy. The potential difference is sometimes called the "electromotive force" and is measured in volts. Therefore, the potential difference in an x-ray circuit is controlled by the kilovolt (peak) setting.

Bushong, "Electricity," p 61; Carlton and McKenna-Adler, "Electricity," p 47; Curry et al., "X-Ray Generators," pp 36–37; Selman, "Electrodynamics: Electric Current," pp 68–70.

47. **(A)** The greatest amplitude is the equivalent of the greatest range of motion. Of all of the tomographic units listed, the hypocycloidal model gives the greatest range of motion during the exposure. Its motion resembles that of a cloverleaf, in comparison with the other three motions, which speak for themselves. The hypocycloidal motion is about five times longer than a conventional linear motion.

Carlton and McKenna-Adler, "Tomography," p 562; Cullinan, "Dedicated Radiographic Equipment and Techniques," p 176; Curry et al., "Body Section Radiography," p 251.

48. **(A)** Two types of radiation are produced at the tungsten target as high-speed electrons that are suddenly decelerated: (1) bremsstrahlung and (2) characteristic. Brems radiation is produced at all energy ranges, from zero to kilovolts (peak). *Brems* radiation is also called "braking" radiation because it is produced when the projectile electrons are slowed down as they pass the nuclei of tungsten atoms. *Characteristic radiation* is only produced at very specific energy levels because it is produced when the projectile electrons strike a K-shell electron, causing ionization of the tungsten atom. When electrons from the outer shells drop down to fill the space left in the K shell, an x ray is emitted, at 69.5 keV, then at other specific energies as the outer electrons continue to drop down to fill the vacant shells. Only the first characteristic x ray produced at 69.5 keV falls within the useful diagnostic range.

Bushong, "X-Ray Production," pp 128–131; Carlton and McKenna-Adler, "X-Ray Production," pp 134–139; Selman, "X-Rays (Roentgen Rays)," pp 170–171.

49. **(A)** According to this spectral distribution curve, the kilovolts (peak) of this x-ray beam is 80 kVp because that is the highest photon energy recorded along the horizontal axis. Looking at the vertical axis of radiation intensity, the majority of the photons being produced are in the 25 to 30

keV range. Even in the most efficient x-ray generators, the average photon energy is usually only about 30 to 40 percent of the kilovolts (peak) (80 × 0.3 = 24 keV; 80 × 0.4 = 32 keV). Therefore, the average energy of this 80-kVp x-ray beam is approximately 30 keV.

Bushong, "X-Ray Production," pp 128–131; Carlton and McKenna-Adler, "X-Ray Production," p 138; Selman, "X-Rays (Roentgen Rays)," pp 170–171.

50. **(B)** One HVL is the amount of filtering material (most likely aluminum) that will reduce the intensity of the beam by one-half. The TVL is the amount of filtering material that will reduce the intensity of the beam to one-tenth its initial intensity. One TVL is equal to 3.3 HVL: (1) 100% ÷ 2 = 50%; (2) 50% ÷ 2 = 25% ; (3) 25% ÷ 2 = 12.5% (3); 12.5% ÷ 1.3 = 10% (3.3). The HVL is important when calculating skin dose to a patient undergoing a diagnostic procedure with exposure to the primary beam. The TVL is more appropriately used for lead shielding in the walls of an x-ray room or for lead aprons worn by radiographers to keep exposure to leakage or scatter radiation to a minimum.

Bushong, "Health Physics," p 497.

51. **(C)** Most EM radiation is categorized by its wavelength, frequency, or energy because the velocity of all EM radiation is constant (speed of light). EM has no mass, and typically the origin is not as important as the photon energy because the energy will determine the possible biologic damage through its ability to ionize.

Carlton and McKenna-Adler, "Radiation Concepts," p 32; Cullinan, "Energy, Atomic Structure and Electromagnetic Radiation," p 8; Selman, "X-Rays (Roentgen Rays)," p 152.

52. **(B)** The filament in a vacuum tube is most likely located on the cathode end of the tube, which is the negative electrode. The filament is the source of electrons that provide a negative energy potential on one side of the tube as compared with the positive (anode) side of the tube, which lacks electrons.

Carlton and McKenna-Adler, "The X-Ray Tube," p 112. Selman, "X-Ray Tubes and Rectifiers," p 205. Curry et al., "Production of X-Rays," p 11.

53. **(A)** The milliamperage selection controls the number of electrons that are boiled off during the preparation or boost stage of x-ray production. How long the electrons flow from cathode to anode is determined by the time selection. The selection of kilovoltage determines the energy of the electrons as they are accelerated from cathode to anode. The higher the potential difference determined by kilovolts (peak), the faster the

electrons will travel and the higher the energy of the x rays that will be produced. The number of electrons, or quantity, is controlled by milli-amperes or current.

Bushong, "X-Ray Emission," p 140; Carlton and McKenna-Adler, "Electricity," p 46; Selman, "X-Rays (Roentgen Rays)," p 164.

54. **(D)** *Radiopaque materials* are materials that will not easily allow x rays to pass through. These materials are usually composed of elements with high atomic numbers, such as calcium-containing bone, barium, iodine, and lead. Radiopaque materials are also more dense, meaning that their atoms are more closely compacted together. *Radiolucent materials* are those that easily allow the passage of x rays, and these are composed of lower atomic numbers and are less dense, such as air or positioning sponges. The terms *transparent* and *translucent* apply to light absorption by materials, not x-ray absorption. For example, a glass window would be transparent, meaning that it allows the majority of light photons to go through, whereas polaroid sunglasses would be translucent, only allowing some light rays to penetrate.

Bushong, "Electromagnetic Radiation," p 52; Cullinan, "Glossary of Related Terminology," p 272.

55. **(B)** A photomultiplier tube is a radiation detection device that gives off light in response to x-ray exposure. Its most useful purpose in diagnostic x-ray equipment is as an AEC device. This is why many radiographers still refer to AEC devices as "phototimers." However, most modern equipment uses an ionization chamber or a solid-state detector for the AEC radiation sensors, so the term phototimer is no longer appropriate.

Bushong, "The X-Ray Unit," p 98; Thompson et al., "X-Ray Machine Operation: The X-Ray Circuit," pp 183–185.

56. **(D)** The diagnostically useful range of x-ray energy levels is from 25 to 150 keV, because 150 kVp is typically the maximum peak energy that can be set on most diagnostic radiographic equipment. Pair production absolutely cannot occur at energies below 1.02 MeV (1020 keV) and therefore is never possible in the diagnostic range. The photoelectric effect occurs at lower-energy levels (usually below 60 keV) and when interacting with tissues of higher atomic number (bone, iodine, barium, and lead). Compton scattering can occur throughout the diagnostic range but is more likely at higher-energy levels and when interactions occur with tissues of lower atomic number (fat, muscle, and water). Classical scattering usually occurs at very low energy levels, usually below the diagnostically useful range, but

can occur with energies generated by diagnostic x-ray equipment.

Bushong, "X-Ray Interaction with Matter," p 155; Carlton and McKenna-Adler, "X-Ray Interactions," p 198; Curry et al., "Basic Interactions Between X-Rays and Matter," p 68.

57. **(B)** The terms *vidicon* and *plumbicon* in an image intensifier refer to the two most common types of camera tubes used to send an image from the output phosphor to the television monitor for viewing. The two main types of phosphors used in image intensifiers are (1) cesium iodide, used for the input phosphor, and (2) zinc cadmium sulfide, used for the output phosphor.

Bushong, "Fluoroscopy," p 327; Carlton and McKenna-Adler, "Fluoroscopy," p 543; Curry et al., "Viewing and Recording the Fluoroscopic Image," p 176.

58. **(A)** The photocathode in an image intensification system is located in the image intensification "tower." The input side of the tower contains the larger input phosphor to intercept the exit beam as x rays exit the patient. The input phosphor serves to convert the exit radiation into light photons. Also located on the input side is the photocathode, placed directly behind the input phosphor. The photocathode serves to convert light photons into electrons. The electrons generated by the photocathode are then focused toward the output side—toward the output phosphor—by the electrostatic lenses. At the output side, the output phosphor converts electrons back into light photons for direct imaging or coupling to a television camera tube.

Bushong, "Fluoroscopy," p 324; Carlton and McKenna-Adler, "Fluoroscopy," pp 536–537; Curry et al., "Fluoroscopic Imaging," pp 166–168.

59. **(B)** To solve this problem, it is first important to be familiar with the HU formula specific for each type of generator. The basic formula is HU = kVp × mA × Time × C. The letter *C* is the rectification constant used for the specific type of generator in question. For a single-phase generator, constant is 1. For a 3-phase, 6-pulse generator, the constant is 1.35. For a 3-phase, 12-pulse generator, the generator constant is 1.41, and for a high-frequency generator, the generator constant is 1.45. Because the generator in this question is a 3-phase, 12-pulse unit, the formula would be as follows:

kVp × mA × Time × 1.41;

72 × 300 x 1 s × 1.41 = 30,456 HU

The first calculation would tell the radiographer how many heat units would be generated by a single exposure using these technical factors. Because the question asked how many of these exposures could be taken before exceeding the maximum heat storage capacity, the radiographer now needs to divide the maximum number (350,000) by 30,456 to find the answer:

$$\frac{350,000}{30,456} = 11.49$$

When the calculation does not yield a whole number, the answer is found by rounding down to the nearest whole number, because rounding up would exceed the maximum number of exposures. Therefore, the correct answer is 11 rapid exposures, because 12 rapid exposures would exceed the maximum heat storage of 350,000.

Bushong, "The X-Ray Tube," pp 122–123; Carlton and McKenna-Adler, "The X-Ray Tube," pp 126–127; Curry et al., "Production of X-Rays," pp 22–25.

60. **(D)** Radiographic equipment manufactured with very small focal spots, sometimes referred to as "fractional focal spots," is mainly used for magnification radiography. The size of the focal spot regulates the recorded detail of the radiograph. The smaller is the focal spot, the better the recorded detail. Because magnification causes recorded detail to decrease, it is desirable to use the smallest FSS possible when performing magnification radiography. Fractional focal spots, less than 0.3 mm, are usually found in dedicated mammography units and special procedure radiographic x-ray tubes where magnification procedures are common. The major disadvantage of small FSSs is the decreased heat-loading capacity. Therefore, for procedures that require a high heat loading, such as tomography or serial rapid exposure imaging, the smaller focal spots are not recommended.

Bushong, "Alternative Film Procedures," p 291; Curry et al., "Geometry of the Radiographic Image," pp 228–229; Selman, "Radiographic Quality," pp 352–353.

SECTION III: IMAGE PRODUCTION AND EVALUATION

61. **(A)** The radiographic contrast of an image receptor is inversely proportional to its latitude. In other words, a film-screen combination with wide latitude would exhibit low contrast. The latitude of an image receptor is basically the range of error allowed to the radiographer when setting technical factors to achieve a diagnostically useful image.

Bushong, "Radiographic Film," p 170; Carlton and McKenna-Adler, "Film/Screen Combinations," p 350; Carroll, "Image Receptor Systems," p 228, 1998.

62. **(A)** Typically, when a particular examination is performed in one radiographic room using single-phase equipment, the radiographer would need to cut the original milliamperage-seconds in half when repeating the same examination in a room using 3-phase, 12-pulse equipment. Therefore, it is necessary to first compute the original milliamperage-seconds:

$$400 \times 0.05 \text{ seconds} = 20 \text{ mAs}$$

Then cut the milliamperage-seconds in half when performing the exam on 3-phase, 12-pulse equipment. The answer would be 10 mAs.

Carlton and McKenna-Adler, "Exposure Conversion Problems," p 514; Carroll, "Machine Phase and Rectification," p 125, 1998.

63. **(A)** When performing an acceptance test to verify the size of the focal spot, the image receptor used should be either a nonscreen holder or an extremity cassette. This is so that the projected blur will be as minimal as possible and so that the most accurate FSS can be determined.

Papp, "Quality Control of Radiographic Equipment," p 80; Cullinan, "Quality Assurance Guidelines," p 258; Hendee, 1979b, p 32; Thompson et al., "Quality Control," p 407.

64. **(B)** When calculating a repeat rate, it is first important to count the number of rejects in the "discard" bin. If there are a total of 20 radiographs in the reject bin, and the radiographer notes that five of these radiographs were rejected because of positioning errors, then the conclusion would be that 5 of 20, or 25 percent, were retakes because of positioning errors. The basic formula for calculating a specific type of error is:

$$\text{Causal repeat rate} = \frac{\text{No. of repeats for a specific cause}}{\text{Total no. of repeats or rejects}} \times 100$$

To calculate the overall repeat rate for the period, the radiographer would need to know the total number of radiographs processed during that same time frame:

$$\text{Percent repeat rate} = \frac{\text{Number of films in reject bin}}{\text{Total number of films processed}} \times 100$$

Knowing the total number of radiographs processed is not an important piece of information in calculating the repeat rate for a specific error.

Carroll, "Quality Control," pp 382–386, 1998; Papp, "Additional Quality Management Procedures," pp 152–154.

65. **(B)** Radiation that is produced at the anode target and then exits the port window is referred to as *primary radiation*. The intensity of the primary beam may be compensated for by using a filter

that varies intensity from one end to the other. Occasionally, radiation may be produced when electrons strike parts of the x-ray tube other than the anode target, and this is referred to as *off-focus radiation*. Off-focus radiation is best controlled by the placement of a lead beam restrictor (collimator) as close to the source as possible. Collimators also help to prevent the production of scatter radiation. However, scatter radiation is produced only when the primary beam strikes a "scattering" object, such as a patient or radiographic table. The best device that can be used to absorb scatter radiation produced in the patient is a grid or grid cassette. An intensifying screen serves to convert x-ray photons into light photons to be used to expose the radiographic film. The purpose of this is to reduce the patient's dose; it does not absorb scatter radiation.

Bushong, "The Grid," p 216; Carlton and McKenna-Adler, "The Grid," p 274; Carroll, "Grids," p 181; Wallace, "Grids and the Bucky," pp 101–102.

66. **(C)** When a focused grid is used beyond the recommended distance range, the result will be grid cutoff at the periphery of the image. This grid cutoff will demonstrate an image with decreased density at the sides and normal density in the center of the image. This is because the center of the grid has grid lines that are placed perpendicular to the film, whereas the grid lines on the sides are canted to allow for divergence of the x-ray beam at a specific distance. This is why using a focused grid upside down will produce the same results as using the grid at the incorrect distance.

Bushong, "The Grid," pp 224–225; Carlton and McKenna-Adler, "The Grid," pp 190–193; Carroll, "Grids," pp 182–186, 1998; Wallace, "Grids and the Bucky," pp 108–111.

67. **(C)** When handling radiographs in the darkroom prior to processing, the radiographer should be cautious to hold the film at the edges and to be careful not to bend the film. When films are handled carelessly, they may be bent around the fingertip, causing a crescent-shaped artifact to appear on the radiograph. Usually this artifact is dark, but it may show up as a crescent-shaped area of decreased density if the pressure is significant.

Carroll, "Film Handling and Duplication Procedures," p 514, 1998; McKinney, "Film Artifacts," p 188; Papp, "Additional Quality Management Procedures," p 162.

68. **(B)** The most common type of automatic processor used for double-emulsion films is the 90-second processor. For single-emulsion films such as a dedicated mammography processor, it is usu-

ally more common to use a 3-minute processor. In a 90-second automatic processor, the film travels through the developer first for 22 seconds, next the fixer for 22 seconds, then the wash bath for 20 seconds, and finally the dryer for 26 seconds. (Carlton says 15 to 20 seconds are needed for clearing time).

Bushong, "Processing the Latent Image," p 179; Carlton and McKenna-Adler, "Radiographic Processing," p 297.

69. **(C)** The FSS and the grid ratio have nothing to do with magnification of the image or size distortion. The two factors that affect size distortion are the SID and the OID. To minimize size distortion, the radiographer should increase the SID or decrease the OID, or both.

Bushong, "Radiographic Quality," p 240; Carlton and McKenna-Adler, "Distortion," pp 420–421; Carroll, "Distance Ratios," p 275, 1998.

70. **(B)** The resolution or resolving ability of a film-screen system is the ability to see very small objects. Resolution is usually measured in line-pairs per millimeter. The greater the line-pair per millimeter value, the higher the resolution of the imaging system. The resolving capability of the naked eye at a typical reading distance is about 5–10 line-pairs per millimeter. Direct exposure x-ray film is capable of recording up to 100 line-pairs per millimeter, but the slowest screens can record only a little over 10 line-pairs per millimeter. In combination, the average spatial resolution for most film-screen combinations would range somewhere between 1 and 10 line-pairs per millimeter.

Bushong, "Intensifying Screens," p 194; Curry et al., "Luminescent Screens," p 123; Papp, "Radiographic Ancillary Equipment," p 105.

71. **(A)** When the optical density on the radiograph is read with a densitometer, essentially the amount of light transmitted through the radiograph is read. The less light that is transmitted, the darker the density on the radiograph. "The ability of a radiograph to stop light is termed opacity." Therefore, by using a logarithmic scale, if the opacity of the radiograph is doubled or increased by a factor of 2, the optical density read by the densitometer has increased by 0.3. "This is because the log of 2 is 0.3." For example, if the optical density reading is 1, only 10 percent, or $\frac{1}{10}$, of the light can be transmitted through the radiograph, and the radiograph is said to have an opacity of 10. If the optical density increases to 1.3, then the opacity has doubled to 20, and only 5 percent of the light can be transmitted. The log relative exposure is basically taking the log value

from doubling the technical factors used to expose the film, either by doubling the milliamperage-seconds or by increasing the kilovolts (peak) by 15 percent.

Bushong, "Radiographic Quality," pp 232–233; Carlton and McKenna-Adler, "Sensitometry," pp 318–319; Papp, "Processor Quality Control," p 49.

72. **(B)** As mentioned in the previous question, the densitometer is used to give a density measurement of the darkness of the radiograph. This is based on how much light can be transmitted through the film and is given a logarithmic value on a scale of 0 to 4. The 0 to 4 scale is calculated using the following formula:

$$\text{Optical density (OD)} = \log_{10}\frac{\text{Incident light}}{\text{Transmitted light}} \text{ or } \log_{10}\frac{I_i}{I_t}$$

If the transmitted light is 10 percent of the incident light, then the optical density reading would be 1. If the transmitted light is 1 percent, then the optical density reading would be 2.

Bushong, "Radiographic Quality," pp 232–233; Carlton and McKenna-Adler, "Sensitometry," pp 318–319; Papp, "Processor Quality Control," p 49.

73. **(A)** Most artifacts leave an area of increased radiographic density on the film that can obscure the image. However, some artifacts, such as dirt in the cassette, actually absorb radiation or light emitted from the screen before it can expose the film, leaving an area of decreased density appearing as white marks. These also can obscure the area of interest on the image. Other types of artifacts that may leave a region of decreased density or white marks are those that actually scratch the emulsion. Some examples of these type of artifacts include (1) when two films are processed too close together and become stuck together, causing *emulsion pick-off;* (2) *guide-shoe marks,* (3) *hesitation marks* that may occur if the transport system fails during processing, and (4) some *crescent or crinkle marks* caused from bending or rough handling of the film (usually crescent marks appear as increased density, but they may appear as light areas if the handling is rough enough to remove parts of the emulsion).

Bushong, "Mammography Quality Control," pp 307–308; Carlton and McKenna-Adler, "Intensifying Screens," p 339; Papp, "Additional Quality Management Procedures," pp 154–162.

74. **(B)** Radiographic film is extremely sensitive to heat and humidity and therefore should be stored in a cool, dry place—ideally, at temperatures below 68°F and at a humidity between 40 percent and 60 percent. This is because high humidity caused by steam or other moisture may increase fog-reducing contrast. A relative humidity below

40 percent is also objectionable because it may lead to static artifacts.

Bushong, "Radiographic Film," p 174; Carlton and McKenna-Adler, "Radiographic Film," p 290; Carroll, "Film Handling and Duplication Procedures," p 512.

75. **(D)** The most common type of film used for radiography is blue-violet sensitive, which can safely be processed in a darkroom using a Kodak Wratten 6-B safelight filter. However, with the introduction of orthochromatic film, which is used with rare earth phosphor cassettes and which is especially sensitive to green light, a Kodak GBX-2 filter is required to process this film safely. The GBX filter is safe for both the typical blue-violet–sensitive film as well as the orthochromatic green-sensitive film. The safelight should be placed at least 3 to 4 ft from the work surface and have a low intensity (7 to 15 W) regardless of the type of film and filter used.

Carlton and McKenna-Adler, "Radiographic Processing," p 307; Carroll, "Film Handling and Duplication Procedures," pp 516–517; Cullinan, "X-Ray Equipment Maintenance," p 244; Papp, "Film Darkrooms," p 16.

76. **(B)** A pi line is so named because it occurs at regularly spaced intervals relative to the circular motion of the transport rollers. Thus, the name "pi" (π) designates the ratio of the circumference of a circle to its diameter. The most common cause of pi lines on a radiograph is dirt deposited on the processor rollers, causing regularly spaced artifacts that run perpendicular to the direction of film travel.

Bushong, "Film Artifacts," p 422; Carroll, "Automatic Processors," pp 505–506, 1998; Papp, "Additional Quality Management Procedures," p 157.

77. **(D)** There are five basic factors that affect the recorded detail on the radiograph: (1) patient motion, (2) OID, (3) FSS, (4) SID, and (5) screen speed. The other technical factors of kilovolts (peak) and milliamperage-seconds affect the visibility of detail because of their affect on density and contrast, but they have no effect on recorded detail. The grid ratio also has no effect on recorded detail. Therefore, the only choice that would contribute to a loss of recorded detail would be patient motion.

Bushong, "Radiographic Technique," p 269; Carlton and McKenna-Adler, "Recorded Detail," p 405; Carroll, "Motion," p 288, 1998.

78. **(A)** The use of high-kilovolt (peak) and low–milliamperage-second technical factors in performing radiographic procedures is thought to extend the life of the x-ray tube because it reduces the amount of heat units produced. It also reduces the patient's exposure. Unfortunately,

there are two major disadvantages to using high-kilovolt (peak) and low–milliamperage-second techniques. One is that the contrast may not be adequate for the type of examination being performed. Another is that the use of insufficient milliamperage-seconds leads to a mottled appearance on the radiograph called *quantum mottle*. This occurs because the milliamperage-second selection has a direct effect on the number of x-ray photons being produced, and if the milliamperage-seconds is too low, there may not be enough x-ray photons to properly expose the film. Quantum mottle is especially significant when rare earth screens are used.

Bushong, "Radiographic Quality," p 230; Carlton and McKenna-Adler, "Intensifying Screens," p 333, and "Minimizing Patient Dose," p 210; Selman, "Radiographic Quality," pp 329, 344, and "X-Ray Tubes and Rectifiers," p 220.

79. **(B)** The two main functions of the automatic processor are to develop the image and to set, or "fix," the image for archival quality. The active ingredients in the first process of development are the reducing agents, which function to reduce the latent image into a manifest image. The reducing agents in an automatic processor are hydroquinone and phenidone. The active ingredient in the fixer is the clearing agent, which functions to clear away the unexposed silver halide crystals, thereby setting a permanent image onto the film. The clearing agent in most automatic processors is ammonium thiosulfate.

Bushong, "Processing the Latent Image," pp 180–182; Carlton and McKenna-Adler, "Radiographic Processing," pp 296–297; Carroll, "Processing Steps and Chemistry," p 482, 1998.

80. **(C)** The anode heel effect is an inherent side effect of most modern radiographic x-ray tubes due to the steep angle of the anode. The steeper the angle of the anode, the more x-ray photons will be absorbed by the heel of the anode. Steep angles are necessary, though, because they provide a greater heat-loading capacity, known as the line focus principle. Because more x rays are absorbed on the anode side of the tube, the anatomic part placed under the anode should be the thinnest body part because this is the least intense area of the x-ray beam. The anode heel effect is especially pronounced when using short SIDs, large film sizes (14 × 17 in.), and when radiographing body parts of widely varying tissue densities, such as the AP femur or AP thoracic spine.

Bushong, "The X-Ray Tube," pp 117–118; Carlton and McKenna-Adler, "Density," pp 374–375; Carroll, "The Anode Bevel," pp 244–245, 1998.

81. **(B)** Increasing the OID from 2 inches to 4 inches would cause increased magnification with a resultant loss of recorded detail. It would also increase contrast because of the air-gap technique principle. Because the part is farther from the image receptor, many scattered photons would be diverged off of the edge of the radiograph and not expose the radiograph, thereby increasing contrast.

Bushong, "Radiographic Quality," pp 239–244; Carroll, "Object-Image Receptor Distance," pp 264–269, 1998; Wallace, "Size Distortion," pp 27–28, 33, and "Methods to Control Scatter," p 123.

82. **(C)** Increasing the image receptor speed from 100 RS to 400 RS would have no effect on magnification. It would increase the radiographic density and might also slightly increase the radiographic contrast. It would also decrease the recorded detail of the image.

Carlton and McKenna-Adler, "Density," p 380; Carroll, "Intensifying Screens," pp 209–211, 1998; Wallace, "Intensifying Screens," pp 160–161.

83. **(B)** Increasing the collimation from a 10 × 12 in. beam to a 4 × 4 in. beam will result in fewer photons reaching the film, causing a reduction in radiographic density. It will also cause fewer scattered photons to be created, causing an increase in radiographic contrast.

Carroll, "Field Size Limitation," pp 138–142, 1998; Wallace, "Methods to Control Scatter," p 118.

84. **(A)** Increasing the grid ratio would also decrease the number of scattered photons reaching the film, thereby decreasing radiographic density and increasing radiographic contrast.

Carlton and McKenna-Adler, "Density," p 380; Carroll, "Grids," pp 185–188, 1998; Wallace, "Grids and the Bucky," pp 112–113.

85. **(D)** The amplitude used during tomography designates the total amount of tube travel. In linear tomography, the amplitude would be the distance from the beginning caudal angle to the ending cephalad angle, or vice versa. The amplitude is very important because it determines the arc degree, which will ultimately affect the slice thickness. If the amplitude necessary to produce a specific thickness is 120 cm of tube travel and the x-ray tube travels at a speed of 20 cm/s, then the exposure time will have to be at least 6 seconds long to achieve a total of 120 cm of tube travel. (120 cm ÷ 20 cm/s = 6 s).

Carlton and McKenna-Adler, "Tomography," pp 562–563; Cullinan, "Tomography," pp 175–183. Curry et al., "Body Section Radiography," pp 242–247.

86. **(C)** When using an AEC device, it is important to know the minimum response time of the unit.

Radiographic examinations requiring very low milliamperage-seconds, such as extremities or infant chest radiographs, should not be taken using an AEC for this reason. The minimum response time multiplied by the milliamperage setting on the machine will determine the smallest amount of milliamperage-seconds that may be used. In this case, the lowest milliamperage-seconds that may be used is 500 × 0.02 s = 10 mAs. The backup timer is also an important factor when the AEC is used. This is a safety feature that must be set to minimize overexposure to the patient in case of a malfunction. The exposure should stop automatically when the backup time (in this case, 200 milliseconds) has been reached regardless of whether the AEC device detects an adequate amount of radiation. A typical backup timer selection is 1 to 2 seconds. A good example of why the backup time is important is when the radiographer mistakenly selects the AEC for a chest stand instead of the Bucky AEC when performing a supine abdomen on the table. The maximum amount of milliamperage-seconds that can be used for this problem can be found by multiplying the milliamperes selected times the selected backup time: 500 × 0.20 s = 100 mAs. For this example, 10 mAs and 100 mAs are possible combinations, but 5 mAs is too small for the minimum response time and the milliamperage setting selected.

Carlton and McKenna-Adler, "Automatic Exposure Controls," p 509; Carroll, "Automatic Exposure Controls," pp 351–354, 1998; Cullinan, "The X-Ray Circuit," pp 23–25.

87. **(B)** When radiographic equipment is tested, there are several types of quality assurance tests that are performed. Some of the most important ones determine the accuracy of the technical factors selected, which may be affected by malfunctions in the x-ray generator. A test for reciprocity, also called linearity, is performed by varying the technical factors of milliamperes and time, producing a consistent milliamperage-seconds and kilovolts (peak) with each exposure. The test for linearity allows for a 10 percent variance between intensity from one exposure to the next. A more stringent test that is performed is called reproducibility, which uses the exact milliamperage station, exposure time, and kilovolts (peak) with multiple exposures. The variance of radiation intensity for reproducibility should not vary by more than 5 percent between successive exposures. The test for HVL also uses identical technical factors, but with alterations in the added filtration. This tests for the effectiveness of the aluminum filtration in the x-ray tube.

Bushong, "Designing for Radiation Protection," p 511; Carroll, "Quality Control," p 391, 1998; Papp, "Quality Control of Radiographic Equipment," p 73.

88. **(B)** Blurring of the radiographic image that causes a decrease in recorded detail may be caused by patient motion, size distortion, large FSS, or poor film-screen contact.

Bushong, "Quality Assurance and Quality Control," p 412; Carlton and McKenna-Adler, "Recorded Detail," p 412; Wallace, "Intensifying Screens," pp 162–163.

89. **(C)** An initial acceptance test should be made on all new radiographic equipment on installation. After that, the focal spot should be tested annually to ensure that there has not been excessive focal spot "blooming." Some blooming, or expansion of the focal spot, is normal with use, but this should not exceed 40 percent of the initial size for focal spot sizes of 0.8 to 1.5 mm. For FSSs smaller than 0.8 mm, the variation can be as much as 50 percent.

Carlton and McKenna-Adler, "Quality Control," p 444–445; Carroll, "Quality Control," pp 400–401, 1998; Gray et al., "X-Ray Tubes and Collimators," p 83; Papp, "Quality Control of Radiographic Equipment," p 81.

90. **(C)** The QC test tool imaged in Figure 5–4 is a wire-mesh device. This device is used to test for film-screen contact. Areas on the wire mesh that appear blurred or demonstrate a loss of recorded detail are indicative of poor film-screen contact.

Bushong, "Quality Assurance and Quality Control," p 412; Carlton and McKenna-Adler, "Quality Control," p 449; Carroll, "Quality Control," p 404, 1998.

91. **(B)** The QC test tool imaged in Figure 5–4 is a wire-mesh device. This device is used to test for film-screen contact. Areas on the wire mesh that appear blurred or demonstrate a loss of recorded detail are indicative of poor-film screen contact.

Bushong, "Quality Assurance and Quality Control," p 412; Carlton and McKenna-Adler, "Quality Control," p 449; Carroll, "Quality Control," p 404.

92. **(A)** It is sometimes necessary to adjust the contrast of a radiograph even when the original radiographic density was adequate. The primary controlling factor is adjusting for radiographic contrast is the kilovolt (peak) selection. If the object is to increase contrast without altering the optimum density, the radiographer should decrease the kilovolt (peak) by 15 percent with a compensating doubling (100 percent increase) of the original milliamperage-seconds. If the object is to decrease contrast, the radiographer should

increase the kilovolts (peak) by 15 percent with a compensating halving (50 percent decrease) of the original milliamperage-seconds.

Carlton and McKenna-Adler, "Contrast," pp 392–397; Carroll, "Kilovoltage-Peak," pp 107–109, 1998; Cullinan, "Technical Factor Selection," p 137; Wallace, "mAs and kVp Relationship," pp 92–95.

93. **(B)** There are two formulas that allow radiographers to calculate the MF on a radiograph. One way is to find the ratio of the image size to the object size: MF = Image size/Object size. If there were not enough information in the problem to use this formula, a second formula using the geometric factors of distance could be used: MF = SID/SID − OID, or MF = SID/SOD. In this case, the SID is 100 cm, and the OID is 7.2 cm. MF = 100/100 −7.2, or MF = 100/92.8; MF = 1.077 (1.08).

Carlton and McKenna-Adler, "Distortion," pp 420–421; Carroll, "Distance Ratio," p 275, 1998; Wallace, "Size Distortion," pp 31–32.

94. **(D)** The ratio of the grid is determined by the height of the lead strips divided by the distance between them: r = h/d. The height of the lead strips in Figure 5–5 is 3.2 mm. The distance between them is 0.20 mm. The ratio then is as follows: r = 3.2/0.20 = 16:1.

Carlton and McKenna-Adler, "The Grid," p 267; Cullinan, "Technical Formulas & Related Data," p 291; Wallace, "Grids and the Bucky," pp 105–106.

95. **(A)** Whenever the kilovolts (peak) routinely exceeds 90, the grid ratio used for that examination or examinations should be high—at least a 12:1 grid ratio is recommended. For dedicated chest units operating above 100 kVp, the standard grid ratio recommended is 16:1. Most Bucky grids used for abdominal radiography between 70 and 80 kVp use an 8:1 grid.

Bushong, "The Grid," p 225; Carroll, "Grids," p 184, 1998.

96. **(C)** When calibrating the operation of various milliamperage settings, a QC test for milliamperage *reciprocity* or *linearity* should be performed. This is done by selecting various milliamperage and timer settings that equal the same total milliamperage-seconds. All of the exposures should have an output radiation intensity that does not vary by more than 10 percent from one milliamperage and timer setting to the next.

Carlton and McKenna-Adler, "Quality Control," p 446; Carroll, "Quality Control," pp 390–391, 1998; Papp, "Quality Control of Radiographic Equipment," pp 78–79.

97. **(C)** Intensifying screens should be cleaned at least quarterly, but they should be cleaned more often in a busy radiology department. The handling of the cassettes in the darkroom will continually expose them to dust and dirt particles. These particles may attenuate the light given off by the phosphor from exposing the film, which will result in low-density artifacts on the radiograph. In mammography, this is especially important because these low-density areas may easily be confused with a specific pathology.

Bushong, "Intensifying Screens," p 201; Carlton and McKenna-Adler, "Intensifying Screens," p 339; Carroll, "Intensifying Screens," p 218, 1998; Papp, "Radiographic Ancillary Equipment," p 106.

98. **(D)** To solve this problem, first calculate the milliamperage-seconds for each set of technical factors:
1. 400 mA × 0.008 s = 3.2 mAs
2. 200 mA × 0.32 s = 64 mAs
3. 400 mA × 0.16 s = 64 mAs
4. 400 mA × 0.08 s = 32 mAs

Next, look at the kilovolts (peak) selected for each set of technical factors and apply the 15 percent kilovolt (peak) rule if necessary:
1. 3.2 mAs at 64 kVp
2. 64 mAs at 64 kVp
3. 64 mAs at 75 kVp
4. 32 mAs at 86 kVp

Remember, when applying the 15 percent kilovolt (peak) rule, if the kilovolts (peak) is increased by 15 percent, it is necessary to decrease the milliamperage-seconds by ½ (50 percent) to maintain radiographic density. If the kilovolts (peak) is decreased by 15 percent, it is necessary to increase the mAs by a factor of 2. Applying this, it is easy to see that choice 3 has twice the milliamperage-seconds of choice 4 and that the kilovolts (peak) in choice 3 is 15 percent less than the kilovolts (peak) in choice 4. The two sets of technical factors with identical radiographic density would then be choices 3 and 4.

Bushong, "X-Ray Production," pp 134–135; Carlton and McKenna-Adler, "Density," pp 372–373; Carroll, "Kilovoltage-Peak," pp 107–110, 1998; Wallace, "mAs and kVp Relationship," pp 92–94.

99. **(C)** Because reducing the size of the beam (collimation) decreases the production of scatter radiation, the number of scattered photons available to expose the film decreases. Consequently, the radiographic density will decrease, and because scatter radiation contributes to "fog," the radiographic contrast will increase when these scattered photons are reduced.

Bushong, "Scatter Radiation and Beam-Restricting Devices," pp 205–206; Carroll, "Field Size Limitation," pp 139–142, 1998; Wallace, "Methods to Control Scatter," p 118.

100. **(A)** Not only the effective atomic number of the tissue, but also how tightly packed the atoms are, affect tissue density or molecules making up that tissue. It is important for the radiographer to understand differences in tissue density so that proper technical factors may be selected for each body part as well as for each individual patient. Bone tissue is considered to be the most compact and thus the densest tissue in the body. Muscle tissue and water are very similar in density in relation to their relative atomic numbers and relative density. Fat is considered to be the least dense of all the soft tissues, and air is the least dense of all types of body tissues.

Bushong, "X-Ray Interaction with Matter," pp 154–158; Carroll, "Interactions of X-Rays within the Patient," pp 59–60, 1998; Wallace, "Radiographic Contrast," pp 75–76.

101. **(D)** There are two main types of filtration in the x-ray tube that help to absorb the low-energy photons from the primary beam, thereby reducing the patient's skin dose. The first type is inherent filtration, which is composed of the Pyrex glass, the beryllium window, and the insulating oil of the x-ray tube. The inherent filtration is usually the aluminum equivalent of 0.50 to 1 mm. Because the total filtration of most x-ray tubes is required by the NCRP to be at least 2.5-mm aluminum equivalent, an additional filter, called added filtration, must also be placed between the x-ray source and the patient. This added filtration is usually made up of aluminum, but it may also consist of copper or other materials that will absorb low-energy photons while allowing the higher-energy photons to penetrate through the filter to expose the patient.

Bushong, "Radiographic Exposure," p 255; Carlton and McKenna-Adler, "Filtration," p 172; Carroll, "Beam Filtration," p 129, 1998.

102. **(D)** A casting material made of fiberglass mesh has become the most popular form of casting a fracture. Because this material is very radiolucent, the majority of the time no increase in technical factors from the original prereduction radiograph is needed. Occasionally, the cast may be especially thick or dense when a very large bone, such as the femur, is set. In this case, the increase in technical factors will be very slight—either a 30 percent increase in milliamperage-seconds or a 5 percent increase in kilovolts (peak)—to produce an optimum radiograph. In some instances, the fiberglass material is also mixed with plaster in equal amounts, in which case the milliamperage-

seconds would need to be increased by 50 percent or the kilovolts (peak) by 8 percent.

Carlton and McKenna-Adler, "Density," p 380; Carroll, "Pathology and Casts," p 171, 1998.

103. **(B)** When spinal radiography for scoliosis surveys is performed, it is sometimes necessary to radiograph the entire spine in one projection. If this is the case, a special cassette with a gradient screen should be used. The gradient screen has a slow-speed, medium-speed, and high-speed phosphor in variance from one end to the other. This is to compensate for the variations in part thickness and tissue density from the cervical spine to the lumbar region.

Carroll, "Intensifying Screens," p 217, 1998.

104. **(A)** The original base used for radiographic film was made of glass, but this quickly became impractical because of its fragility. The next generation of bases used for the radiographic emulsion was cellulose nitrate, but this also was found to be impractical because the edges tended to curl and it was highly flammable. The next generation of film base, introduced in 1924, was cellulose acetate, known as "safety x-ray film." The modern radiographic film base is made of polyester. It is very practical because of its flexibility for use in automatic processors and because of its supreme archival quality (long shelf life).

Bushong, "Radiographic Film," pp 166–167; Carlton and McKenna-Adler, "Radiographic Film," pp 280–281; Carroll, "Recording the Permanent Image," p 22, 1998.

105. **(C)** When a radiographer is consistently using both single-phase and 3-phase equipment to perform diagnostic radiography, it is important to become familiar with technical adjustments between them. Because 3-phase equipment produces a voltage ripple that is nearly constant, the x-ray intensity is greater than that in single-phase equipment. Therefore, when changing from single-phase to 3-phase, 6-pulse, 66 percent of the original milliamperage-second value is required to produce the same radiographic density. When adjusting from single-phase to 3-phase, 12-pulse or high-frequency equipment, 50 percent of the original milliamperage-second value is required. In this example, the original milliamperage-second value was as follows: 800 mA × $\frac{1}{16}$ s = 50 mAs, so the milliamperage-seconds will need to be decreased to 25. The only answer that will produce a milliamperage-seconds of 25 is choice C: 400 mA × $\frac{1}{16}$ s = 25 mAs. The following chart demonstrates how to adjust factors from one type of radiographic equipment to another:

When converting Generator Phase		To maintain Density, multiply mAs by a
From:	**To:**	**Conversion Factor of:**
Singleϕ	3ϕ6p	0.6
Singleϕ	3ϕ12p/ HF	0.5
3ϕ6p	Singleϕ	1.6
3ϕ6p	3ϕ12p / HF	0.8
3ϕ12p / HF	Singleϕ	2.0
3ϕ12p / HF	3ϕ6p	1.2

Carlton and McKenna-Adler, "Exposure Conversion Problems," p 514; Carroll, "Machine Phase and Rectification," pp 124–125, 1998; Cullinan, "The X-Ray Tube," p 46.

106. **(A)** A quality assurance test for reproducibility requires several exposures using identical technical factors. Each exposure should fall within 5 percent of the average beam intensity. To solve this problem, first find 5 percent of 77 mR: 77 × 0.05 = 3.85 (approximately 4). All of the values for each exposure should then fall within ±4 mR of 77, or between 73 and 81 mR. Therefore, choices 1 and 2 fall within the acceptable limits, but choice 3, which is 85 mR, is outside the acceptance limits for the reproducibility test.

Bushong, "Designing for Radiation Protection," p 511; Carroll, "Quality Control," p 391, 1998; Papp, "Quality Control of Radiographic Equipment," p 73.

107. **(C)** Low humidity in the darkroom will cause static appearing as tree shapes, crown shapes, or smudges. As mentioned in question 67, rough handling of the film may cause bending of the emulsion around the handler's fingers. This may cause an area of increased density resembling a crescent (half-moon) shape. This artifact is also called a crinkle mark. It usually shows up dark, but it may also appear as a low-density artifact if the handling is especially rough. Dirt on the processor rollers also causes artifacts of increased density, but these are usually more random in nature. The same is true for dirt in the intensifying screens, although these artifacts always appear as areas of decreased radiographic density because they tend to absorb the light given off by the screen before it can expose the film.

Carroll, "Film Handling and Duplication Procedures," p 514, 1998; McKinney, "Film Artifacts," p 188; Papp, "Additional Quality Management Procedures," p 162.

108. **(A)** The only two factors listed that affect magnification are the geometric factors of distance: SID and OID. To calculate the MF for each set of technical factors, use the following formula: SID/SID − OID or SID/SOD. The MF for each of the four choices would be as follows:

	SID	OID	SID/SOD	MF
A.	100	25	100/75	1.33
B.	150	30	150/120	1.25
C.	120	20	120/100	1.20
D.	200	40	200/160	1.25

Of the four choices, choice A has the greatest magnification with 1.33.

Carlton and McKenna-Adler, "Distortion," pp 420–421; Carroll, "Distance Ratios," p 272, 1998; Wallace, "Size Distortion," pp 31–33.

109. **(A)** The latitude of a grid refers to its ability to allow some room for error with alignment to the x-ray beam without causing excessive grid cutoff. Grids that have the greatest amount of centering and distance latitude generally have a low grid ratio, and focused grids have the greatest latitude of all of the grid types. This is because they are specially designed to converge with the natural divergence of the x-ray beam. Parallel or linear grids always produce some type of grid cutoff because the lead strips are not canted, or angled, as a focused grid is. Grid cutoff with a parallel (linear) grid will be even more pronounced at shorter SIDs and therefore should only be used at longer SIDs. The rhombic, or crosshatched, grid has the least centering and distance latitude of all of the grid types.

Bushong, "The Grid," p 225; Carlton and McKenna-Adler, "The Grid," pp 269–270.

110. **(D)** The patient in Figure 5–7 has areas of increased subject density caused by Paget's disease. This increase in subject density will require an increase in technical factors. There is a difference of opinion among authors as to which technical factor (either milliamperage-seconds or kilovolts [peak]) would be the most suitable choice to adjust for pathological changes in tissue density. There is also disagreement as to how much of an increase or decrease there should be for a particular pathology. However, the only choice that requires an increase in technical factors is choice D.

Carlton and McKenna-Adler, "The Pathology Problem," pp 254–259; Carroll, "Pathology and Casts," pp 164–167, 1998; Wallace, "Radiographic Technique Charts," pp 212–213.

SECTION IV: RADIOGRAPHIC PROCEDURES AND RELATED ANATOMY

111. **(A)** The circle of Willis is a highly complex arterial structure located in the base of the brain that serves to join the anterior and posterior blood supply to the brain. It is formed by the anastomosis, or linking together, of several major arteries. It is of critical importance to the brain because it provides a means of collateral circulation. This collateral circulation may limit the damage to one of the major arteries caused by a blockage or hemorrhage from either pathology or trauma.

Ballinger, Vol 2, p 595; Bontrager, "Angiography," p 686; Kelley and Petersen, "Brain," p 67; Tortorici, "Cerebral Angiography," p 222, 1995.

112. **(C)** The side of interest that is best demonstrated in an oblique projection of the ribs is either the side down if the patient is supine, or the side up if the patient is prone. The best positions that will demonstrate injuries to the right axillary ribs would be either the RPO or the LAO.

Ballinger, Vol 1, pp 430–431; Cornuelle and Gronefeld, "Bony Thorax," pp 258–259.

113. **(A)** Air is quite commonly seen in the colon, rectum, and the fundus of the stomach. This is due to gas that is created in both the stomach and the large intestine. Gas in the small intestine, on the other hand, is very uncommon. If it is seen on an abdominal radiograph, it is usually an indication that there is an obstruction or an infection, such as ileus, somewhere in the alimentary canal.

Bontrager, "Small Bowel Series," p 455; Cornuelle and Gronefeld, "The Abdomen: Digestive System," p 62; Eisenberg and Dennis, "Gastrointestinal System," pp 138–142.

114. **(C)** A routine parietoacanthial (Waters) projection will not demonstrate the sphenoid sinus. Therefore, choices A, B, and D may be immediately eliminated. Only the open-mouth parietoacanthial (Waters) projection and the SMV projection clearly demonstrate the sphenoid sinus.

Ballinger, Vol 2, pp 382–385; Bontrager, "Paranasal Sinuses," p 388. Cornuelle and Gronefeld, "Paranasal Sinuses," pp 372–375.

115. **(A)** To place the right kidney parallel for demonstration in profile on the radiograph, the patient needs to be rotated toward the left side so that the patient's right side is elevated 30° off of the table (LPO position).

Ballinger, Vol 2, p 172; Cornuelle and Gronefeld, "Urinary System," p 432. Bontrager, "Intravenous Urography," p 523.

116. **(C)** When a lateral projection is performed during skull radiography, both the MSP and the IOML are adjusted parallel with the plane of the cassette. The IOML should also be adjusted parallel to the long axis of the cassette. The interpupillary line should be adjusted perpendicular to the plane of the cassette.

Ballinger, Vol 2, p 238; Bontrager, "Cranium," p 351; Cornuelle and Gronefeld, "Skull," p 342.

117. **(A)** There are two accepted methods of locating breast tumors: (1) the clock method and (2) the quadrant method. The quadrant method is easiest and therefore is the most commonly used localization method. Most carcinomas of the breast are found in the UOQ, making the craniocaudal and mediolateral oblique projections critical for correct positioning.

Bontrager, "Mammography," p 531; LiVolsi et al., p 380; Wentz, p 58.

118. **(D)** If the patient's condition does not allow him or her to extend the forearm for a routine AP projection of the elbow, then the radiographer must compromise by radiographing the elbow in acute flexion using two separate frontal projections. Both the AP and the PA projection are performed by placing the patient's humerus in contact with the cassette. The AP projection requires a perpendicular central ray centered 2 inches superior to the olecranon process. The anatomy demonstrated in the AP projection is the olecranon process and distal humerus. For the PA projection, the patient position remains the same, but the central ray is angled perpendicular to the flexed forearm, entering 2 inches distal to the olecranon process. The anatomy demonstrated in the PA projection is the proximal radius and ulna, which would also include the olecranon process. The coronoid process is not well demonstrated in either projection.

Ballinger, Vol 1, pp 108–109; Bontrager, "Elbow," p 140.

119. **(C)** The scapular Y projection of the shoulder is mainly performed to demonstrate the relationship between the humeral head and the glenoid fossa for possible dislocations. It is not the ideal projection to demonstrate either the humeral head for fractures or the glenoid fossa. The AC joints are also not well demonstrated with this projection.

Ballinger, Vol 1, pp 142–143; Bontrager, "Shoulder: Trauma Routine," p 162.

120. **(B)** The best positions to demonstrate the hepatic flexure of the colon during a BE examination are the LPO and the RAO. The side up is always better visualized when the patient is in the

supine position (AP projection), and the side down is always better visualized when the patient is in the prone position (PA projection).

Ballinger, Vol 2, pp 135, 140; Bontrager, "Barium Enema," pp 473, 475.

121. **(D)** For best demonstration of the knee joint in the AP projection, the central ray should be directed ½ inch distal to the apex of the patella. In hypersthenic patients, it may also be advisable to angle 5° cephalad, and for asthenic patients, an angle of 5° caudal will better open up the joint space.

Ballinger, Vol 1, pp 240–241; Bontrager, "Knee," p 206.

122. **(D)** The clavicle articulates medially with the sternum at the sternoclavicular (SC) joint and laterally with the scapula at the AC joint. It does not articulate with the humerus. Therefore, choices A, B, and C may be eliminated.

Ballinger, Vol 1, p 122; Bontrager, "Shoulder Girdle: Clavicle," p 149.

123. **(D)** Performing cholangiography during a surgical procedure can be done to diagnose biliary disease that may be causing obstructions of either the biliary ducts or the sphincter of Oddi. The most common cause of obstruction in the biliary vessels is from biliary calculi. The procedure has become quite common during most biliary tract surgery.

Ballinger, Vol 2, p 76; Bontrager, "Gallbladder and Biliary Ducts," p 490.

124. **(B)** Unlike the other divisions of the vertebral column, not all cervical vertebrae are alike. In fact, C1 and C2 are called atypical vertebrae because they are either missing parts that are found in a typical vertebra or they have additional anatomic parts that are not found in a typical vertebra. However, all cervical vertebrae have in common the presence of three foramina, one for the passage of the spinal cord (the vertebral foramen) and two for the passage of vertebral vessels and nerves (transverse foramina).

Ballinger, Vol 1, pp 315–317; Bontrager, "Cervical Vertebrae," pp 252–253; Cornuelle and Gronefeld, "Vertebral Column," pp 270–271.

125. **(B)** The suffix -*plasia* translates to formation or development. It is often used to describe abnormal growths in terms such as *hyperplasia,* which means excessive growth or development, or *dysplasia,* which means bad or difficult growth.

Eisenberg and Dennis, "Introduction to Pathology," pp 5–6; Laudicina, "Introduction to Pathology," p 8; Linn-Watson, "Pathology Principles," p 4.

126. **(A)** The roof of the mouth, sometimes called the "hard palate," is comprised of the maxillae and the palatine bones. The mandible makes up the entire "jaw bone," and the vomer forms the inferosuperior portion of the nasal septum.

Ballinger, Vol 2, pp 230–231; Bontrager, "Facial Bones," pp 333–335; Cornuelle and Gronefeld, "Facial Bones and Paranasal Sinuses," pp 358–361.

127. **(B)** It is very important for radiographers to recognize the differences in patients' sizes and shapes according to their category of body habitus. This is because variations in body habitus have a great effect on the location of certain abdominopelvic organs. Certain organs, such as the liver and the kidneys, remain fairly predictable in their location from one body habitus to another. However, some organs, such as the stomach and the gallbladder, can vary in both their vertical and their transverse positions from asthenic to hypersthenic body habitus. The skills of a radiographer become critical when localizing these two organs specifically.

Ballinger, Vol 1, pp 41–42; Bontrager, "Upper Gastrointestinal System," p 420; Cornuelle and Gronefeld, "The Abdomen," p 60.

128. **(C)** The hyoid bone is a bone that is suspended by the styloid from the styloid process of the temporal bone and sits just below the level of the mandible in the neck. Its purpose is to stabilize the tongue and articulate with other muscles of the throat. The cricoid is not a bone, but rather a projection of cartilage that is situated just superior to the thyroid cartilage, or "Adam's apple," of the neck. The thyroid is also not a bone, but it is a gland in the endocrine system that is situated posteriorly to the thyroid cartilage.

Ballinger, Vol 2, p 232; Bontrager, "Chest," p 58; Cornuelle and Gronefeld, "Facial Bones and Paranasal Sinuses," p 362.

129. **(D)** The periosteum is the outer dense, fibrous portion of bone that covers the entire shaft of the bone except at the articulating surfaces. The periosteum serves as a point of attachment for both ligaments and tendons, but concerning the joints, it is continuous with the hyaline (articular) cartilage. The bursae are fluid-filled sacs that are positioned between tissues surrounding some diarthrodial joints.

Cornuelle and Gronefeld, "Musculoskeletal System," p 83.

130. **(D)** *Peritonitis* is defined literally as inflammation of the peritoneum. It is usually caused from a bacterial infection in the peritoneal cavity, either from a perforation somewhere in the gastrointestinal (GI) tract or as a complication of invasive surgery. *Ascites* is a collection of fluid in the abdominal cavity and may be caused by several

types of disease processes, such as cirrhosis of the liver or metastases. *Gastroenteritis* is an infection of the stomach and intestines, and *jaundice* is a complication of liver dysfunction in which the bilirubin is not properly broken down and thus escapes into the bloodstream, giving the patient yellowish-colored skin.

Bontrager, "Lower Gastrointestinal System," p, 448; Scanlon and Sanders, "The Digestive System," p 369.

131. **(A)** The most anterior bone of the carpal bones is the pisiform, which can usually be felt in the medial surface of the palm of the hand. Also, the hamate, which has a hooklike process that projects anteriorly, can sometimes be palpated on the medial surface of the palm of the hand.

Ballinger, Vol 1, pp 60–61; Bontrager, "Hand and Wrist," p 104; Cornuelle and Gronefeld, "Upper Limb (Extremity)," p 103.

132. **(C)** The knee joint is formed by the articulation between the distal femur and the proximal tibia. The patella also articulates with the femur on its posterior surface. The fibula does not form part of the knee joint because it does not articulate with the distal femur.

Bontrager, "Lower Limb: Leg, Knee and Distal Femur," p 180; Cornuelle and Gronefeld, "Lower Limb (Extremity)," p 175.

133. **(B)** The best imaging method to diagnose discrepancies of bone length in the lower extremities is a scanogram. The scanogram is performed with the use of a ruler that is radiographed alongside the lower extremity by dividing the cassette into thirds and by first radiographing the hip joint, then the knee joint, and finally the ankle joint at the bottom third. The ruler can be imaged either with a 14 × 17 in. cassette in diagnostic radiography or with the use of a CT scanner. The scanogram is also called "orthoroentgenography" because it may be used by orthopedic surgeons prior to treating the limb discrepancy.

Bontrager, "Orthoroentgenography," pp 612–614; Cornuelle and Gronefeld, "Lower Limb (Extremity)," pp 180–181.

134. **(B)** When a decubitus radiograph of the abdomen is performed, the object is to demonstrate free air. This air is most likely to be located more superior in the abdomen, just under the diaphragm. Therefore, it is not necessary to try and include the symphysis pubis for a frontal projection of the abdomen in the decubitus position. It is also not necessary to include the side down—in this case, the left side of the body—because the free air will rise to the side up, in this case, the right side. The left lateral decubitus position is the one most often used to demonstrate free air in the abdomen be-

cause the air in the fundus of the stomach may obscure free air in the abdomen on a right lateral decubitus.

Ballinger, Vol 2, p 41. Bontrager, "Abdomen," p 96. Cornuelle & Gronefeld, "The Abdomen," p 77.

135. **(B)** A hysterosalpingogram is a procedure that is done to evaluate the uterus and fallopian tubes. The patient is injected with contrast through the cervix to check for patency of the oviducts, which may be a cause of infertility. In some instances, the procedure may actually be therapeutic because the contrast agent opens up the stenosed oviduct. Following injection of the patient under fluoroscopy, the radiologist may request that an overhead radiograph be taken. If this is required, the radiograph should be centered 2 inches superior to the symphysis.

Ballinger, Vol 2, pp 200–201; Cornuelle and Gronefeld, "The Abdomen," p 73.

136. **(C)** The most prominent point of the greater trochanter lies at approximately the same level of the symphysis pubis. The most superior aspect of the greater trochanter lies at approximately 1 inch superior to the upper border of the symphysis pubis.

Ballinger, Vol 1, p 275; Bontrager, "Proximal Femur and Pelvic Girdle," p 224.

137. **(C)** Sutures are fused joints between two bones and are commonly found in the adult skull. Sutures are considered to be totally immovable joints and are therefore classified as synarthrodial. Diarthrodial joints are freely movable joints and usually contain a bursal sac filled with synovial fluid. Examples of diarthrodial joints include the knee, hip, and shoulder joints. Amphiarthrodial joints are partially movable joints that are separated by a layer of fibrous cartilage, such as the intervertebral disk and the symphysis pubis. A gompharthrodial joint is a misnomer in that the proper term is "gomphoses." A joint that is classified as gomphosis is a special type of articulation in which one bone with a conical process fits firmly into a socketlike portion of the other bone. This is the type of joint seen in the teeth of the mandible and maxillae.

Bontrager, "Arthrology," p 10; Cornuelle and Gronefeld, "Musculoskeletal System," p 89; Scanlon and Sanders, "The Skeletal System," p 124.

138. **(B)** A properly positioned lateral projection of the humerus is performed with the patient's arm placed in internal rotation. This should demonstrate the epicondyles superimposed on the image, and the lesser tubercle of the proximal humerus should be demonstrated in profile on the medial side of the humeral head.

Ballinger, Vol 1, p 117; Bontrager, "Humerus," p 144; Cornuelle and Gronefeld, "Upper Limb (Extremity)," pp 142–143.

139. **(B)** The cuboid bone is one of the tarsal bones of the foot and is best demonstrated in the AP medial oblique projection. This projection also should clearly demonstrate the third through the fifth metatarsus completely free of superimposition, the tuberosity of the fifth metatarsus, and the trabecular markings of the phalanges, metatarsus, and tarsus. This is why it is usually the routine oblique projection taken.
    Ballinger, Vol 1, p 200; Bontrager, "Foot," p 194; Cornuelle and Gronefeld, "Lower Limb (Extremity)," p 189.

140. **(D)** If the thoracic spine is not adjusted to place the horizontal plane parallel with the plane of the image receptor in the lateral projection, then an angulation of 10° to 15° cephalad may be required to better open up the intervertebral disk spaces. The thoracic spine should be made level by placing radiolucent supports under the lower thorax and waist.
    Ballinger, Vol 1, p 359; Bontrager, "Thoracic Spine," p 276; Cornuelle and Gronefeld, "Vertebral Column," p 300.

141. **(C)** If the pisiform and triquetrum are of primary interest when radiographing the wrist, an additional oblique projection may be required with the hand in semisupination. This is the AP oblique position and is very effective at separating the pisiform from the triquetrum.
    Ballinger, Vol 1, p 88; Cornuelle and Gronefeld, "Upper Limb (Extremity)," p 126.

142. **(C)** The symphysis pubis is classified as an amphiarthrodial, or partially movable, joint. It can also be further classified as a cartilaginous connective joint, not as a fibrous connective joint. An example of a fibrous connective, amphiarthrodial joint is the articulation between the distal tibia and fibula.
    Bontrager, "Arthrology," pp 10–11; Scanlon and Sanders, "The Skeletal System," p 124; Cornuelle and Gronefeld, "Musculoskeletal System," p 89.

143. **(C)** and 144. **(C)** This axial projection of the knee joint is also known as the "tunnel" method. The primary anatomy of interest in this projection is the intercondyloid fossa. There are three accepted methods of obtaining this image, and all three require that the central ray be directed perpendicular to the long axis of the tibia; however, the tibia may be positioned.
    Ballinger, Vol 1, pp 250–255; Bontrager, "Knee: Intercondylar Fossa," pp 210–211; Cornuelle and Gronefeld, "Lower Limb (Extremity)," pp 204–207.

145. **(D)** The main function of the respiratory system is to supply oxygen to the body and also to rid the body of excess carbon dioxide. The lungs do this by inhaling oxygen from the air and through absorption on the microscopic level in the capillaries of the alveoli. Oxygen is then sent to the heart via the pulmonary veins. The heart then takes over to send the oxygenated blood to the rest of the body through the largest artery in the body, the aorta. Without oxygen, the tissues of the body will quickly die. In fact, brain tissue will begin to die in as little as 4 minutes if deprived of oxygen. This is why it is so critical to begin CPR as quickly as possible when a victim has undergone either respiratory or cardiac arrest.
    Cornuelle and Gronefeld, "Respiratory System," p 30; Scanlon and Sanders, "Respiratory System," p 334; Spence, "The Respiratory System," p 511.

146. **(D)** The spinal cord is protected all along the length of the vertebral column on its anterior side by the vertebral bodies and on its posterior side by the posterior arch of the vertebrae. This large opening formed by the shape of the vertebral body and posterior arch is called the vertebral foramen. The intervertebral foramina are small openings that provide passageways for individual spinal nerves that branch off of the spinal cord. The transverse foramina are also much smaller openings that exist only in the cervical spine to provide passageways for spinal nerves and arteries. The obturator foramina are the two large foramina found in the ischial bones of the pelvis.
    Bontrager, "Vertebral Column," p 250; Cornuelle and Gronefeld, "Vertebral Column," p 269; Tortora and Grabowski, "The Skeletal System: The Axial Skeleton," p 186.

147. **(A)** Radiologists prefer to view AP projection images for diagnosis by hanging those images so that the patient appears to be facing the viewer. The right side of the patient's body should always be to the viewer's left, and the patient's left side should always be to the viewer's right. For lateral projections, the radiographs are usually placed from the perspective of how the x-ray tube sees the patient. The only exception to these two general rules is when a decubitus image is placed on the viewbox for interpretation. In this case, the radiologist usually requires the side up to be placed up and the side down is placed down, just as the x-ray tube viewed the patient.
    Ballinger, Vol 1, pp 5–7; Bontrager, "Positioning Principles," p 54; Cornuelle and Gronefeld, "Introduction to Radiography," p 24.

148. **(A)** To aid in peristalsis after a barium meal, the patient should be placed in the RAO or the right

lateral position. Either of these positions is the favored when the patient is recumbent during fluoroscopy of the upper gastrointestinal tract because gravity will help to draw the contents of the stomach into the duodenum.

Ballinger, Vol 2, p 106.

149. **(C)** The pancreas is the accessory organ of digestion that functions to balance the insulin and glucagon circulating in the bloodstream. If these two chemicals are out of balance, the patient is said to be either hypoglycemic (low blood sugar) or hyperglycemic (high blood sugar). Both conditions could be a sign of pathology of the pancreas, most likely diabetes. The liver controls the breakdown and disposal of red blood cells, which produce bile. The gallbladder stores the bile produced by the liver, and the kidney is responsible for disposing of all the waste products found in the bloodstream.

Ballinger, Vol 2, p 35; Cornuelle and Gronefeld, "Biliary System," p 490; Tortora and Grabowski, "The Endocrine System," pp 549–551.

150. **(D)** The centering point for a lateral projection of the nasal bones should be ¾ inch distal to the nasion. The radiographer should center at the zygoma for a lateral projection of the facial bones. Bontrager says ½ inch inferior to the nasion.

Ballinger, Vol 2, p 315; Bontrager, "Nasal Bones," p 367; Cornuelle and Gronefeld, "Facial Bones and Paranasal Sinuses," p 382.

151. **(D)** The vomer articulates inferiorly with the maxillae and palatine bones. It articulates superiorly with both the ethmoid and sphenoid bone, and it also articulates with the septal cartilage.

Bontrager, "Facial Bones," p 335; Cornuelle and Gronefeld, "Facial Bones and Paranasal Sinuses," pp 358–361.

152. **(C)** Lordotic and kyphotic curvatures of the spine are anterior and posterior curvatures and are therefore best demonstrated on a lateral projection. Scoliotic curvatures of the spine are lateral curvatures and are best demonstrated on either an AP or a PA weight-bearing projection.

Ballinger, Vol 1, p 396; Bontrager, "Scoliosis Series," p 295; Cornuelle and Gronefeld, "Vertebral Column," p 269.

153. **(C)** The shoulder girdle does not refer to the shoulder joint, but rather the bones that support the shoulder joint. It is formed by the clavicle and scapula and serves to attach the upper limb to the trunk. The shoulder joint is formed by the humerus and the scapula.

Ballinger, Vol 1, p 122; Bontrager, "Shoulder Girdle: Clavicle," p 149; Cornuelle and Gronefeld, "Shoulder Girdle," p 150.

154. **(A)** This AP projection of the elbow was taken with the hand in supination. It can be evaluated by the clear visualization of the olecranon fossa (number 5) and by the fact that the radial head and the coronoid process of the ulna are slightly obscured by one another. The external oblique projection is done specifically to demonstrate the radial head free of superimposition, and the internal oblique projection is performed to demonstrate the coronoid process in profile. A PA projection radiograph of the elbow would be very difficult for the patient and would most likely not show a clear image of the olecranon fossa, as seen in Figure 5–9.

Ballinger, Vol 1, p 101; Bontrager, "Elbow," p 136; Cornuelle and Gronefeld, "Upper Limb (Extremity)," p 134.

155 **(A)** and 156 **(C)** The anatomic part identified by the number 1 is the lateral epicondyle, by 2 the capitellum, by 3 the radial head, by 4 the radial tuberosity, by 5 the olecranon fossa, by 6 the medial epicondyle, and by 7 the trochlea.

Ballinger, Vol 1, p 101; Bontrager, "Elbow," p 136; Cornuelle and Gronefeld, "Upper Limb (Extremity)," p 134.

157. **(B)** There are three bones in the middle ear hat serve to pass sound waves from the tympanic membrane to the structures of the inner ear. These three bones are the malleus, incus, and stapes. The cochlea is a cartilaginous structure found in the inner ear that passes sound waves through fluid and sends this signal to the auditory nerve.

Ballinger, Vol 2, pp 228–229; Bontrager, "Temporal Bone," p 392; Cornuelle and Gronefeld, "Skull," pp 327–328.

158. **(C)** Most adult humans have only five lumbar vertebrae. Some adults may have an additional vertebra that articulates with the sacrum. This sixth lumbar vertebra is sometimes referred to as a transitional vertebra, or *lumbarization. Sacralization* is where the body of L5 fuses to the body of S1.

Cornuelle and Gronefeld, "Vertebral Column," p 272; Eisenberg and Dennis, "Skeletal System," p 66; Linn-Watson, "Skeletal System," pp 29–30.

159. **(C)** If the patient's teeth are obscuring the odontoid process in the AP open-mouth projection of the cervical spine, the patient's chin is tucked too much. The adjustment would be to extend the patient's neck to align the mastoid process and the upper row of teeth in the same plane. If the patient's posterior occiput is obscuring the odontoid process, the chin needs to be depressed.

Greathouse, "Cervical Spine," Vol 1, p 349; McQuillen-Martensen, "Radiographic Critique of the Cervical & Thoracic Vertebrae," p 325.

160. **(B)** Failure to dorsiflex the foot for an AP medial oblique projection of the ankle will result in inaccurate demonstration of the lateral malleolus. The foot should be flexed at least 90° for the best demonstration of the distal fibula. If the foot is not fully flexed, the calcaneus may partially obscure the lateral malleolus of the fibula.

Ballinger, Vol 1, p 231; McQuillen-Martensen, "Radiographic Critique of the Lower Extremity," p 238.

161. **(C)** The most common anatomic structure to use for critique of rotation on a PA projection of the chest is the SC joints. The SC joints should be symmetrical on a correctly positioned frontal projection of the chest. The heart size may be altered by rotation, but it is not an acceptable means of critiquing for correct positioning, because the altered heart size may be due to pathology. Counting the number of ribs seen on a PA projection of the chest is a valuable critique for acceptable inspiratory effort from the patient during the exposure. A good inspiration chest radiograph should demonstrate 10 pairs of posterior ribs on the PA projection.

Ballinger, Vol 1, p 455; Bontrager, "Chest," p 67; McQuillen-Martensen, "Radiographic Critique of the Chest and Abdomen," p 42.

162. **(C)** The most common cause of failure to demonstrate the lower cervical vertebrae and upper thoracic on a shoot-through lateral projection of the cervical spine is superimposition of the shoulders. If this is the case, the shoulders will need to be depressed. This may be accomplished by having the patient pull on a sheet or strap that is wrapped around the patient's feet, or by having a nonradiation worker pull gently on the arms during the exposure. Also, taking the exposure on expiration will also help to lower the shoulders. Scatter may also be a problem due to the thickness of the part; this is why it is recommended that if any technical factor is adjusted, usually the milliamperage-seconds should be increased, not the kilovolts (peak). The recommended increase for proper demonstration of the lower cervical spine is a 100 percent increase, or doubling, of the milliamperage-seconds rather than a 50 percent increase.

Ballinger, Vol 1, p 350; Bontrager, "Trauma and Mobile: Cervical Spine," p 572; Cornuelle and Gronefeld, "Vertebral Column," p 281; McQuillen-Martensen, "Radiographic Critique of the Cervical and Thoracic Vertebrae," p 329.

163. **(A)** The placement of the acetabulum and the symphysis pubis will not change regardless of the placement of the feet for an AP projection of the pelvis. The most noticeable change in anatomy when the lower extremities are inverted is the vi-sualization of the femoral necks, although the SI joints are better visualized when the lower extremities are inverted 15°. When the patient is recumbent and the legs are allowed to rotate laterally in a relaxed position, the femoral necks will be obscured because of foreshortening.

Ballinger, Vol 1, p 276; McQuillen-Martensen, "Radiographic Critique of the Hip and Pelvis," p 306.

164. **(A)** The most common reasons, other than pathology, for failure to demonstrate the patella on the AP projection are (1) insufficient penetration due to a lack of kilovolts (peak) and (2) insufficient radiographic density due to either a lack of kilovolts (peak) or a lack of milliamperage-seconds. An insufficient SID would not be the cause of inadequate demonstration of the patella, although an excessive SID might. An AP projection of a patient's knee that measures less than 5 inches does not require a grid, and a kilovolt (peak) range between 60 and 70 kVp is usually sufficient. If the patient's knee is greater than 5 inches, a grid with a minimum kilovolts (peak) of 70 is usually required to absorb the excess scatter.

Ballinger, Vol 1, pp 240–241; Bontrager, "Knee," p 206; McQuillen-Martensen, "Radiographic Critique of the Lower Extremity," p 251.

165. **(C)** When positioning a patient for a lateral projection of the elbow, it is very important to ensure that the wrist, elbow, and shoulder joints lie in the same plane. If the axilla is not in the same plane as the elbow joint, the humeral epicondyles will not be superimposed as required, and the result will be distortion of the anatomy of interest. An unobstructed view of the radial head is seen on the AP lateral oblique projection, and a profile of the coronoid process is obtained by the AP medial oblique projection.

Ballinger, Vol 1, p 102; Bontrager, "Elbow," p 139; Cornuelle and Gronefeld, "Upper Limb (Extremity)," p 138; McQuillen-Martensen, "Radiographic Critique of the Upper Extremity," pp 147–149.

166. **(D)** Most lateral knee radiographs are positioned for a mediolateral projection. In larger patients, or those with a wider pelvis, this results in magnification of the medial condyle, which may cause superimposition over the knee joint. To correct this, the radiographer can try angling the central ray 5° to 7° cephalad. This angle should project the magnified condyle above the knee joint. The knee should only be flexed between 20° and 30°.

Ballinger, Vol 1, p 243; Cornuelle and Gronefeld, "Lower Limb (Extremity)," pp 202–203; McQuillen-Martensen, "Radiographic Critique of the Lower Extremity," pp 264–265.

167. **(D)** Knowing the patient's body habitus is important for radiographers, especially when radiographing anatomy that may be altered significantly from one body type to another. A good example of this is the stomach. The stomach appears very high and transverse in a hypersthenic patient as compared with the average (sthenic) patient. This means that the radiographer will have to center higher and closer to the midline in demonstrate the entire stomach. The accepted centering point for a PA projection of the stomach for a sthenic patient is at approximately the level of L2 and 1 inch left of the vertebral column. For a hypersthenic patient, the adjustment should be 2 inches higher and closer to the midline.

Ballinger, Vol 2 pp 102–103; Bontrager, "Upper GI Series," p 441; Cornuelle and Gronefeld, "Digestive System," p 464.

168. **(A)** *Hydronephrosis* is a condition that literally means "water in the kidney." The kidney has become distended with fluid due to a blockage somewhere in the urinary tract, typically in the renal pelvis or the proximal ureter. To adequately visualize the ureters, the patient should be placed in the prone position when the initial AP projection radiographs demonstrate this pathology.

Ballinger, Vol 1, p 170; Cornuelle and Gronefeld, "Urinary System," p 424.

169. **(D)** Even when radiographing infants, an AP projection chest radiograph should adequately demonstrate 10 posterior ribs. If there are not at least 10 posterior ribs demonstrated, it may mean that the exposure was not taken on inspiration. This feature is critical because the inadequate demonstration of 10 pairs of ribs may mimic pathology, especially in the neonate.

Ballinger, Vol 1, p 455; Bontrager, "Chest," p 72; Cornuelle and Gronefeld, "Respiratory System," p 37; McQuillen-Martensen, "Radiographic Critique of the Chest and Abdomen," p 45.

170. **(A)** When an air-contrast BE examination is performed, there should not be any barium demonstrated in the stomach, so choice C may be eliminated. With the patient lying on the right side, air will rise to the side up, or left side, and barium will settle on the side down. This means that air will be demonstrated in the medial ascending colon and the lateral descending colon, and barium will be demonstrated in the lateral ascending colon and medial descending colon.

Ballinger, Vol 2, p 143; Bontrager, "Barium Enema," p 477; Cornuelle and Gronefeld, "Digestive System," p 481.

SECTION V: PATIENT CARE

171. **(D)** Breach of confidentiality is a form of invasion of privacy and is a very serious charge. Public revelation of a patient's medical records without that patient's consent may lead to this charge. Most health-care institutions establish strict policies concerning patient confidentiality whereby if confidentiality has been breached the employee may be terminated. Also, the patient may take legal action against the employee and the institution. All health-care professionals should exercise extreme caution when discussing any patient's medical history and be sure to include in the conversation only those health-care professionals who have a direct involvement with that patient's care.

American Society of Radiologic Technologists (ASRT), Code of Ethics, Principle 9; Ehrlich and McCloskey, "The Radiographer as a Member of the Health Care Team," pp 51–53; Wilson, "Basic Concepts of Medical Law," p 147.

172. **(B)** When CPR is performed on an adult patient, the pulse should be assessed using the carotid artery in the neck. It is safer to assess the pulse of an infant under age 1 at the brachial artery in the upper arm. With your thumb on the outside of the arm, gently press your fingers until you feel the pulse.

American Heart Association, 1997, "Pediatric Basic Life Support," pp 6–7.

173. **(B)** *Emia* is the suffix meaning "blood condition." *Leukemia* is an abnormal condition of white blood cells, *leuk/o* meaning "white"; its most common connotation is malignancy of the white blood cells. *Anemia* combines the prefix *an-*, which means "without or lack of," and the suffix *-emia*, which translates to "a deficiency of red blood cells, or erythrocytes." Patients who are anemic may have the condition as a result of a low-iron diet, or it may be as a result of recent trauma in which the patient suffered a large blood loss. *Hypoglycemia* denotes a low blood sugar and *hyperglycemia* an excessive blood sugar, two conditions usually associated with diabetes.

Gylys and Wedding, "Blood and Lymphatic System," p 185; Mace and Kowalczyk, "The Hemopoietic System," p 337; Taber's Cyclopedic Medical Dictionary, pp 96–100.

174. **(A)** There are several variations of reactions to contrast media from mild to moderate to severe. Some examples of mild symptoms include a warm sensation, reddening of the face, sneezing or coughing, and nausea and vomiting. These types of initial reactions are quite common in

ionic contrast media, but most patients will not suffer any of these ill effects with nonionic contrast media. The patient should be monitored if these mild symptoms appear because they may be early warning signals for more severe symptoms, which include swelling of the tongue leading to difficulty swallowing and difficulty breathing, edema, and eventually respiratory or cardiac arrest. Severe reactions are not common and occur only in about 1 in 14,000 cases, and fatal reactions are very rare, occurring in about 1 in 40,000 cases.

Adler and Carlton, "Contrast Media," p 318, Table 19–8; Ehrlich, and McCloskey, "Dealing with Acute Situations," p 234; Torres, "Medical Emergencies in Diagnostic Imaging," pp 93–94.

175. **(A)** Prior to "scrubbing in," the health-care professional first puts on shoe covers, a hair net, and then a face mask. After properly scrubbing the hands and forearms, a sterile gown is put on with the help of a second health-care professional. Finally, the sterile gloves should be put on last.

Adler and Carlton, "Aseptic Techniques," pp 221–229; Ehrlich and McCloskey, "Infection Control," pp 172–180; Kowalczyk and Donnett, "Infection Control and Aseptic Technique," pp 98–99.

176. **(B)** Barium sulfate is mixed and forms a colloidal suspension, not a solution. Therefore, the body cannot easily absorb it if it happens to seep into a body cavity. It is for this reason that barium sulfate should *never* be used in the GI tract whenever there is a suspicion of GI tract perforation. Instead, a water-soluble contrast agent such as water-based iodine should be used instead.

Adler and Carlton, "Contrast Media," pp 304–306; Ehrlich and McCloskey, "Preparation and Examination of the Gastrointestinal Tract," p 253; Kowalczyk and Donnett, "Medication Administration," p 190.

177. **(B)** When inserting an enema tip for a BE, it is important to insert it far enough that it will stay inserted throughout the procedure, but no more than 3 to 4 inches inside the rectum.

Adler and Carlton, "Nonaseptic Techniques," pp 248–249; Torres, "Patient Care during Imaging Examinations of the Gastrointestinal System," p 138.

178. **(D)** Of the four major groups of microorganisms (bacteria, fungi, protozoa, and viruses), bacteria are the most resistant to aseptic techniques. The most resistant of all bacteria are the types that form spores. Spores surround the bacteria to protect it from an unfavorable environment. Once the destructive agent is removed from the environment, the bacteria will once again become active. Thus, many types of asepsis are ineffective against the spore-type bacteria.

Adler and Carlton, "Infection Control," pp 196–197; Ehrlich and McCloskey, "Infection Control," p 138. Torres, "Infection Control," p 23.

179. **(C)** Children are very intimidated by adults, especially strangers. To make them feel more comfortable, it is important to get down to their level and be friendly and positive. This will allow them to develop trust in the health-care provider before beginning any procedure. The health-care provider should never talk in a loud or intimidating voice and should not attempt to touch the child until trust has been developed.

Adler and Carlton, "Patient Preparations," p 129; Ehrlich and McCloskey, "Professional Communications," pp 70–71; Kowalczyk and Donnett, "Age-Related Considerations," pp 44–47.

180. **(B)** When preparing a site for an invasive procedure, it is important to start cleansing in the center and move outward in a circular motion. This motion should be repeated a second time using a sterile gauze sponge to remove the soap and water. This type of preparation is important for preparing patients for invasive radiological procedures such as arthrograms and myelograms.

Ehrlich and McCloskey, "Infection Control," p 172, Box 6–2; Torres, "Surgical Asepsis," pp 78–79.

181. **(C)** Aside from the universal, or standard, precautions set forth by the Centers for Disease Control and Prevention (CDC), there are other category-specific types of isolation. One such example is enteric isolation precautions, which are designed to prevent the spread of infection from possible exposure to fecal material.

Adler and Carlton, "Infection Control," p 210; Kowalczyk and Donnett, "Infection Control and Aseptic Technique," p 88, Table 5–1.

182. **(A)** Entry into the GI tract through a normal orifice, such as the nose, mouth, or anus, is not considered a sterile procedure. Although medical asepsis requiring the placement of clean, disposable items should be used, a sterile preparation procedure is not *necessary*. However, entry into other body systems, such as by puncture of the skin or by catheterization of the urethra or blood vessels, is an invasive procedure requiring surgical asepsis. This means that the site of catheterization or puncture should be properly prepared, and health-care provider should wear sterile gloves.

Adler and Carlton, "Aseptic Techniques," pp 232–235; Kowalczyk and Donnett, "Tubes, Catheters and Vascular Access Lines," p 153.

183. **(B)** Hypoglycemia is sometimes a complication of diabetes in which the patient has received too much insulin and is now experiencing low blood

sugar. Usually the patient is familiar with the early warning signs of hypoglycemia, such as weakness, dizziness, and extremity tremors, and can treat himself or herself by ingesting either fruit juice or any food containing sugar. Hypoglycemia may be a problem with diabetic patients who are NPO pending a radiographic examination. This is why diabetic patients should be given first priority on the fluoroscopic schedule whenever possible. Hypoglycemia can quickly lead to insulin shock, so it must be treated immediately.

Adler and Carlton, "Medical Emergencies," p 261; Ehrlich and McCloskey, "Dealing with Acute Situations," pp 235–236; Kowalczyk and Donnett, "Patient Care in Critical Situations," pp 214–215.

184. **(B)** Diuretics are drugs that increase or stimulate urine output. Common examples would be caffeine and furosemide (Lasix). Diuretics are often administered to relieve hypertension or excessive edema. Emetics promote vomiting, and cathartics or laxatives promote defecation.

Adler and Carlton, "Pharmacology," p 284; Ehrlich and McCloskey, "Medications and Their Administration," p 188, Table 7–1.

185. **(B)** Log rolling a patient is an accepted method of moving a patient with a suspected spinal cord injury because this motion will cause the least amount of movement and twisting in the spinal column. It is not recommended for patients who are only suspected of having a head injury or an extremity fracture.

Ehrlich and McCloskey, "Dealing with Acute Situations," p 229; Kowalczyk and Donnett, "Emergency Medicine," p 223.

186. **(A)** When communicating with pediatric patients, it is not only important to get down on their level to talk to them, but also establishing trust is absolutely essential if the radiographer desires cooperation. For this reason, the radiographer should be totally honest and tell the child in his or her terms what the procedure may feel like. Do not say that a needle stick "won't hurt," or that you will only have to do the procedure one time, or take one film. This will only make the child less likely to cooperate if any of these statements prove to be false. Also, do not try to bribe the child into cooperating. This is also an ineffective method, especially if you have not been honest with the child concerning the rest of the procedure.

Adler and Carlton, "Patient Preparations," p 129; Ehrlich and McCloskey, "Professional Communications," pp 70–71; Kowalczyk and Donnett, "Age-Related Considerations," pp 44–47.

187. **(C)** All of these concerns—allergies, medications, and radiosensitivity of human tissues—should be

of concern to radiographers for *all* patients. However, when radiographing elderly patients, the radiographer should take special care when handling the patient's skin. This is because many elderly patients have brittle, dry, or even paper-thin skin that can easily tear. Be careful not to pull, grab, or bump the patient too harshly. In addition, the elderly patient's bones are very brittle; therefore, extreme care should be taken whenever handling this type of patient.

Ehrlich and McCloskey, "Professional Communications," p 72; Kowalczyk and Donnett, "Age-Related Considerations," pp 54–55; Torres, "Care of Patients with Special Problems," pp 116–117.

188. **(D)** Intravenous administration of contrast media is the most likely route that will induce a reaction. Even contrast media that have been administered into an artery are not as likely to cause an adverse reaction. This could be due to the fact that osmosis, or escape of contrast media into surrounding tissues, is more likely to occur through a vein than through any other lumen.

Ehrlich and McCloskey, "Dealing with Acute Situations," p 234; Torres, "Medical Emergencies in Diagnostic Imaging," pp 93–94.

189. **(B)** Because barium sulfate is a suspension, and the main function of the colon is to absorb excess water from waste. If the barium is not properly evacuated following the enema examination, it may become hardened in the colon, causing constipation and possibly an obstruction. This is why upon completion of the BE examination, all patients should be advised to drink plenty of fluids, and some elderly patients with a history of constipation may be advised to follow up with laxatives and cleansing enemas as well.

Adler and Carlton, "Contrast Media," pp 304–306; Ehrlich and McCloskey, "Preparation and Examination of the Gastrointestinal Tract," p 253; Kowalczyk and Donnett, "Medication Administration," p 190.

190. **(D)** A *tort* is a civil, wrongful act committed against a person or property. Tort is the most common type of lawsuit brought against healthcare workers and is more commonly referred to in health care as "malpractice." There are four aspects of medical malpractice that must be proved for a plaintiff (patient) to be successful in a potential lawsuit: (1) Was there a *duty to care?* (2) Was there a *breach of that duty?* (3) Was *injury caused* to the patient? and (4) Was *injury a direct result* of that *breach* of duty? Torts may be intentional, due to gross negligence, or unintentional. Most medical malpractice lawsuits are unintentional torts. Common examples would be failure to provide a safe environment for the patient,

failure to properly educate a patient, or failure to properly carry out orders. The Latin term *res ipsa loquitur* means that the thing speaks for itself. A good example of a lawsuit based on *res ipsa loquitur* doctrine would be an abdominal radiograph displaying forceps left in the patient after surgery, resulting in death of that patient. The legal doctrine *respondeat superior* means that the person in charge is responsible for all subordinates who may have caused injury to a patient even though that person was not directly involved with the patient's care. The legal term *assault* means "threatening to do harm or injury," such as "Mrs. Jones, if you don't hold still for this x ray, I will be forced to strap you down."

Kowalczyk and Donnett, "Medical Ethics and Legalities," pp 66–68; Wilson, "Basic Concepts of Medical Law," p 144.

191. **(B)** The NG tube is used to provide nutrition to a patient through a tube inserted into the nose that leads to the stomach. A Hickman catheter is a type of central-line venous catheter inserted into the subclavian vein for purposes of drug administration, chemotherapy, or parenteral nutrition. A nasal cannula is used to administer oxygen through the nose and is the most common means of oxygen administration.

Adler and Carlton, "Vital Signs and Oxygen," p 188; Ehrlich and McCloskey, "Dealing with Acute Situations," p 221; Kowalczyk and Donnett, "Patient Care in Critical Situations," p 201.

192. **(C)** The abbreviation MI stands for myocardial infarction, which literally translates to "death in the heart muscle, or heart attack." The abbreviation CVA stands for cerebrovascular accident, more commonly known as a "stroke." The abbreviation HA stands for headache, and the abbreviation TIA stands for transient ischemic attack, sometimes referred to as "ministroke."

Gylys and Wedding, "Cardiovascular System," p 154; Mosby's Medical Nursing and Allied Health Dictionary, "Appendix 2," p 1769.

193. **(A)** *Atelectasis* is a medical term meaning "insufficient or incomplete dilation or expansion." It translates to mean "collapsed lung." Atelectasis is quite common in neonates and one of the primary reasons for requesting a chest radiograph.

Eisenberg and Dennis, "Respiratory System," pp 47–48; Mace and Kowalczyk, "The Respiratory System," p 132.

194. **(D)** The normal pulse rate for an adult is between 80 to 100 beats per minute. If the pulse is over 100 beats per minute, the patient is said to have tachycardia, or a rapid pulse rate. If the

pulse rate is under 80 beats per minute, the patient is said to have bradycardia, or a slow pulse rate.

Adler and Carlton, "Vital Signs and Oxygen," pp 180–181; Ehrlich and McCloskey, "Patient Care and Assessment," p 122.

195. **(B)** When a radiographic examination of the colon is performed on a patient with a colostomy, the usual placement of the enema tip is in the stoma, or artificial opening into the colon. The normal lower intestinal procedure may have to be altered depending on the placement of the stoma.

Adler and Carlton, "Nonaseptic Techniques," pp 253–254; Ehrlich and McCloskey, "Preparation and Examination of the Gastrointestinal Tract," pp 253–256; Torres, "Barium Studies of the Upper Gastrointestinal Tract," pp 139–140.

196. **(A)** All health-care professionals should be following standard precautions as set forth in the guidelines by the CDC. This includes frequent hand washing between procedures and patients, as well as wearing protective devices such as gloves, gowns, masks, and so forth, especially when handling contaminated items that may have come in contact with blood or body fluids such as linens. All used needles should be properly disposed of but *never* should be recapped after use because this may result in an accidental needle stick. If a needle is attached to a syringe, then the entire syringe should be disposed of in a sharps-guard container.

Kowalczyk and Donnett, "Infection Control & Aseptic Technique," p 86; Ehrlich, "Appendix G," p 332.

197. **(D)** The patient on a clear-liquid diet is not allowed to ingest any solid foods other than gelatin. Dry toast is considered a solid food and is therefore restricted in a clear-liquid diet. This type of diet is often required for 24 hours following surgery and prior to certain types of radiological examinations.

Adler and Carlton, "Nonaseptic Techniques," p 248; Ehrlich and McCloskey, "Preparation and Examination of the Gastrointestinal Tract," p 244.

198. **(C)** When a radiographer performs chest compressions on an adult victim, the victim's sternum should be depressed between 1½ to 2 inches. For infant CPR, the compression should be between ½ to 1 inch, and for a child between ages 1 and 8, the compression should be between 1 to 1½ inches

Adler and Carlton, "Medical Emergencies," p 265; American Heart Association, "Adult Basic Life Sup-

port," 1997, pp 4–12; Kowalczyk and Donnett, "Patient Care in Critical Situations," p 206.

199. **(B)** The diastolic pressure is the blood pressure during diastole, or the relaxation phase of the heart. It is the time when there is the least amount of pressure in the blood vessels as blood is circulated. When taking a patient's blood pressure, the systolic pressure is on top, and the diastolic pressure is on the bottom. The normal range of diastolic pressure should fall between 60 and 90 mm Hg. Blood pressure below 60 mm Hg would indicate hypotension, and a diastolic pressure above 90 mm Hg would indicate hypertension.

Adler and Carlton, "Vital Signs and Oxygen," p 186; Ehrlich and McCloskey, "Patient Care and Assessment," p 127; Kowalczyk and Donnett, "Patient Assessment and Assistance," p 112.

200. **(D)** There are many types of drugs available in the radiology department in case of emergency. One of the most common types of emergencies seen in the radiology department is an allergic reaction to contrast media. An antihistamine should be administered in this case to counteract any histamines produced in the patient from the reaction. An analgesic is a pain medication. A cathartic is a drug that induces defecation, and a diuretic increases urine production.

Adler and Carlton, "Pharmacology," p 283; Ehrlich and McCloskey, "Medications and Their Administration," pp 186–187; Kowalczyk and Donnett, "Medication Administration," p 173.

BIBLIOGRAPHY

Adler, AM, and Carlton, RR: Introduction to Radiography and Patient Care. WB Saunders, Philadelphia, 1993.

American Heart Association (AHA): Basic Life Support for Healthcare Providers. Author, Dallas, TX, 1997.

American Society of Radiologic Technologists (ASRT): Code of Ethics. Author, Albuquerque, NM, 1997.

Ballinger, PW: Merrill's Atlas of Radiographic Positions and Radiologic Procedures, ed 8. 3 vols. Mosby-Year Book, St. Louis, 1995.

Bontrager, KL: Textbook of Radiographic Positioning and Related Anatomy, ed 4. Mosby-Year Book, St. Louis, 1997.

Burns, EF: Radiographic Imaging: A Guide to Producing Quality Radiographs. WB Saunders, Philadelphia, 1992.

Bushong, S: Radiologic Science for Technologists: Physics, Biology and Protection, ed 6. St. Louis, Mosby-Year Book, 1997.

Carlton, RR, and McKenna-Adler, A: Principles of Radiographic Imaging: An Art and a Science, ed 2. Delmar, Albany, 1996.

Carroll, QB: Fuchs's Radiographic Exposure, Processing and Quality Control, ed 6. Charles C Thomas, Springfield, IL, 1998.

Centers for Disease Control and Prevention: Infection Control Standards & Guidelines for Healthcare Workers. Author, Atlanta, 1997.

Cornuelle, AG, and Gronefeld, DH: Radiographic Anatomy & Positioning: An Integrated Approach. Appleton & Lange, Stamford, CT, 1998.

Cullinan, AM: Producing Quality Radiographs, ed 2. Lippincott, Philadelphia, 1994.

Curry, TS, et al: Christensen's Physics of Diagnostic Radiology, ed 4. Lea & Febiger, Philadelphia, 1990.

Dennis, CA, and Eisenberg, RL: Applied Radiographic Calculations, WB Saunders, Philadelphia, 1993.

Dowd, SB, and Tilson, ER: Practical Radiation Protection and Applied Radiobiology, ed 2. WB Saunders, Philadelphia, 1999.

Ehrlich, RA, and McCloskey, ED: Patient Care in Radiography, ed 5. Mosby, St. Louis, 1999.

Eisenberg, RL, and Dennis, CA: Comprehensive Radiographic Pathology, ed 2. Mosby, St. Louis, 1995.

Eisenberg, RL, et al: Radiographic Positioning. Little Brown and Co., Boston, 1989.

Garza, D, and Becan-McBride, K: Phlebotomy Handbook, ed 3. Appleton & Lange, Norwalk, CT, 1993.

Gould, BE: Pathophysiology for the Health Related Professions. WB Saunders, Philadelphia, 1997.

Gray, JE, et al: Quality Control in Diagnostic Imaging. University Park Press, Baltimore, 1983.

Greathouse, JS: Radiographic Positioning & Procedures, 3 vols. Delmar, Albany, NY, 1998.

Gurley, LT, and Callaway, WJ: Introduction to Radiologic Technology, ed 4. Mosby, St. Louis, 1996.

Gylys, BA, and Wedding, ME: Medical Terminology: A Systems Approach, ed 3. FA Davis, Philadelphia, 1995.

Hendee, WR: Medical Radiation Physics: Roentgenology, Nuclear Medicine and Ultrasound, ed 2. Year Book Medical Publishers, Chicago, 1979.

Hiss, SS: Understanding Radiography, ed 3. Charles C Thomas, Springfield, IL, 1993.

Ireland, SJ: Integrated Mathematics of Radiographic Exposure. Mosby, St. Louis, 1994.

Kelley, LL, and Petersen, CM: Sectional Anatomy for Imaging Professionals, Mosby, St. Louis, 1997.

Kowalczyk, N, and Donnett, K: Integrated Patient Care for the Imaging Professional. Mosby, St. Louis, 1996.

Laudicina, P: Applied Pathology for Radiographers. WB Saunders, Philadelphia, 1989.

Linn-Watson, TA: Radiographic Pathology. WB Saunders, Philadelphia, 1996.

LiVolsa, VA, et al: Pathology, ed 3. Harwal Publishing, Philadelphia, 1994.

Mace, JD, and Kowalczyk, N: Radiographic Pathology, ed 2. Mosby-Year Book, St. Louis, 1994.

Mallett, M: Anatomy and Physiology for Students of Medical Radiation Technology. Burnell, Mankato, MN, 1981.

Malott, JC, and Fodor, J: The Art and Science of Medical Radiography, ed 7. Mosby, St. Louis, 1993.

McKinney, WEJ: Radiographic Processing and Quality Control. Lippincott, Philadelphia, 1988.

McQuillen-Martenseng, K: Radiographic Critique. WB Saunders, Philadelphia, 1996.

Memmler, RL, and Wood, DL: The Human Body in Health & Disease, JB Lippincott, Philadelphia, 1983.

Mosby's Medical, Nursing and Allied Health Dictionary, ed 3. Mosby, St. Louis, 1993.

National Council on Radiation Protection and Measurements (NCRP): Limitation of Exposure to Ionizing Radiation. Report No. 116. Author, Bethesda, MD, 1993.

NCRP: Medical X-ray Electron Beam and Gamma-Ray Protection for Energies up to 50 MeV (Equipment Design, Performance and Use). Report No. 102. Author, Bethesda, MD, 1989.

NCRP: Quality Assurance for Diagnostic Imaging. Report No. 99. Author, Bethesda, MD, 1988.

NCRP: Radiation Protection for Medical and Allied Health Personnel. Report No. 105. Author, Bethesda, MD, 1989.

Obergfell, AM: Law and Ethics in Diagnostic Imaging and Therapeutic Radiology. WB Saunders, Philadelphia, 1995.

Papp, J: Quality Management in the Radiologic Sciences. Mosby, St. Louis, 1998.

Scanlon, VC, and Sanders, T: Essentials of Anatomy and Physiology, ed 2. FA Davis, Philadelphia, 1991.

Selman, J: The Fundamentals of X-ray and Radium Physics, ed 8. Charles C Thomas, Springfield, IL, 1994.

Sheldon, H: Boyd's Introduction to the Study of Disease, ed 10. Lea & Febiger, Philadelphia, 1988.

Snopek, AM: Fundamentals of Special Radiographic Procedures, ed 3. WB Saunders, Philadelphia, 1992.

Spence, AP: Basic Human Anatomy, ed 3. Benjamin/Cummings, Redwood City, CA, 1990.

Springhouse Medication Administration & I.V. Therapy Manual: Process & Procedures. Author, Springhouse Corp., Springhouse, PA, 1988.

Statkiewicz-Sherer, MA, et al: Radiation Protection in Medical Radiography, ed 3. Mosby, St. Louis, 1998.

Sweeney, RJ: Radiographic Artifacts: Their Cause and Control. Lippincott, Philadelphia, 1983.

Taber's Cyclopedic Medical Dictionary, ed 18. FA Davis, Philadelphia, 1996.

Tamparo, CD, and Lewis, MA: Diseases of the Human Body, ed 2. FA Davis, Philadelphia, 1995.

Thompson, MA, et al: Principles of Imaging Science and Protection. WB Saunders, Philadelphia, 1994.

Torres, LS: Basic Medical Techniques and Patient Care in Imaging Technology, ed 5. Lippincott, Philadelphia, 1997.

Tortora, GJ, and Grabowski, SR: Principles of Anatomy and Physiology, ed 7. Harper Collins, New York, 1993.

Tortorici, MR: Concepts in Medical Radiographic Imaging: Circuitry, Exposure and Quality Control. WB Saunders, Philadelphia, 1992.

Tortorici, MR, and Apfel, PJ: Advanced Radiographic and Angiographic Procedures. FA Davis, Philadelphia, 1995.

Travis, EL: Primer of Medical Radiobiology, ed 2. Year Book, Chicago, 1989.

Wallace, JE: Radiographic Exposure: Principles & Practice. FA Davis, Philadelphia, 1995.

Wentz, G, and Parsons, WC: Mammography for Radiologic Technologists, ed 2. McGraw-Hill, New York, 1996.

Wilson, BG: Ethics and Basic Law for Medical Imaging Professionals. FA Davis, Philadelphia, 1997.

Wolbarst, AB: Physics of Radiology. Appleton & Lange, Norwalk, CT, 1993.

SIMULATION TEST #5

NAME_____
　　　　　Last　　　　　　　　　　　　　　　　First　　　　　　　　　　Middle

ADDRESS _____
　　　　　Street

_____
　　　　City　　　　　　　　　　　　　　　　State　　　　　　　　　Zip

· ·

MAKE
ERASURES
COMPLETE

PLEASE USE NO. 2 PENCIL ONLY.

↓ BEGIN HERE

**Radiation Protection
and Radiobiology**

			Image Production and Evaluation	
01 Ⓐ Ⓑ Ⓒ Ⓓ	21 Ⓐ Ⓑ Ⓒ Ⓓ	41 Ⓐ Ⓑ Ⓒ Ⓓ		61 Ⓐ Ⓑ Ⓒ Ⓓ
02 Ⓐ Ⓑ Ⓒ Ⓓ	22 Ⓐ Ⓑ Ⓒ Ⓓ	42 Ⓐ Ⓑ Ⓒ Ⓓ		62 Ⓐ Ⓑ Ⓒ Ⓓ
03 Ⓐ Ⓑ Ⓒ Ⓓ	23 Ⓐ Ⓑ Ⓒ Ⓓ	43 Ⓐ Ⓑ Ⓒ Ⓓ		63 Ⓐ Ⓑ Ⓒ Ⓓ
04 Ⓐ Ⓑ Ⓒ Ⓓ	24 Ⓐ Ⓑ Ⓒ Ⓓ	44 Ⓐ Ⓑ Ⓒ Ⓓ		64 Ⓐ Ⓑ Ⓒ Ⓓ
05 Ⓐ Ⓑ Ⓒ Ⓓ	25 Ⓐ Ⓑ Ⓒ Ⓓ	45 Ⓐ Ⓑ Ⓒ Ⓓ		65 Ⓐ Ⓑ Ⓒ Ⓓ
06 Ⓐ Ⓑ Ⓒ Ⓓ	26 Ⓐ Ⓑ Ⓒ Ⓓ	46 Ⓐ Ⓑ Ⓒ Ⓓ		66 Ⓐ Ⓑ Ⓒ Ⓓ
07 Ⓐ Ⓑ Ⓒ Ⓓ	27 Ⓐ Ⓑ Ⓒ Ⓓ	47 Ⓐ Ⓑ Ⓒ Ⓓ		67 Ⓐ Ⓑ Ⓒ Ⓓ
08 Ⓐ Ⓑ Ⓒ Ⓓ	28 Ⓐ Ⓑ Ⓒ Ⓓ	48 Ⓐ Ⓑ Ⓒ Ⓓ		68 Ⓐ Ⓑ Ⓒ Ⓓ
09 Ⓐ Ⓑ Ⓒ Ⓓ	29 Ⓐ Ⓑ Ⓒ Ⓓ	49 Ⓐ Ⓑ Ⓒ Ⓓ		69 Ⓐ Ⓑ Ⓒ Ⓓ
10 Ⓐ Ⓑ Ⓒ Ⓓ	30 Ⓐ Ⓑ Ⓒ Ⓓ	50 Ⓐ Ⓑ Ⓒ Ⓓ		70 Ⓐ Ⓑ Ⓒ Ⓓ
11 Ⓐ Ⓑ Ⓒ Ⓓ	31 Ⓐ Ⓑ Ⓒ Ⓓ	51 Ⓐ Ⓑ Ⓒ Ⓓ		71 Ⓐ Ⓑ Ⓒ Ⓓ
12 Ⓐ Ⓑ Ⓒ Ⓓ	32 Ⓐ Ⓑ Ⓒ Ⓓ	52 Ⓐ Ⓑ Ⓒ Ⓓ		72 Ⓐ Ⓑ Ⓒ Ⓓ
13 Ⓐ Ⓑ Ⓒ Ⓓ	33 Ⓐ Ⓑ Ⓒ Ⓓ	53 Ⓐ Ⓑ Ⓒ Ⓓ		73 Ⓐ Ⓑ Ⓒ Ⓓ
14 Ⓐ Ⓑ Ⓒ Ⓓ	34 Ⓐ Ⓑ Ⓒ Ⓓ	54 Ⓐ Ⓑ Ⓒ Ⓓ		74 Ⓐ Ⓑ Ⓒ Ⓓ
15 Ⓐ Ⓑ Ⓒ Ⓓ	35 Ⓐ Ⓑ Ⓒ Ⓓ	55 Ⓐ Ⓑ Ⓒ Ⓓ		75 Ⓐ Ⓑ Ⓒ Ⓓ
16 Ⓐ Ⓑ Ⓒ Ⓓ	36 Ⓐ Ⓑ Ⓒ Ⓓ	56 Ⓐ Ⓑ Ⓒ Ⓓ		76 Ⓐ Ⓑ Ⓒ Ⓓ
17 Ⓐ Ⓑ Ⓒ Ⓓ	37 Ⓐ Ⓑ Ⓒ Ⓓ	57 Ⓐ Ⓑ Ⓒ Ⓓ		77 Ⓐ Ⓑ Ⓒ Ⓓ
18 Ⓐ Ⓑ Ⓒ Ⓓ	38 Ⓐ Ⓑ Ⓒ Ⓓ	58 Ⓐ Ⓑ Ⓒ Ⓓ		78 Ⓐ Ⓑ Ⓒ Ⓓ
19 Ⓐ Ⓑ Ⓒ Ⓓ	39 Ⓐ Ⓑ Ⓒ Ⓓ	59 Ⓐ Ⓑ Ⓒ Ⓓ		79 Ⓐ Ⓑ Ⓒ Ⓓ
20 Ⓐ Ⓑ Ⓒ Ⓓ	40 Ⓐ Ⓑ Ⓒ Ⓓ	60 Ⓐ Ⓑ Ⓒ Ⓓ		80 Ⓐ Ⓑ Ⓒ Ⓓ

**Equipment
Operation and
Maintenance** (before 31)

081 Ⓐ Ⓑ Ⓒ Ⓓ

Radiographic Procedures and Related Anatomy

111 Ⓐ Ⓑ Ⓒ Ⓓ

141 Ⓐ Ⓑ Ⓒ Ⓓ

Patient Care

171 Ⓐ Ⓑ Ⓒ Ⓓ

082 Ⓐ Ⓑ Ⓒ Ⓓ   112 Ⓐ Ⓑ Ⓒ Ⓓ   142 Ⓐ Ⓑ Ⓒ Ⓓ   172 Ⓐ Ⓑ Ⓒ Ⓓ
083 Ⓐ Ⓑ Ⓒ Ⓓ   113 Ⓐ Ⓑ Ⓒ Ⓓ   143 Ⓐ Ⓑ Ⓒ Ⓓ   173 Ⓐ Ⓑ Ⓒ Ⓓ
084 Ⓐ Ⓑ Ⓒ Ⓓ   114 Ⓐ Ⓑ Ⓒ Ⓓ   144 Ⓐ Ⓑ Ⓒ Ⓓ   174 Ⓐ Ⓑ Ⓒ Ⓓ
085 Ⓐ Ⓑ Ⓒ Ⓓ   115 Ⓐ Ⓑ Ⓒ Ⓓ   145 Ⓐ Ⓑ Ⓒ Ⓓ   175 Ⓐ Ⓑ Ⓒ Ⓓ
086 Ⓐ Ⓑ Ⓒ Ⓓ   116 Ⓐ Ⓑ Ⓒ Ⓓ   146 Ⓐ Ⓑ Ⓒ Ⓓ   176 Ⓐ Ⓑ Ⓒ Ⓓ
087 Ⓐ Ⓑ Ⓒ Ⓓ   117 Ⓐ Ⓑ Ⓒ Ⓓ   147 Ⓐ Ⓑ Ⓒ Ⓓ   177 Ⓐ Ⓑ Ⓒ Ⓓ
088 Ⓐ Ⓑ Ⓒ Ⓓ   118 Ⓐ Ⓑ Ⓒ Ⓓ   148 Ⓐ Ⓑ Ⓒ Ⓓ   178 Ⓐ Ⓑ Ⓒ Ⓓ
089 Ⓐ Ⓑ Ⓒ Ⓓ   119 Ⓐ Ⓑ Ⓒ Ⓓ   149 Ⓐ Ⓑ Ⓒ Ⓓ   179 Ⓐ Ⓑ Ⓒ Ⓓ
090 Ⓐ Ⓑ Ⓒ Ⓓ   120 Ⓐ Ⓑ Ⓒ Ⓓ   150 Ⓐ Ⓑ Ⓒ Ⓓ   180 Ⓐ Ⓑ Ⓒ Ⓓ
091 Ⓐ Ⓑ Ⓒ Ⓓ   121 Ⓐ Ⓑ Ⓒ Ⓓ   151 Ⓐ Ⓑ Ⓒ Ⓓ   181 Ⓐ Ⓑ Ⓒ Ⓓ
092 Ⓐ Ⓑ Ⓒ Ⓓ   122 Ⓐ Ⓑ Ⓒ Ⓓ   152 Ⓐ Ⓑ Ⓒ Ⓓ   182 Ⓐ Ⓑ Ⓒ Ⓓ
093 Ⓐ Ⓑ Ⓒ Ⓓ   123 Ⓐ Ⓑ Ⓒ Ⓓ   153 Ⓐ Ⓑ Ⓒ Ⓓ   183 Ⓐ Ⓑ Ⓒ Ⓓ
094 Ⓐ Ⓑ Ⓒ Ⓓ   124 Ⓐ Ⓑ Ⓒ Ⓓ   154 Ⓐ Ⓑ Ⓒ Ⓓ   184 Ⓐ Ⓑ Ⓒ Ⓓ
095 Ⓐ Ⓑ Ⓒ Ⓓ   125 Ⓐ Ⓑ Ⓒ Ⓓ   155 Ⓐ Ⓑ Ⓒ Ⓓ   185 Ⓐ Ⓑ Ⓒ Ⓓ
096 Ⓐ Ⓑ Ⓒ Ⓓ   126 Ⓐ Ⓑ Ⓒ Ⓓ   156 Ⓐ Ⓑ Ⓒ Ⓓ   186 Ⓐ Ⓑ Ⓒ Ⓓ
097 Ⓐ Ⓑ Ⓒ Ⓓ   127 Ⓐ Ⓑ Ⓒ Ⓓ   157 Ⓐ Ⓑ Ⓒ Ⓓ   187 Ⓐ Ⓑ Ⓒ Ⓓ
098 Ⓐ Ⓑ Ⓒ Ⓓ   128 Ⓐ Ⓑ Ⓒ Ⓓ   158 Ⓐ Ⓑ Ⓒ Ⓓ   188 Ⓐ Ⓑ Ⓒ Ⓓ
099 Ⓐ Ⓑ Ⓒ Ⓓ   129 Ⓐ Ⓑ Ⓒ Ⓓ   159 Ⓐ Ⓑ Ⓒ Ⓓ   189 Ⓐ Ⓑ Ⓒ Ⓓ
100 Ⓐ Ⓑ Ⓒ Ⓓ   130 Ⓐ Ⓑ Ⓒ Ⓓ   160 Ⓐ Ⓑ Ⓒ Ⓓ   190 Ⓐ Ⓑ Ⓒ Ⓓ
101 Ⓐ Ⓑ Ⓒ Ⓓ   131 Ⓐ Ⓑ Ⓒ Ⓓ   161 Ⓐ Ⓑ Ⓒ Ⓓ   191 Ⓐ Ⓑ Ⓒ Ⓓ
102 Ⓐ Ⓑ Ⓒ Ⓓ   132 Ⓐ Ⓑ Ⓒ Ⓓ   162 Ⓐ Ⓑ Ⓒ Ⓓ   192 Ⓐ Ⓑ Ⓒ Ⓓ
103 Ⓐ Ⓑ Ⓒ Ⓓ   133 Ⓐ Ⓑ Ⓒ Ⓓ   163 Ⓐ Ⓑ Ⓒ Ⓓ   193 Ⓐ Ⓑ Ⓒ Ⓓ
104 Ⓐ Ⓑ Ⓒ Ⓓ   134 Ⓐ Ⓑ Ⓒ Ⓓ   164 Ⓐ Ⓑ Ⓒ Ⓓ   194 Ⓐ Ⓑ Ⓒ Ⓓ
105 Ⓐ Ⓑ Ⓒ Ⓓ   135 Ⓐ Ⓑ Ⓒ Ⓓ   165 Ⓐ Ⓑ Ⓒ Ⓓ   195 Ⓐ Ⓑ Ⓒ Ⓓ
106 Ⓐ Ⓑ Ⓒ Ⓓ   136 Ⓐ Ⓑ Ⓒ Ⓓ   166 Ⓐ Ⓑ Ⓒ Ⓓ   196 Ⓐ Ⓑ Ⓒ Ⓓ
107 Ⓐ Ⓑ Ⓒ Ⓓ   137 Ⓐ Ⓑ Ⓒ Ⓓ   167 Ⓐ Ⓑ Ⓒ Ⓓ   197 Ⓐ Ⓑ Ⓒ Ⓓ
108 Ⓐ Ⓑ Ⓒ Ⓓ   138 Ⓐ Ⓑ Ⓒ Ⓓ   168 Ⓐ Ⓑ Ⓒ Ⓓ   198 Ⓐ Ⓑ Ⓒ Ⓓ
109 Ⓐ Ⓑ Ⓒ Ⓓ   139 Ⓐ Ⓑ Ⓒ Ⓓ   169 Ⓐ Ⓑ Ⓒ Ⓓ   199 Ⓐ Ⓑ Ⓒ Ⓓ
110 Ⓐ Ⓑ Ⓒ Ⓓ   140 Ⓐ Ⓑ Ⓒ Ⓓ   170 Ⓐ Ⓑ Ⓒ Ⓓ   200 Ⓐ Ⓑ Ⓒ Ⓓ

PART 3

SCALED SCORES FOR EXAMINATIONS

DETERMINING SCALED SCORE FOR EXAMINATIONS

The total number of Incorrect responses are indicated by the odd-numbered rows (1, 3, 5, and 7). The corresponding scaled score is indicated by the even-numbered rows (2, 4, 6, and 8).

1	2	3	4	5	6	7	8
1	100	51	80	101	55	151	30
2	100	52	79	102	54	152	29
3	100	53	79	103	54	153	29
4	100	54	78	104	53	154	28
5	99	55	78	105	53	155	28
6	99	56	77	106	52	156	27
7	99	57	77	107	52	157	27
8	99	58	76	108	51	158	26
9	99	59	76	109	51	159	26
10	99	60	*75	110	50	160	25
11	99	61	*75	111	50	161	25
12	99	62	74	112	49	162	24
13	99	63	74	113	49	163	24
14	98	64	73	114	48	164	23
15	98	65	73	115	48	165	23
16	97	66	72	116	47	166	22
17	97	67	72	117	47	167	22
18	96	68	71	118	46	168	21
19	96	69	71	119	46	169	21
20	95	70	70	120	45	170	20
21	95	71	70	121	45	171	20
22	94	72	69	122	44	172	19
23	94	73	69	123	44	173	19
24	93	74	68	124	43	174	18
25	93	75	68	125	43	175	18
26	92	76	67	126	42	176	17
27	92	77	67	127	42	177	17
28	91	78	66	128	41	178	16
29	91	79	66	129	41	179	16
30	90	80	65	130	40	180	15
31	90	81	65	131	40	181	15
32	89	82	64	132	39	182	14
33	89	83	64	133	39	183	14
34	88	84	63	134	38	184	13
35	88	85	63	135	38	185	13
36	87	86	62	136	37	186	12
37	87	87	62	137	37	187	12
38	86	88	61	138	36	188	11
39	86	89	61	139	36	189	11
40	85	90	60	140	35	190	10
41	85	91	60	141	35	191	9
42	84	92	59	142	34	192	8
43	84	93	59	143	34	193	7
44	83	94	58	144	33	194	6
45	83	95	58	145	33	195	5
46	82	96	57	146	32	196	4
47	82	97	57	147	32	197	3
48	81	98	56	148	31	198	2
49	81	99	56	149	31	199	1
50	80	100	55	150	30	200	0

*A scaled score of 75% or above is required for passing the examination.

(Revised with permission from Allied Health & Science Publishers; Robert DeAngelis, author.)

DETERMINING SCORES FOR EACH SECTION
Shaded area indicates number of incorrect answers. Unshaded area indicates percentage section score.

Section I.   Radiation Protection and Radiobiology

0	1	2	3	4	5	6	7	8	9	10	11	12	13	14	15
10	9.7	9.3	9.0	8.7	8.3	8.0	7.7	7.3	7.0	6.7	6.3	6.0	5.7	5.3	5.0
16	17	18	19	20	21	22	23	24	25	26	27	28	29	30	
4.7	4.3	4.0	3.7	3.3	3.0	2.7	2.3	2.0	1.7	1.3	1.0	0.7	0.3	0	

Section II.   Equipment Operation and Maintenance

0	1	2	3	4	5	6	7	8	9	10	11	12	13	14	15
10	9.7	9.3	9.0	8.7	8.3	8.0	7.7	7.3	7.0	6.7	6.3	6.0	5.7	5.3	5.0
16	17	18	19	20	21	22	23	24	25	26	27	28	29	30	
4.7	4.3	4.0	3.7	3.3	3.0	2.7	2.3	2.0	1.7	1.3	1.0	0.7	0.3	0	

Section III.   Image Production and Evaluation

0	1	2	3	4	5	6	7	8	9	10	11	12	13	14	15	16	17
10	9.8	9.6	9.4	9.2	9.0	8.8	8.6	8.4	8.2	8.0	7.8	7.6	7.4	7.2	7.0	6.8	6.6
18	19	20	21	22	23	24	25	26	27	28	29	30	31	32	33	34	35
6.4	6.2	6.0	5.8	5.6	5.4	5.2	5.0	4.8	4.6	4.4	4.2	4.0	3.8	3.6	3.4	3.2	3.0
36	37	38	39	40	41	42	43	44	45	46	47	48	49	50			
2.8	2.6	2.4	2.2	2.0	1.8	1.6	1.4	1.2	1.0	0.8	0.6	0.4	0.2	0			

Section IV.   Radiographic Procedures and Related Anatomy

0	1	2	3	4	5	6	7	8	9	10	11	12	13	14	15
10	9.8	9.7	9.5	9.3	9.2	9.0	8.8	8.7	8.5	8.3	8.2	8.0	7.8	7.7	7.5
16	17	18	19	20	21	22	23	24	25	26	27	28	29	30	31
7.3	7.2	7.0	6.8	6.7	6.5	6.3	6.2	6.0	5.8	5.7	5.5	5.3	5.2	5.0	4.8
32	33	34	35	36	37	38	39	40	41	42	43	44	45	46	47
4.7	4.5	4.3	4.2	4.0	3.8	3.7	3.5	3.3	3.2	3.0	2.8	2.7	2.5	2.3	2.2
48	49	50	51	52	53	54	55	56	57	58	59	60			
2.0	1.8	1.7	1.5	1.3	1.2	1.0	0.8	0.7	0.5	0.3	0.2	0			

Section V.   Patient Care

0	1	2	3	4	5	6	7	8	9	10	11	12	13	14	15
10	9.7	9.3	9.0	8.7	8.3	8.0	7.7	7.3	7.0	6.7	6.3	6.0	5.7	5.3	5.0
16	17	18	19	20	21	22	23	24	25	26	27	28	29	30	
4.7	4.3	4.0	3.7	3.3	3.0	2.7	2.3	2.0	1.7	1.3	1.0	0.7	0.3	0	

(Revised with permission from Allied Health & Science Publishers; Robert DeAngelis, author.)

INDIVIDUAL EVALUATION SHEET FOR AVERAGE SECTION SCORE

	2.5	3.0	3.5	4.0	4.5	5.0	5.5	6.0	6.5	7.0	7.5	8.0	8.5	9.0	9.5	10
Section I RADIATION PROTECTION AND RADIOBIOLOGY																
Section II EQUIPMENT OPERATION AND MAINTENANCE																
Section III IMAGE PRODUCTION AND EVALUATION																
Section IV RADIOGRAPHIC PROCEDURES AND RELATED ANATOMY																
Section V PATIENT CARE																

TOTAL % RAW SCORE _____

CORRELATED SCALED SCORE _____

Any section score with a percentage below 75 indicates the need for further study.

(Revised with permission from Allied Health & Science Publishers; Robert DeAngelis, author.)

INSTRUCTOR EVALUATION SHEET FOR DETERMINING CLASS AVERAGE

STUDENT'S NAME	Section I	Section II	Section III	Section IV	Section V	% Raw Score	Correlated Scaled Score
CLASS AVERAGE							

(Revised with permission from Allied Health & Science Publishers; Robert DeAngelis, author.)